Adolescent Emotional Development and the
of Depressive Disorders

Adolescent Emotional Development and the Emergence of Depressive Disorders

Edited by

Nicholas B. Allen

Lisa B. Sheeber

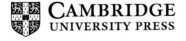

CAMBRIDGE
UNIVERSITY PRESS

CAMBRIDGE UNIVERSITY PRESS
Cambridge, New York, Melbourne, Madrid, Cape Town,
Singapore, São Paulo, Delhi, Mexico City

Cambridge University Press
The Edinburgh Building, Cambridge CB2 8RU, UK

Published in the United States of America by Cambridge University Press, New York

www.cambridge.org
Information on this title: www.cambridge.org/9781107406599

First published 2008
First paperback edition 2012

A catalogue record for this publication is available from the British Library

Library of Congress Cataloguing in Publication Data
Adolescent emotional development and the emergence of depressive disorders / edited by Nicholas
B. Allen, Lisa B. Sheeber.
    p. ; cm.
    Includes bibliographical references.
    ISBN 978-0-521-86939-3 (hardback)
1. Depression in adolescence–Etiology. 2. Emotions in adolescence. 3. Adolescent psychology.
I. Allen, Nicholas B. II. Sheeber, Lisa B. [DNLM: 1. Adolescent Psychology. 2. Adolescent Development.
3. Cognition. 4. Depressive Disorder. 5. Emotion. 6. Puberty–psychology.
WS 462 A24114 2008]
RJ506.D4A37 2008
618.92′8527–dc22

                                                                            2008029664

ISBN 978-0-521-86939-3 Hardback
ISBN 978-1-107-40659-9 Paperback

Additional resources for this publication at www.cambridge.org/9781107406599

To our teachers, Ian M. Campbell and James H. Johnson

Contents

Color plate section is between pages 144 and 145. The figures are also available for download from www.cambridge.org/9781107406599

Contributors

Nicholas B. Allen
Department of Psychology and ORYGEN Research Centre
University of Melbourne
Parkville, Victoria
Australia

Joan Rosenbaum Asarnow
Semel Institute for Neuroscience and Human Behavior
University of California, Los Angeles
Los Angeles, CA
USA

Jeanne Brooks-Gunn
Teachers College and College of Physicians and Surgeons
Columbia University
New York, NY
USA

Ronald E. Dahl
Departments of Psychiatry, Pediatrics, and Psychology
University of Pittsburgh
Pittsburgh, PA
USA

Joanne Davila
Department of Psychology
Stony Brook University
Stony Brook, NY
USA

Laura M. DeRose
Derner Institute of Advanced Psychological Studies
Adelphi University
Garden City, NY
USA

Lea R. Dougherty
Department of Psychology
Stony Brook University
Stony Brook, NY
USA

Nancy Eisenberg
Department of Psychology
Arizona State University
Tempe, AZ
USA

Erika E. Forbes
Western Psychiatric Institute and Clinic (WPIC)
University of Pittsburgh
Pittsburgh, PA
USA

Wyndol Furman
Department of Psychology
University of Denver
Denver, CO
USA

Paul Gilbert
Mental Health Research Unit
Kingsway Hospital
Derby
UK

Julia A. Graber
Department of Psychology
University of Florida
Gainesville, FL
USA

Danielle M. Hessler
Department of Psychology
University of Washington
Seattle, WA
USA

Erin C. Hunter
Department of Psychology
University of Washington
Seattle, WA
USA

Chris Irons
Mental Health Research Unit
Kingsway Hospital
Derby
UK

Lynn Fainsilber Katz
Department of Psychology
University of Washington
Seattle, WA
USA

Amanda Kesek
Department of Psychology
University of Toronto
Toronto, Ontario
Canada

Daniel N. Klein
Department of Psychology
Stony Brook University
Stony Brook, NY
USA

Annette M. La Greca
Department of Psychology
University of Miami
Coral Gables, FL
USA

Rebecca S. Laptook
Department of Psychology
Stony Brook University
Stony Brook, NY
USA

Reed W. Larson
Department of Human and Community Development
University of Illinois
Urbana, IL
USA

Primrose Letcher
Department of Paediatrics
University of Melbourne
Parkville, Victoria
Australia

Peter M. Lewinsohn
Oregon Research Institute
Eugene, OR
USA

Marc D. Lewis
Department of Human Development and Applied Psychology
Ontario Institute for Studies in Education
University of Toronto
Toronto, Ontario
Canada

Christine McDunn
Department of Psychology
University of Denver
Denver, CO
USA

James W. McKowen
Department of Psychology
Boston University
Boston, MA
USA

Christopher S. Monk
Department of Psychology
University of Michigan
Ann Arbor, MI
USA

Amanda Sheffield Morris
Human Development and Family Science
Oklahoma State University
Tulsa, OK
USA

Thomas M. Olino
Department of Psychology
Stony Brook University
Stony Brook, NY
USA

Tomáš Paus
Brain and Body Centre
University of Nottingham
University Park
Nottingham
UK

Daniel S. Pine
National Institute of Mental Health
Bethesda, MD
USA

Ann V. Sanson
Department of Paediatrics
University of Melbourne
Parkville, Victoria
Australia

John R. Seeley
Oregon Research Institute
Eugene, OR
USA

Lisa B. Sheeber
Oregon Research Institute
Eugene, OR
USA

Rebecca Siegel
Department of Psychology
University of Miami
Coral Gables, FL
USA

Jennifer S. Silk
Western Psychiatric Institute and Clinic (WPIC)
University of Pittsburgh
Pittsburgh, PA
USA

Diana Smart
Australian Institute of Family Studies
Melbourne, Victoria
Australia

Martha C. Tompson
Department of Psychology
Boston University
Boston, MA
USA

Julie Vaughan
Department of Psychology
Arizona State University
Tempe, AZ
USA

Brennan J. Young
Department of Psychology
University of Denver
Frontier Hall
Denver, CO
USA

Philip David Zelazo
Department of Psychology
University of Toronto
Toronto, Ontario
Canada

Acknowledgments

We would like to express our appreciation to our funders, the National Institute of Mental Health (MH065340) and the Colonial Foundation, whose support enables our research on adolescent depression. As well, we wish to thank Christina Elmore, Laurie Levites, and Judith Thompson for their careful proofing and assembly of this volume.

The importance of affective development for the emergence of depressive disorders during adolescence

Nicholas B. Allen and Lisa B. Sheeber

One of the most striking aspects of the epidemiology of depressive disorders across the lifespan is the rapid rise in the incidence of depression that is observed in early adolescence (Lewinsohn *et al.*, 1993, 1998). A recent meta-analysis of epidemiological studies estimated the prevalence of unipolar depressive disorders to be approximately 5.6% in adolescents as compared with 2.8% in children below age 13 (Costello *et al.*, 2006). Lifetime estimate rates for adolescents, ranging from 15–20%, are comparable with those of adults (Birmaher *et al.*, 1996). Further, longitudinal data indicate that an episode of depression is a substantial risk factor for subsequent episodes, both within adolescence and into adulthood (Birmaher *et al.*, 1996; Harrington & Vostanis, 1995). This increased vulnerability likely reflects the adverse impact of depressive episodes on neurobiological and cognitive development (Harrison, 2002; Vythilingam *et al.*, 2002) as well as on emotional, social, and occupational functioning (Bardone *et al.*, 1996; Rohde *et al.*, 1994).

These data indicate the important public health significance of adolescent depressive syndromes. Moreover, they direct our attention to the likelihood that some causative mechanism, or mechanisms, underlie this population-wide increase in vulnerability, and in so doing highlight the need to understand the relationships between early adolescent development and the psychopathological processes that give rise to depressive conditions. Explicating these relationships will yield important insights not only for understanding depressive disorders during adolescence (a critically important life stage if we are to provide effective prevention and early intervention), but likely also for understanding vulnerability throughout the life span. In other words, the developmentally driven changes that occur during early adolescence and result in an increased cohort-wide vulnerability to depression may provide clues as to

Adolescent Emotional Development and the Emergence of Depressive Disorders, ed. Nicholas B. Allen and Lisa B. Sheeber. Published by Cambridge University Press. © Cambridge University Press 2009.

the salient individual differences that render individuals more vulnerable to depression during other phases of life.

Emotional development during early adolescence

In this book we take the perspective that understanding the developmental changes occurring in *affective* functioning during the transition from childhood to early adolescence will enable a comprehensive and integrated picture of how vulnerability to depressive disorders is transformed during this stage of life. Not only is depression increasingly conceptualized as a disorder of affective functioning, but affective development is inextricably linked with cognitive, biological, sexual, and interpersonal processes also undergoing rapid and marked development during this period. Hence, the focus on affective development facilitates a broad and integrative exploration of the developmental roots of vulnerability to depressive disorder.

Adolescence is characterized by significant increases in negative emotionality, greater sensitivity to peer-related social interactions, greater reward-seeking, and greater engagement with long-term and socially complex goals (Nelson *et al.*, 2005). While these changes promote the skills necessary for greater independence from the family and the establishment of developmentally important peer and romantic relationships, they are also hypothesized to create greater vulnerability to emotional and behavioral dysregulation (Spear, 2000; Steinberg, 2005).

The defining neurobiological change of early adolescence is puberty. Although biological researchers have traditionally viewed puberty from an endocrine perspective, more recent developments have emphasized the neural control of hormone secretion and the extensive brain remodeling that is associated with puberty (Sisk & Foster, 2004). In particular, brain regions associated with affective processing (particularly a ventral network of structures that includes the amygdala/hippocampus, ventral striatum, and hypothalamus), are densely innervated by gonadal steroid receptors (Nelson *et al.*, 2005; Sisk & Foster, 2004). These steroids also play a role in regulating many of the neurotransmitter systems associated with affective and social responsiveness, including dopamine, serotonin, endogenous opioids, oxytocin, and vasopression (De Vries *et al.*, 1992; Epperson *et al.*, 1999; McCarthy, 1995; McEwen, 2001; Osterlund & Hurd, 2001; Rubinow & Schmidt, 1996). Furthermore, gonadal steroids have their own direct effects on affective processes (Baulieu, 1998; McEwen, 2001). For example, higher levels of gonadal steroids are associated with increased affective responses to infant stimuli in parents (Fleming *et al.*, 1997, 2002). Also, both human and animal studies support a link between gonadal hormones (especially testosterone) and sensitivity to social status (Book *et al.*, 2001; Rowe *et al.*, 2004). Thus, although the main function of puberty may be to increase sensitivity to sexual stimuli and increase sexual motivation (Sisk & Forster, 2004), it may also serve to increase affective reactivity to non-sexual stimuli, perhaps reflecting a more general reorientation to the social and emotional aspects of the environment (Nelson et al., 2005).

Consistent with this hypothesis, findings from other studies suggest that puberty is associated with increased emotionality and reward-seeking. For example, significant associations have been documented between pubertal stage and measures of sensation seeking and risk-taking (Martin et al., 2002). By contrast, age did not show an association with these variables. Similarly, Steinberg (1987) found that pubertal status predicted the frequency and intensity of parent–adolescent conflict more strongly than did chronological age, which may reflect, in part, greater negative affect on the part of the adolescent. Puberty has also been shown to predict risk for depression more strongly than age (Angold et al., 1999).

Adolescents are also substantially more sociable than younger children (Steinberg & Sheffield Morris, 2001), spending up to a third of their waking hours in the company of their peers (Hartup & Stevens, 1997). This sociability, as well as the more effortful and deliberate formation of relationships characterizing this age group, is at least in part driven by the increased affective salience of socially related events (Larson & Richards, 1994; Steinberg & Sheffield Morris, 2001). The social world that children encounter during the transition to adolescence, moreover, is increasingly broad, hierarchical, and complex (Brown, 2004). One-on-one relationships become more intimate and trusting (Steinberg & Sheffield Morris, 2001), and romantic relationships emerge, prompted by new motivational systems, sexual development, and cultural imperatives (Steinberg et al., 2006). Small groups of between three and ten members become important (Brown & Klute, 2003), and adolescents may also start to associate with larger crowds consisting of people who have established the same basic identity as each other (e.g. goths, nerds, skaters). Thus dyadic relationships are nested in dynamic group structures that are themselves nested in broader crowd structures, resulting in a more layered and complex social system than exists in the pre-adolescent years.

Adolescent relationships are also inherently unstable (Brown, 2004; Hardy et al., 2002). Fewer than half of adolescent friendships endure over the period of a year (Connolly et al., 2000; Degirmencioglu et al., 1998), and romantic relationships are similarly short-lived, especially in early adolescence (Connolly et al., 2000; Connolly & Goldberg, 1999; Feiring, 1996). The tenuousness and complexity of adolescent relationships occur in the context of adolescents' increased sensitivity to acceptance and rejection by peers (Brown, 2004; Larson & Richards, 1994; Nelson et al., 2005; O'Brien & Bierman, 1988). This combination makes adolescence a period of particularly high interpersonal stress, associated especially with the establishment and maintenance of the kind of social reputation that will enhance social acceptance and reduce the likelihood of rejection and ostracism.

Adolescence is also characterized by the maturation of a set of core executive and self-regulatory skills, although on a different trajectory to the aforementioned puberty-related affective and motivational changes (Steinberg, 2005). In particular, the development of these self-regulatory skills is characterized by slower and more gradual maturation that continues into early adulthood. This maturation is thought to be associated with significant remodeling in brain regions associated with social cognition, response inhibition, monitoring, emotion regulation, and the capacity for abstract, reflective, and hypothetical thinking (Nelson *et al.*, 2005; Paus, 2005). Notably, these changes have been hypothesized to both protect and increase vulnerability to depression. On the one hand, adolescents may be vulnerable as a function of being motivated toward increasingly rewarding and potentially risky activities before they have an adaptive regulatory architecture in place. This is particularly the case given the powerful negative emotions they may experience when such rewards are not realized. So, for example, their emotional equilibrium may be uniquely challenged by the vicissitudes of early romantic relationships, rendering them prone to negative affectivity and depressive symptoms (see Furman, McDunn, & Young, Chapter 16 and La Greca, Davila, & Siegel, Chapter 17, this volume) to a greater extent than they will be a few years later. On the other hand, some aspects of these developing regulatory competencies may actually increase vulnerability to distress and depression. In particular, the increased capacity to engage with abstract and temporally distal rewards may potentiate risk for depression in that pursuit of these rewards is more easily frustrated or thwarted than is the pursuit of more proximal and concrete ones (Davey *et al.*, 2008). The difficulties inherent in engaging with abstract rewards can be seen, for example, in adolescents' increasing concern about reputation and their distress at potential threats to their social standing (see Gilbert and Irons, Chapter 11, this volume).

Finally, significant changes also begin to occur in the nature of family and social relations. One of the primary developmental tasks for families of adolescents is renegotiating relationships such that the necessarily asymmetrical power structure evident between children and their parents starts to become more balanced, as adolescents are increasingly allowed more autonomy and input into family and personal decision-making (Gutman & Eccles, 2007; Steinberg, 2001). These changes in parent–adolescent relationships necessarily mean that external contributors to adolescent affective and behavioral regulation, in the form of parental support and structure, are reduced at the same time that increased emotionality and reward-seeking create additional regulatory demands.

This brief review of some of the salient factors impinging on emotional development during early adolescence illustrates the range of developmental changes potentially contributing to vulnerability to depressive disorder: (1) puberty-driven increases in reward seeking and social sensitivity, (2) immaturity of the neurobiological systems underlying emotion and self-regulation, (3) reductions in parental supervision and increases in family conflict, (4) increased cognitive capacity to affectively engage with abstract, temporally distant, and socially embedded goals and (5) increased importance of, and instability in, peer relationships. Surprisingly, however, although adolescence is a time of increased stress, most adolescents negotiate these changes successfully (Arnett, 1999). This implies that the increased prevalence of depressive disorder during adolescence must be a result of these developmental processes interacting with other individual, environmental, and cultural vulnerabilities to result in depressive symptoms. Examining the interaction between developmental processes during adolescence and pre-existing vulnerability factors therefore has the potential to offer unique insights into the etiology of depressive disorders. It is the desire to enhance our understanding of these interactions that has motivated the preparation and design of this volume.

The structure of this volume

This volume has, to our knowledge, a unique structure. We have identified a series of critical domains relevant to adolescent emotional development, and within each of these domains we have included one chapter from a leading developmentalist (or group thereof) describing the normative adolescent developmental processes relevant to that domain. These chapters are paired with chapters written by clinicians and clinical researchers, who explore the relationship between developmental processes in that domain and vulnerability to depressive disorders. Each chapter addresses gender and cultural differences as well as risk for bipolar disorder within their relevant domain, to the extent that the literature allows. By utilizing such a structure, we hope to not only create a set of up-to-date and comprehensive reviews of the issues relevant to adolescent emotional development and the emergence of depressive disorders, but also to create a "conversation" between the developmental and clinical perspectives on these issues for the reader.

In the first section following this introduction we include a pair of chapters describing the changes in *emotional experience and the prevalence of depressive disorder* during the transition from childhood to adolescence. First Reed Larson and Lisa Sheeber describe the normative changes in the daily emotional experience and behavior during this developmental transition, with an emphasis on findings from studies using experience-sampling methodologies. They describe adolescence as a time of increasing negative affect, examine the contributions of stress, puberty, and cognitive development to this increase, and explore how these normative changes may relate to depressive disorder. The chapter by John Seeley and Peter M. Lewinsohn draws on data from the

Oregon Adolescent Depression Project, which is one of the most important epidemiological studies of the causes and consequences of depressive disorders during adolescence. They describe not only the epidemiological changes in depression that occur during the transition from childhood to adolescence, but also the implications of these disorders for lifetime risk for mental health problems.

The second section explores *adolescent brain development*. Tomáš Paus first describes how research in structural and functional neuroimaging has shed new light on our understanding of brain development during adolescence, and also specifically explores the issue of sex differences in adolescent brain development. Given that the rise of depression during adolescence is particularly notable in females, sex differences in brain development is one domain that might provide clues to the emergence of these sex differences in vulnerability. Erika Forbes, Jennifer Silk, and Ron Dahl then explore the links between brain development and adolescent depression. They note the striking overlap between the neural systems undergoing development during adolescence, and those associated with depression. As well as exploring the impact of brain development on risk for depression, they also consider the important, but under-researched topic of the impact of adolescent depression on brain development and future functioning.

The third section of the book addresses *pubertal and sexual development*. Laura DeRose and Jeanne Brooks-Gunn first explore the association between both pubertal stage and pubertal timing and affect. Julia Graber then explores the impact of these processes on risk for depressive disorders. Although both these reviews find evidence of an association between pubertal development and vulnerability to distressing affect and depressive disorder, they also make it clear that puberty, as a normative developmental process, is not pathogenic in and of itself. Rather, it plays a role in potentiating the effects of other vulnerability factors. Both chapters also identify priorities for future research.

The next section deals with *cognitive development*. Amanda Kesek, Philip David Zelazo, and Marc Lewis describe the development of executive cognitive functions and their implications for emotion regulation. Their chapter specifically explores the relationship between the development of the prefrontal cortex and these executive abilities. They describe how as these brain structures develop, adolescents are increasingly able to use complex rule hierarchies to guide their behavior. Christopher Monk and Daniel Pine then explore the relationship between cognitive development and depression, and they describe how cognitive function can be used to bridge the symptoms of depression to brain function.

The next section is the first to explicitly explore individual differences that might impact on both emotional development and risk for depression. Developmental researchers have long used *temperament* to describe the fundamental dimensions of individual differences across the life span. Ann Sanson,

Primrose Letcher, and Diana Smart first explore the specific characteristics of temperament that are relevant to adolescent socio-emotional functioning. They describe the degree of stability and change in temperament from childhood through to adolescence, how temperament provides the basis for emerging personality differences, and the implications of temperamental differences for both healthy and unhealthy development. Dan Klein, Lea Dougherty, Rebecca Laptook, and Thomas Olino then explore the relationship of temperament to risk for mood disorders. They conclude that temperament is a well-established risk factor, and explore some of the potential mediators and moderators of this relationship, including gender, stress, and neurobiological processes.

Familial processes are explored in the next section. Erin Hunter, Danielle Hessler, and Lynn Fainsilber Katz examine the role of the family in the affective development of adolescents, with a particular emphasis on the role of socialization processes during both childhood and adolescence. Martha Tompson, James McKowan, and Joan Asarnow then explore the relationship between family processes and mood disorder, including a specific discussion of the impact of parental mood disorder on both family processes and adolescent risk. They conclude that the adolescent in a distressed family environment will have more difficulty navigating the developmental tasks of the adolescent period and developing a positive and effective sense of self, potentially resulting in increased risk for depression. With the onset of depression, youth may also have increasingly conflictual, and less rewarding interactions with family members.

Many of the brain and cognitive changes occurring during adolescence are thought to potentiate significant changes in social cognition and behavior, which are the focus of the next two sections. Developmental changes in *social and moral emotions*, such as shame, guilt and empathy/sympathy, are explored in the next section. Nancy Eisenberg and Amanda Sheffield Morris describe the development of these emotions and their relationship to a range of socio-emotional outcomes in non-clinical samples. Paul Gilbert and Chris Irons then address the emergence of shame, self-criticism and self-compassion during adolescence, and explore their implications for depressive disorders.

The next section deals with social behavior in the form of *peer and romantic relationships*. Wyndol Furman, Christine McDunn, and Brennan Young describe the impact of these social relationships on affective experience and affect regulation. They conclude that despite the salience of these relationships during adolescence, the particular pathways by which they impact emotional development are not yet well delineated. Annette La Greca, Joanne Davila, and Rebecca Siegel then explore the significance of the adolescent social context for the development and maintenance of depression. As in the previous chapter, they outline how despite the clear association between peer processes and depression, more research is needed on the particular mechanisms by which these associations emerge.

We (the editors) provide a final chapter exploring the implications of the material presented in the book for a developmentally informed account of depression during adolescence. First, we consider the possibility of developing a more integrative perspective on adolescent development and risk for depression, and explore some recent examples of such perspectives, including one of our own. Finally, implications for future research directions, prevention, and early intervention are explored. We are hopeful that the material presented in the volume will stimulate further empirical and conceptual work on the relationships between development and psychopathology during adolescence, and that these developments will be translated into effective, evidence-based approaches to preventing and treating adolescent depression and promoting healthy youth development.

REFERENCES

Angold, A., Costello, E. J., Erkanli, A., & Worthman, C. M. (1999). Pubertal changes in hormone levels and depression in girls. *Psychological Medicine, 29*(5), 1043–1053.

Arnett, J. J. (1999). Adolescent storm and stress, reconsidered. *American Psychologist,* **54**(5), 317–326.

Bardone, A. M., Moffitt, T., Caspi, A., & Dickson, N. (1996). Adult mental health and social outcomes of adolescent girls with depression and conduct disorder. *Development and Psychopathology,* 8(4), 811–829.

Baulieu, E. E. (1998). Neurosteroids: a novel function of the brain. *Psychoneuroendocrinology,* 23(8), 963–987.

Birmaher, B., Ryan, N. D., Wiliamson, D. E. *et al.* (1996). Childhood and adolescent depression: A review of the past 10 years. Part 1. *Journal of the American Academy of Child & Adolescent Psychiatry,* **35**, 1427–1439.

Book, A. S., Starzyk, K. B., & Quinsey, V. L. (2001). The relationship between testosterone and aggression: a meta-analysis. *Aggression and Violent Behavior,* **6**(6), 579–599.

Brown, B. B. (2004). Adolescents' relationships with peers. In R. M. Lerner & L. D. Steinberg (Eds.), *Handbook of Adolescent Psychology* (2nd edn, pp. 363–394). Hoboken, NJ: John Wiley & Sons.

Brown, B. B., & Klute, C. (2003). Friendships, cliques, and crowds. In G. R. Adams & M. D. Berzonsky (Eds.), *Blackwell Handbook of Adolescence* (pp. 330–348). Malden, MA: Blackwell.

Connolly, J., & Goldberg, A. (1999). Romantic relationships in adolescence: the role of friends and peers in their emergence and development. In W. Furman, B. Brown, & C. Feiring (Eds.), *The Development of Romantic Relationships in Adolescence* (pp. 266–290). New York, NY: Cambridge University Press.

Connolly, J., Furman, W., & Konarski, R. (2000). The role of peers in the emergence of heterosexual romantic relationships in adolescence. *Child Development,* **71**(5), 1395–1408.

Costello, E. J., Erkanli, A., & Angold, A. (2006). Is there an epidemic of child or adolescent depression? *Journal of Child Psychology and Psychiatry and Allied Disciplines,* **47**(12), 1263–1271.

Davey, C., Yucel, M., & Allen, N.B. (2008). The emergence of depression in adolescence: development of the prefrontal cortex and the representation of reward. *Neuroscience and Biobehavioral Reviews*, **32**, 1–19.

De Vries, G.J., Crenshaw, B.J., & al-Shamma, H.A. (1992). Gonadal steroid modulation of vasopressin pathways. *Annals of the New York Academy of Science*, **652**, 387–396.

Degirmencioglu, S.M., Urberg, K.A., Tolson, J.M., & Richard, P. (1998). Adolescent friendship networks: continuity and change over the school year. *Merrill-Palmer Quarterly*, **44**(3), 313–337.

Epperson, C.N., Wisner, K.L., & Yamamoto, B. (1999). Gonadal steroids in the treatment of mood disorders. *Psychosomatic Medicine*, **61**(5), 676–697.

Feiring, C. (1996). Concepts of romance in 15-year-old adolescents. *Journal of Research on Adolescence*, **6**(2), 181–200.

Fleming, A.S., Ruble, D., Krieger, H., & Wong, P.Y. (1997). Hormonal and experiential correlates of maternal responsiveness during pregnancy and the puerperium in human mothers. *Hormones and Behavior*, **31**(2), 145–158.

Fleming, A.S., Corter, C., Stallings, J., & Steiner, M. (2002). Testosterone and prolactin are associated with emotional responses to infant cries in new fathers. *Hormones and Behavior*, **42**(4), 399–413.

Gutman, L.M., & Eccles, J.S. (2007). Stage-environment fit during adolescence: trajectories of family relations and adolescent outcomes. *Developmental Psychology*, **43**(2), 522–537.

Hardy, C.L., Bukowski, W.M., & Sippola, L.K. (2002). Stability and change in peer relationships during the transition to middle level school. *Journal of Early Adolescence*, **22**(2), 117.

Harrington, R., & Vostanis, P. (1995). Longitudinal perspectives and affective disorder in children and adolescents. In I.M. Goodyer (Ed.), *The Depressed Child and Adolescent* (pp. 311–341). Cambridge, UK: Cambridge University Press.

Harrison, P.J. (2002). The neuropathology of primary mood disorder. *Brain*, **125**, 1428–1449.

Hartup, W.W., & Stevens, N. (1997). Friendships and adaptation in the life course. *Psychological Bulletin*, **121**(3), 355–370.

Larson, R.E., & Richards, M.H. (1994). *Divergent Realities: The Emotional Lives of Mothers, Fathers, and Adolescents*. New York, NY: Basic Books.

Lewinsohn, P.M., Hops, H., Roberts, R.E., Seeley, J.R., & Andrews, J.A. (1993). Adolescent psychopathology: I. Prevalence and incidence of depression and other DSM-III-R disorders in high school students. *Journal of Abnormal Psychology*, **102**(1), 133–144.

Lewinsohn, P.M., Rohde, P., & Seeley, J.R. (1998). Major depressive disorder in older adolescents: prevalence, risk factors, and clinical implications. *Clinical Psychology Review*, **18**(7), 765–794.

Martin, C.A., Kelly, T.H., Rayens, M.K. *et al.* (2002). Sensation seeking, puberty and nicotine, alcohol and marijuana use in adolescence. *Journal of the American Academy of Child and Adolescent Psychiatry*, **41**(12), 1495–1502.

McCarthy, M.M. (1995). Estrogen modulation of oxytocin and its relation to behavior. *Advances in Experimental Medicine and Biology*, **395**, 235–245.

McEwen, B.S. (2001). Invited review: Estrogens effects on the brain: multiple sites and molecular mechanisms. *Journal of Applied Physiology*, **91**(6), 2785–2801.

Nelson, E. E., Leibenluft, E., McClure, E. B., & Pine, D. S. (2005). The social re-orientation of adolescence: a neuroscience perspective on the process and its relation to psychopathology. *Psychological Medicine*, **35**(2), 163–174.

O'Brien, S. F., & Bierman, K. L. (1988). Conceptions and perceived influence of peer groups: interviews with preadolescents and adolescents. *Child Development*, **59**(5), 1360–1365.

Osterlund, M. K., & Hurd, Y. L. (2001). Estrogen receptors in the human forebrain and the relation to neuropsychiatric disorders. *Progress in Neurobiology*, **64**(3), 251–267.

Paus, T. (2005). Mapping brain maturation and cognitive development during adolescence. *Trends in Cognitive Science*, **9**(2), 60–68.

Rohde, P., Lewinsohn, P. M., & Seeley, J. R. (1994). Are adolescents changed by an episode of major depression? *Journal of the American Academy of Child and Adolescent Psychiatry*, **33**(9), 1289–1298.

Rowe, R., Maughan, B., Worthman, C. M., Costello, E. J., & Angold, A. (2004). Testosterone, antisocial behavior, and social dominance in boys: pubertal development and biosocial interaction. *Biological Psychiatry*, **55**(5), 546–552.

Rubinow, D. R., & Schmidt, P. J. (1996). Androgens, brain, and behavior. *American Journal of Psychiatry*, **153**(8), 974–984.

Sisk, C. L., & Foster, D. L. (2004). The neural basis of puberty and adolescence. *Nature and Neuroscience*, **7**(10), 1040–1047.

Spear, L. P. (2000). The adolescent brain and age-related behavioral manifestations. *Neuroscience and Biobehavioral Reviews*, **24**(4), 417–463.

Steinberg, L. (1987). Impact of puberty on family relations: effects of pubertal status and pubertal timing. *Developmental Psychology*, **23**(3), 451–460.

Steinberg, L. (2001). We know some things: parent-adolescent relationships in retrospect and prospect. *Journal of Research on Adolescence*, **11**(1), 1–19.

Steinberg, L. (2005). Cognitive and affective development in adolescence. *Trends in Cognitive Science*, **9**(2), 69–74.

Steinberg, L., & Sheffield Morris, A. (2001). Adolescent development. *Annual Review of Psychology*, **52**, 83–110.

Steinberg, L., Dahl, R., Keating, D. *et al.* (2006). The study of developmental psychopathology in adolescence: integrating affective neuroscience with the study of context. In D. Cicchetti & D. Cohen (Eds.), *Developmental Psychopathology, Volume 2, Developmental Neuroscience* (pp. 710–741). Hoboken, NJ: John Wiley & Sons.

Vythilingam, M., Heim, C., Newport, J. *et al.* (2002). Childhood trauma associated with smaller hippocampal volume in women with major depression. *American Journal of Psychiatry*, **159**(12), 2072–2080.

2

The daily emotional experience of adolescents: are adolescents more emotional, why, and how is that related to depression?

Reed W. Larson and Lisa B. Sheeber

Some time ago, one of us (LS) recruited a healthy comparison sample for an adolescent depression study via neighborhood canvassing. Armed with clipboards and name badges my staff and I knocked on doors and explained to the bewildered occupants that we were seeking adolescents who were *not* depressed to participate in a scientific investigation. To me, having grown up in an urban east coast environment, the most notable part of the public response was that people opened their doors to us. Second though, was the near unanimity with which the residents joked that "non-depressed adolescents" was a contradiction in terms. Weren't we aware that adolescents were a depressed and moody lot, subject to the vagaries of their raging hormones?

By reputation adolescence is an emotional period. In surveys, adults describe the typical adolescent as subject to strong and unpredictable emotional shifts, including not just to depression and anxiety, but also to exuberance and elation (Farkas & Johnson, 1997; Hess & Goldblatt, 1957). Moreover, if the teachings of Aristotle and Confucius (among others) are any indication, this reputation of adolescents for moodiness is a cross-cultural phenomenon that has characterized adults' views of youth for millennia (Larson, 1991).

A wide range of factors might reasonably be thought to make adolescence a period of increased emotionality. Adolescence is characterized by significant biological, contextual, interpersonal, and cognitive changes. Among these, puberty has most often been credited as a source of emotional lability in adolescents – puberty is hypothesized to influence teenagers' moods through either the direct effect of hormones, or the indirect effects of physical changes on teens' social relationships (DeRose & Brooks-Gunn, see Chapter 4, this volume). Another possible factor is that adolescents spend less time in the familiar, supervised, and narrow world of family and more time in the unpredictable,

Adolescent Emotional Development and the Emergence of Depressive Disorders, ed. Nicholas B. Allen and Lisa B. Sheeber. Published by Cambridge University Press. © Cambridge University Press 2009.

less controlled, and less secure world of peers (Csikszentmihalyi & Larson, 1984; Larson & Richards, 1991). Early adolescence, moreover, is characterized by a confluence of normative stressors (i.e. school transitions, budding romantic interests), accompanied by a higher rate of daily hassles and stressful events such as conflicts with family and friends, school difficulties, and romantic break-ups (Larson & Ham, 1993). Not only does this broadening of children's worlds subject them to more situations that might elicit emotions – the excitement of first kisses and the misery of first break-ups – but adolescents' increased autonomy means that they are progressively more responsible for regulating their own affective responses (Steinberg *et al.*, 2006). Finally, adolescents' greater emotionality could also be attributable to cognitive developments in this age period that render them more vulnerable to self-consciousness and apprehension as well as more able to empathize with, and hence take on the emotional experiences of others (Larson & Asmussen, 1991; Eisenberg *et al.*, see Chapter 10, this volume).

But is the stereotype that adolescents are excessively emotional true? Acceptance of an exaggerated or otherwise inaccurate depiction of adolescents is a disservice and could lead parents, teachers, and other professionals to dismiss distressing and impairing levels of emotionality as "adolescence." In fact, such dismissiveness may contribute to the low rates with which families of depressed adolescents seek treatment (Flament *et al.*, 2001; Lewinsohn *et al.*, 1995). We need to better understand how emotionality might be inter-related with problem behaviors such as substance use and eating disorders that increase at this developmental stage (Steinberg *et al.*, 2006). In particular, it is important to understand how this emotionality might be related to the increase in depressive symptomatology and disorder, which epidemiological studies consistently find with entry into adolescence (Seeley & Lewinsohn, see Chapter 3, this volume). Might emotional distress or lability contribute to depression?

This chapter reviews evidence from a program of research conducted by the first author and colleagues that has examined normative developmental changes in emotionality, drawing on data from adolescents' hour-to-hour experiences obtained with the Experience Sampling Method (ESM). We address three principal questions that were central to this research: (1) Do adolescents experience wider emotional swings than people in younger and older age groups? (2) If so, how are these emotions related to puberty, stress, and cognitive changes? And (3) what relation might there be between adolescents' daily emotions and the increased rates of depression during this age period?

A methodology for sampling adolescents' daily experiences

The Experience Sampling Method is designed to study emotions as they are experienced in daily life. Participants in ESM studies carry a pager (or other electronic device) and are signaled at random moments across the waking

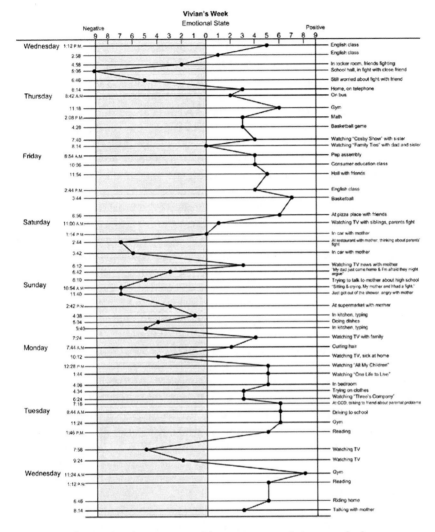

Figure 2.1. The emotional states reported by one teenager during a week of
participating in ESM research. Reprinted with permission from Larson & Richards, 1994a.

hours of the day, typically for one week. When signaled, participants respond
to a brief inventory of questions regarding their current situation (activity,
who with, location), their subjective state, and anything else an investigator
wants to know about their momentary experience (Hektner *et al.*, 2007).

In order to understand this methodology and get a feel for the nature of the
data it yields, it is useful to examine the reports provided by an individual
youth. Figure 2.1 summarizes the reports provided by an 8th grader named

Vivian. On the right side, one can see the situations she reported being in each time she was signaled; the bullets inside the chart show the emotional state she reported. Values for her emotional states were based on her ratings for three 7-point semantic differential items (happy–unhappy, friendly–angry, cheerful–irritable). Together these items form an affect scale, which provides a general index of how she reported feeling at the moment she was signaled.

What is immediately apparent is that Vivian is an emotional adolescent, or at least that she had an emotional week. At 5:06 pm on the first day, she reported being at the extreme negative end of the scales (feeling "very" unhappy, angry, and irritable). The explanation she gave was that her female friends were in a fist fight, which made her distraught. Yet by 8:14 pm that same evening, she was back on the positive side of the scale, and she remained there until Saturday when she went into a negative state that lasted for the rest of the weekend. Vivian attributed this negative emotion to a conflict that was unfolding between her parents. As the next week started, we see additional strong fluctuations in her emotions between negative and positive.

The first question we will be addressing is whether the "moodiness" reflected in Vivian's report is typical of and specific to adolescence. That is, do adolescents experience wider emotional swings than people in younger and older age groups? The primary data we have used to address this and other questions come from the Youth and Adolescence Study (YAS), in which the ESM was used with a randomly selected sample of 483 working- and middle-class European–American 5th–9th graders (Larson & Lampman-Petraitis, 1989). A subset of 220 of these youth also provided ESM data 4 years later when they were in the 9th–12th grades (Larson *et al.*, 2002). These findings will be supplemented by those obtained in studies of 262 5th–8th grade poor- and working-class African–American students (Richards *et al.*, 2004) and 100 middle-class 8th graders in India (Verma & Larson, 1999), as well as those by other investigators. The mothers and fathers of the Indian youth as well as of a subsample of the YAS youth ($n = 55$) provided ESM data at the same time as their children.

The strength of this methodology is the systematic random sampling of daily experience as it occurs. Across studies, participants completed a report in response to approximately 80% of the random signals sent to them. Thus the method provided a sampling of most of the teenagers' daily experiences. There were missed signals, and when we quizzed youth about each missed report the most frequent explanations were forgetting the pager at home and preoccupation in an activity. The adolescents' retrospective reports on what they felt at the moment of missed signals suggested that no particular categories of emotional experience were systematically excluded (Larson, 1989). The fact that these reports were made as experiences occur is also important. Numerous psychological studies have shown that people are not good at recalling emotionally valenced past experiences (Kahneman & Riis, 2005).

It is also important to note that this method assesses subjective or conscious emotions, which researchers consider to be somewhat distinct from emotions assessed through facial expressions or physiological monitors. Research findings with adults suggests that these three sources of data – self-report, observed expression, and physiological indicators – deal with separate and only marginally inter-correlated emotional domains (e.g. Bradley & Lang, 2000). The subjective, conscious domain of emotions is important because it represents individuals' lived experience: that is, the feelings of which they are aware and that shape their daily reality. We have found, moreover, that ESM reports on the affect scale are related to depressive symptoms, teachers' ratings of mood levels, school grades, and other measures of psychosocial adjustment (Csikszentmihalyi & Larson, 1987; Hektner *et al.*, 2007; Larson & Ham, 1993).

Differences in emotional experiences across age groups

The stereotype of adolescents as emotional or moody involves implicit comparisons to people at other age periods. Our first question is whether 'moodiness,' as reflected in individuals' overall averages, variability, and rates of positive and negative emotions, is more characteristic of adolescents than adults or children.

Are adolescents moodier than adults?

We have carried out three studies that compare the daily emotions experienced by adolescents to those of adults. All present a common picture that is consistent with the hypothesis that adolescents are more emotional. In the first study, we compared two unrelated samples of adolescents and adults and found that there was greater variability in adolescents' reported moods than in those of adults (Larson *et al.*, 1980). The adolescents reported extreme emotions more frequently than did the adults, including both more negative and positive emotions. The two samples did not differ in their average state on the scale from positive to negative valence, but the adolescents had wider fluctuations above and below this mean. Because these two samples were not matched in any way, however, the findings were not fully persuasive. It is possible that the adults (blue- and white-collar workers at area businesses) were a subdued lot who were not comparable to the high school students on other dimensions.

Our second study, using data from YAS, was more definitive. In this case we had the mothers and fathers of 55 young adolescents provide ESM data. Teens and their parents were signaled at the same times as each went about their daily activities. As in the prior study, we found that though teens and adults did not differ markedly in the average negative-positive valence of their

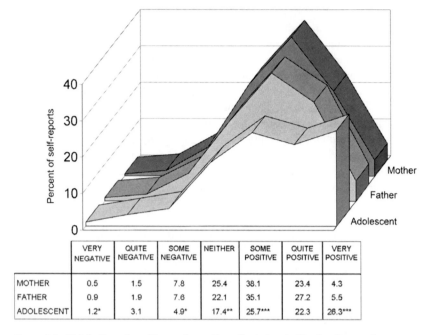

	VERY NEGATIVE	QUITE NEGATIVE	SOME NEGATIVE	NEITHER	SOME POSITIVE	QUITE POSITIVE	VERY POSITIVE
MOTHER	0.5	1.5	7.8	25.4	38.1	23.4	4.3
FATHER	0.9	1.9	7.6	22.1	35.1	27.2	5.5
ADOLESCENT	1.2*	3.1	4.9*	17.4**	25.7***	22.3	26.3***

Figure 2.2. Distribution of positive and negative affect reported by family members. Asterisks show the two-tailed significance of comparisons between adolescents and their same-sex parents. None of the comparisons between mothers and fathers were significant. Reprinted with permission from Larson & Richards, 1994b.

emotional states, the young adolescents demonstrated much greater variance than their parents in the range of their emotional swings (Larson & Richards, 1994a, b). To examine this further, we computed the percentage of time that each individual reported experiencing each of seven gradations from extreme negative to extreme positive emotion. As shown in Figure 2.2, the adolescents reported significantly more occasions when they felt extreme negative and positive affect, while their parents reported more occasions when their emotions were toward the middle of the scale, in the neutral and moderate range (Larson & Richards, 1994a, b). The differences were substantial, particularly with regard to extreme positive emotions. The youth reported feeling "very" happy approximately five times more often (26.3%) than did their parents (mothers: 4.3%; fathers: 5.5%). These basic differences between adolescents and parents were replicated in the third study, with 100 middle-class families in northern India. The 8th graders in this study reported extreme positive and negative emotions significantly more frequently than did their mothers and fathers (Verma & Larson, 1999).

A skeptic could ask whether these findings might reflect differences in how teens and adults use the rating scales. Maybe adults feel the same states, but rate them as less extreme. To provide a check against that possibility, we asked both the teens and parents in the YAS sample to use the same rating scales to identify the emotions they perceived in a set of faces, chosen to represent different levels of happy and unhappy emotions (Larson & Richards, 1994a). We found that there was no difference in their average ratings for these faces, suggesting that both were using the scales to indicate comparable levels of emotion. It is also informative that in the ESM data, parents reported *more* extreme scores than their children on self-rating scales that dealt, not with emotions, but with other dimensions of experience. Parents rated themselves as feeling very "interested," "in control," and "hurried" more often during their daily lives. So adults are not inhibited about using the extremes of the scales. For dimensions relevant to parents' lives – motivation, command, and pressure – adults *do* report strong states. These findings strengthen the case that the adolescents' reports of more extreme emotions represent actual differences in their lived experience.

Taken together, these three studies provide substantial support for the thesis that adolescents experience wider emotional swings than adults. It is important to stress that the emotional swings of adolescents include not just more frequent strong negative emotions than adults, but also more strong positive emotions: times when they use the extreme superlative ends of the scale to describe how they feel. So, if we define "moodiness" as wide emotional fluctuations, the stereotype is true; adolescents are more moody than adults. But their average emotional state is not more morose than that of adults. Both youth and adults report many more occasions of positive emotions than negative emotions, a ratio that is associated with positive well-being (Fredrickson & Losada, 2005).

Are adolescents moodier than pre-adolescents?

But are these wide emotional fluctuations distinctive to adolescence? Or might they merely reflect continuity in a pattern of emotions from childhood? Because the YAS sample bridged the transition from elementary into middle school, it provided a good opportunity to examine whether daily emotional experience changed as the youth entered adolescence.

What the data showed was a downward shift in the average affective state across this period from 5th to 9th grade. The width of the statistical variance on our bipolar emotional scales did not differ substantially as a function of age; that is to say, adolescents did not evidence appreciably wider emotional swings than pre-adolescents (Larson & Lampman-Petraitis, 1989). However, there was a notable change across this period in the average valence of reported mood states, with dysphoric moods increasing linearly with age.

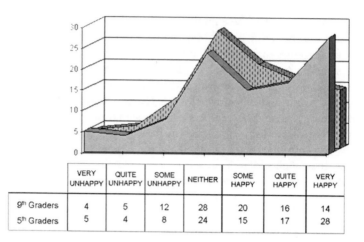

	VERY UNHAPPY	QUITE UNHAPPY	SOME UNHAPPY	NEITHER	SOME HAPPY	QUITE HAPPY	VERY HAPPY
9th Graders	4	5	12	28	20	16	14
5th Graders	5	4	8	24	15	17	28

Figure 2.3. Differences in the frequency of gradations of unhappiness and happiness between 5th and 9th grade. Reprinted with permission from Larson *et al.* (2002).

As depicted in Figure 2.3, this change was characterised by a decrease in the frequency of extreme positive emotions and an increase in the frequency of mildly negative ones (i.e. feeling "somewhat" unhappy, irritable, angry) among the 8th and 9th grade youth. As with the comparison of adolescents and their parents discussed above, the possibility that findings were attributable to age differences in use of the affect scales was ruled out by the finding that younger and older did not differ in how they rated the emotions depicted in the pictures of faces (Larson & Lampman-Petraitis, 1989).

Notably, this basic age trend was consistent across gender, and ethnicity/ race. Girls and boys in the YAS showed the same downward shift over the period from 5th–9th grade. Girls' average reported emotional states were somewhat more positive than boys across the age period, a difference due to girls reporting higher levels of feeling cheerful and friendly than boys. However, both sexes showed the same dramatic decline in rates of extreme positive emotions and an increase in the rates of negative emotions (Larson & Lampman-Petraitis, 1989). A similar downward shift in emotional states also was found to occur between 5th and 8th grade in the study of urban African–American students (Larson *et al.*, 2002). To our knowledge there have not been studies that have examined these age changes for other ethnic groups, or in other nations. Nonetheless, the replication across two large samples suggests a measure of robustness to the findings, at least within the American developmental experience.

Our data suggest, then, that although adolescents' typical states are not more morose than adults', they are more morose than pre-adolescents'. It is important to point out, however, that the young adolescents in these two samples (the 7th–9th graders) reported positive emotions much more often than they reported negative emotions. The preponderance of positive affect that is associated with mental health remains the norm. Thus, while entry into the adolescent years was associated with more frequent occasions of unhappiness, anger, and distress, negative emotion by no means dominated their lives. In the next section, we examine the nature of youths' emotional experiences as adolescence unfolds into and during the high school years.

Trends across adolescence

If early adolescence is a time when negative affect increases, what happens in middle adolescence? Does negative affect increase further? Or does the pattern of daily emotions start to look more like that of adulthood, with reduced variability in emotional states? A subset of the YAS sample ($n = 220$) participated in a follow-up assessment 4 years after the original study, providing an opportunity to examine the trajectory of emotional experiences during the high school years. Attrition was greater among boys, and among youth with lower GPAs, higher self-reported depression scores, and higher rates of negative affect at Time 1. It should be noted, however, that these differences were not large. For example, among youth whose average affect at Time 1 was in the lowest one third, 38% did not participate at Time 2 as compared with 30% for the other youth.

The primary finding of this investigation was that the downward trend in affect did not continue throughout the high school years (Larson *et al.*, 2002). The increase in dysphoric affect stopped at tenth grade, and leveled out after that point. This trajectory was the same across gender. Consistent with the Time 1 data, girls' average affect at Time 2 was somewhat more positive than that of the boys (Figure 2.4). In particular, girls reported greater cheerfulness and friendliness, especially when signaled in social contexts (Larson & Pleck, 1999). Another longitudinal ESM study suggested a similar leveling out of a downward change in affect in the high school years (Csikszentmihalyi & Hunter, 2003; Moneta *et al.*, 2001); and studies using questionnaire measures of affective states suggest that rates of negative affect begin to decrease in the post high school years (Chen *et al.*, 1998; Holsen *et al.*, 2000). Together, these studies indicate that the transition to adolescence is associated with a normative increase in the rate of daily negative emotion that slows down and plateaus in mid- to late-adolescence.

These patterns, however, represent the group norm, and do not reflect the variability that occurred among the teens. First, not all youth showed the downward shift in emotions across this 4-year span from middle school to high school. Sixty-three percent of youth reported lower average affect across their ESM reports at Time 2 than Time 1; approximately half of these (34%) showed downward shifts in average affect that were substantial (i.e. greater

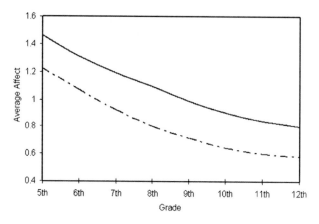

Figure 2.4. **Estimated time trends in mean affect across grades for girls and boys.**

than 0.5 SD from their Time 1 mean). As attrition was greater among more distressed youth, these values may somewhat under-estimate the extent of the change.

These results, then suggest that mid-adolescence – the high school period – represents a kind of nadir of normative emotional experience. Rates of negative emotions did not increase across this period, but they did not diminish either. Furthermore, in the YAS data the high variability in adolescents' daily emotions did not begin to contract toward the pattern we found for adults. It is important to recognize, however, that even at this nadir, the emotional states of most youth in the YAS sample was still positive most of the time. Though adolescents reported more frequent negative emotions (19.6% of reports) at the Time 2 assessment, than they had 4 years earlier (12.7%), the ratio of positive to negative emotion was still strongly in the positive direction (Larson *et al.*, 2002).

In summary, it appears that adolescents have a wider emotional range than do adults, such that they experience more extreme positive and more extreme negative emotions with greater frequency. This range, however, does *not* discriminate them from pre-adolescents. Rather, the distinguishing feature relative to younger children is a diminishing of extreme positive and an increase in negative affect. In the next section, we address our second question regarding the factors that contribute to this negative affect.

What factors relate to the distressed emotions of adolescence?

Is the early adolescent increase in negative emotions related to puberty, as is commonly believed, or might other variables like stress and cognitive change play a role? The YAS data provided an opportunity to examine the relationships of these three factors to the emotions of adolescence. We focus specifically on the Time 1 data, because they allowed us to see associations during the age period of greatest change in emotional patterns.

Puberty

In the YAS, puberty was assessed using a self-report scale of physical development on which youth indicate their level of genital and pubic hair development relative to drawings indicating Tanner stages for their sex (Morris *et al.*, 1980). Reports on these scales have been found to be highly correlated with physician's ratings. The adolescents also provided an estimate of the degree to which their pubertal development was "on time," early, or late. Age was controlled for in the analyses in order to examine the independent association between pubertal stage and emotions.

Overall, the findings failed to bear out the expectation that pubertal development would be correlated with emotionality (Richards & Larson, 1993). In particular, there was no evidence that either greater pubertal development or adolescents' perceptions of the timing of their pubertal development were associated with more negative average states on the affect scale for either boys or girls (Richards & Larson, 1993). Isolated relationships between pubertal development and other affective states did emerge. In particular, there were associations, for both boys and girls, with feeling "in love" more often. This relationship makes sense given the evolutionary function of puberty – to make youth into reproductive creatures. More advanced development also was associated with boys feeling "tense" and "frustrated" more often and with girls feeling frustrated *less* frequently. Most of the infrequent associations between puberty and daily experience occurred for the younger participants (in the 5th and 6th grades). The general pattern, then suggests that the relationships between puberty and negative emotions or other patterns of emotions are limited at most. This general lack of relationship was also replicated in the sample of African–American youth.[1]

Though contrary to "popular opinion," these results are largely consistent with the body of literature that has developed using questionnaire measures of emotions in conjunction with more precise measures of hormones and puberty. Overall, this research indicates that associations between pubertal stage and emotionality are small in magnitude and appear to be strongest at the height of pubertal change (DeRose and Brooks-Gunn, see Chapter 4, this volume; Graber & Brooks-Gunn, 1996). This questionnaire research also suggests that stress may be a more important factor.

Stress

The transition into adolescence is characterized by a "pile up" of life changes, and the cumulative stress of these changes is thought to tax adolescents' emotional and coping resources (Graber & Brooks-Gunn, 1996; Simmons *et al.*, 1987). Might the increase in negative emotions during adolescence be attributable to this increase in daily stress? The evidence that young adolescents' rates of stressful experiences are associated with their reports of depressive symptomatology is suggestive in this regard (Brooks-Gunn & Warren, 1989).

The ESM data provided the opportunity to evaluate the relationships between stressful experience and emotions measured during daily life. These relationships were examined at both time points (T1 5th to 9th grade; T2 9th–12th grade). Reports of stressful events were provided by both the adolescents and their parents. Adolescents who experienced a greater number of stressful events reported negative affect a greater proportion of the time than did those who experienced fewer negative events (Greene & Larson, 1991; Larson & Ham, 1993; Larson *et al.*, 2002). Family-related stressors were particularly salient in this regard. Similar results emerged in the sample of African–American middle-school students. In this sample, negative life events were associated, in particular, with youths' reports of angry affect. A recent ESM study of Dutch adolescents found that adolescents who experienced a greater number of negative events reported more negative affect and less positive affect than did their peers (Schneiders *et al.*, 2006). In this study, the nature of the mood response was influenced by the social context of the stressor, with depressive and anxious mood being associated with family and school events, respectively.

As these data are cross-sectional and correlational, caution is needed in making conclusion about the mechanisms accounting for the association. Certainly, experiencing adverse events would be expected to result in more negative mood states, and longitudinal research using questionnaire measures of affect substantiate such a predictive relationship over time (Compas, 1987; Simmons *et al.*, 1987). It should also be recognized that the relations between stress and emotional states may be mediated by other variables, such as the sleep disruptions associated with stress (Fuligni & Hardway, 2006). Furthermore, the possibility that these correlational findings result, at least in part, from reverse causality, should also be considered. Evidence indicates that adolescents experiencing depressive symptoms are more likely to generate stressors, especially of an interpersonal nature (Cole *et al.*, 2006; Rudolph *et al.*, 2000). Further research is needed to estimate the size and mechanisms of reciprocal influence.

Before moving on to the role of cognition, however, there is one more finding that is particularly provocative. In the YAS we found that the association between stressful events and negative affect interacted significantly with age, such that the association was much stronger among the adolescents (7th–9th grade) than among the pre-adolescents (5th–6th graders; Larson & Ham, 1993). A number of factors could explain this interaction. For one thing, adolescents' reduced reliance on adult supports may leave them more dependent on their own resources and, hence, more vulnerable to the emotional impact of stressful events. Also, as described in the next section, changes in adolescents' cognitive abilities may contribute to this unexpected finding.

Cognitive changes

It has long been argued that adolescents acquire new ways of thinking. They are more able to think abstractly, use propositional reasoning, and think deeply about dynamic systems and how they interact (Keating, 2004; Kesek *et al.*, see Chapter 8, this volume). There are also changes in how adolescents think about self and others in social contexts. They are more able to perceive and imagine other's points of view (Selman, 2003) and empathize with them (Eisenberg *et al.*, see Chapter 10, this volume).

Data from the YAS sample suggest that these changes may be related to adolescent increases in negative affect. Each time participants in the study were signaled, they were asked, "If you were feeling a lot of something, why did you feel that way?," and responses to this question were coded into categories. Striking differences emerged in the explanations provided by the adolescents (7th–9th grades), as compared with the pre-adolescents (5th–6th graders). Adolescents were more likely to attribute their emotions to events occurring in peer and romantic relationships. Twice the proportion of their negative emotions was attributed to factors in these relationships (Larson & Asmussen, 1991). Peer and romantic relationships, moreover, continued to be a frequent explanation for strong emotions at Time 2, during high school (Wilson-Shockley, 1995; see also Furman, McDunn, & Young, Chapter 16, this volume; La Greca, Davila, & Seigel, Chapter 17, this volume). It appeared they were becoming more invested in and emotionally sensitive to the peer world.

What is most notable, however, is the cognitive complexity of the explanations the older youth provided for their negative emotions. The younger group most often explained their negative emotions in terms of the immediate situation, (e.g. "mad, because I hate cleaning my rabbit's cage"; "frustrated, because I hate spelling"; "bored, I was just standing in line"). Their emotions were attributed to concrete situations in the present moment. In contrast, the adolescents' explanations for their negative emotions were more likely to incorporate abstract concepts, include actual or imagined events outside the here and now, and involve considerations of others' perspectives (Larson & Asmussen, 1991). Their accounts were less tied to tangible circumstances and more tied to the psychological meanings of events within dynamic interpersonal systems.

Adolescents' explanations for their negative emotions involved many of the cognitive developments that scholars attribute to adolescence. They involved the ability to reason about abstract psychological concepts ("when Mike and I fought last night I felt that I was losing a piece of myself") and reason about hypothetical future contingencies ("worried and nervous, because Tom is supposed to ask me out. I hope I don't goof"). They entailed inferences about what others may be feeling or thinking ("he's trying to make me feel guilty"), including empathy for the experiences of others. Adolescents' explanations also entailed the ability to reason about complex interpersonal systems that include several peers and their subjective realities ("jealous, because a girl I like likes Sean"). Although recent "theory of mind" research shows that younger children are able to demonstrate some capability for understanding others' points of view in controlled laboratory situations, there is little evidence that they use this reasoning frequently during daily life. They are not likely, for example, to think in terms of "a piece of myself," let alone worry about losing it. Nor are they as invested in the types of strong peer and romantic relationships that were the context for many of these negative feelings.

These explanations suggest that adolescents' new cognitive skills may make them more vulnerable to daily events than they were a few years earlier. But why should developing new skills render adolescents more vulnerable? One might expect that these new cognitive skills would allow them to better anticipate and avoid stressful situations, as well as to cope with them when they occur. Perhaps, however, ignorance is bliss. Rosenblum & Lewis (2003) argue that the emergence of new thinking skills means that emotions may be elicited by abstract ideas, anticipated events, and recalled events. Adolescents may hence be more prone than younger children to ruminating about adverse experiences, past and present. Moreover, their improved ability to take others' perspectives may render adolescents more vulnerable to experience distress brought about by events occurring to others (see Eisenberg *et al.*, Chapter 10, this volume). Larson & Asmussen (1991) suggest that these new skills make them more susceptible to hurt across a wider plane of time and interpersonal space.

Finally, one needs to consider that adolescents are not quite "finished products" as regards cognitive development. As described by Kesek and colleagues (see Chapter 8, this volume), it has become increasingly apparent that development in executive control (and the neurological systems hypothesized to underlie it), continues through young adulthood. Hence, in the short term, the broadening of the adolescents' world, socially and cognitively, may render them vulnerable to events and negative emotions, before they have the capacity for effective regulation.

How do normative patterns in adolescents' daily emotions relate to depression?

An underlying assumption of this chapter, indeed of this volume, is that normative patterns of emotional experience in adolescence are relevant to understanding affective psychopathology. Our final question, therefore, is how the normative patterns in daily emotion that we have been discussing may relate to the emergence of a broader array of psychological symptoms. We consider two issues. First, in what ways might the increased experience of negative affect in early adolescence relate to depressive symptoms and disorder, which increase at this same age period? Second, how might other factors, such as the pile up of life stress and/or individual differences, feed into this equation? Existing ESM findings only scratch the surface in addressing these issues, but they provide tantalizing hints for future research.

The association between daily emotions and adolescents' increased depression

A beginning point for this discussion is the robust finding of ESM studies that youth experiencing high rates of negative affect are more likely to manifest symptoms of depression. In YAS, rates of negative affect were consistently correlated with scores on the Child Depression Inventory across the pre-adolescent, early adolescent, and middle adolescent years, with no significant difference in these associations between boys and girls (Larson et al., 1990, 2002). Other ESM studies, including a study using a clinical sample (Merrick, 1992), have found that adolescents with elevated scores on measures of depressive symptomatology experience more negative affect (i.e. anger, sadness, anxiety), less positive affect (happiness, perceived well-being), and greater emotional variability (Barber et al., 1998; Silk et al., 2003; Verma & Larson, 1999; Whalen et al., 2001). Depressed youth also reported lower hour-to-hour levels of arousal and energy, and greater levels of subjective distress (Barber et al., 1998; Whalen et al., 2001). These findings establish that daily negative affect and depression are consistently correlated.

The fact that rates of negative affect and depression both show a normative increase in early adolescence, and then plateau in mid-adolescence, suggests a further level of correspondence between the two phenomena. One explanation for this parallel age pattern might be that adolescents' greater negative affect, when potentiated by intrapersonal or situational characteristics, may engender the broader pattern of depressive symptoms (like sleep dysfunction, disturbed eating, pessimism, and suicidal ideation), apparent in depressive disorder. For example, poor emotion-regulation skills or interpersonal difficulties fed by irritable or dysphoric affect could exacerbate the normative affective changes in vulnerable youth. Relatedly, shared genetic vulnerability between temperamental negative emotionality and depressive disorder (Hettema et al., 2006) may also contribute to this confluence.

Marked gender differences in these corresponding age patterns also need to be considered. Though negative affect increases in early adolescence for both girls and boys, researchers have consistently shown that depressive symptomatology and disorder increase primarily for girls (Seeley & Lewinsohn, see Chapter 3, this volume). Why might the age trends show more correspondence for girls than boys? One explanation may lie in the finding that girls are more likely to ruminate on depressed mood (Barber *et al.*, 1998), and it is possible that this ruminative process amplifies negative moods and contributes to the generation of these other symptoms.

Another, almost contradictory, gender difference is that girls in ESM studies report more *positive* average daily emotions than boys (Figure 2.4; see also Barber *et al.*, 1998; Larson & Lampman-Petraitis, 1989). Thus, although girls are more prone to depressive symptoms, they also have a higher balance of positive daily affective states. This contradiction is partly explained by the finding that, as girls enter the adolescent years, they show wider emotional swings than they did earlier (Larson *et al.*, 2002). They become more likely to be extremely happy at one interval of time and despondent at another (as illustrated by Vivian in Figure 2.1), and it is possible that these negative swings are accompanied by or generative of depressive symptoms. Further research is needed to assess these gender differences and how they are related to developmental trajectories for depression.

From normative description to dynamic processes

One factor likely to play a role in these developmental trajectories is the experience of stress. Based on the findings reported earlier, we hypothesize a pathway from the normative pile up of stress in early adolescence to increased negative emotion to depression (with this last link stronger for girls). This pile up, combined with greater vulnerability created by age-related cognitive development, may be the critical factors that initiate the sequence in the pathway.

The possibility of individual differences in how youth respond to stress and negative affect, however, also needs to be considered. There is, of course, an extensive literature documenting biological and environmental characteristics that predispose individuals to affective disturbance. As youth move into adolescence, these individual factors may influence not only the nature and frequency of stressful experiences, but also their ability to respond adaptively to them. Hence, depression-prone youth may generate stressful experiences and also be more likely to respond to them in non-adaptive ways, while more resilient youth may have resources that enable them to avoid or attenuate the impact of these experiences.

What is called for, then, is better integration of knowledge and approaches from the study of normative development with those used to examine individual differences. Studies are needed that use longitudinal designs to allow examination of the interaction between the normative changes of adolescence and these individual factors. The perspective provided by ESM helps us think about these interactions as processes that occur in the contexts of daily lives. Let us give two examples of research that are suggestive of these processes.

The first example uses data from recent studies to illustrate differences in how depressed vs. non-depressed adolescents respond to acute negative events. First, in an ESM study of mood reactivity to daily events, high risk adolescents (defined by a cluster of difficulties including elevated depression scores) were shown to be more reactive to negative events than were their peers. They responded to negative events with both greater reductions in positive affect and greater increases in negative affect (Schneiders *et al.*, 2006). Moreover, these results were most pronounced in adolescents who had experienced greater levels of recent life stress. Second, an ESM study conducted by Silk and colleagues (2003) provided evidence that depressed adolescents had greater difficulty shifting out of negative affect states than did non-depressed peers. Similar findings have been reported from a third study using observational measures of negative affect during parent–child interactions (Sheeber *et al.*, 2000). The Silk study also found that depressed adolescents were more likely than peers to respond to negative emotion with disengagement (e.g. avoidance, wishful thinking) and involuntary engagement (e.g. rumination; impulsive behavior), responses that were correlated with difficulty shifting out of sad and angry emotional states.

Together, these results indicate that depressed adolescents are more likely to respond to daily events with negative affect, especially if they are experiencing a pile up of stressful events, and that they recover from these states less quickly. They suggest a process whereby individual differences render certain individuals more susceptible to sustained negative affect, which might in turn develop into depressive disorder.

The second example illustrates the role that context might play in mediating the relationship between daily experience and depression. In a series of analyses of the ESM studies described above, Larson found that the time adolescents spent alone appeared to have a dynamic relationship with both mood and mood regulation (Larson, 1990, 1997; Larson & Csikszentmihalyi, 1978; Larson *et al.*, 1982). First, they found that when alone, teens experience greater loneliness and dysphoria; however, at the next ESM report *after* being alone, they report feeling more positive than they did on other similar occasions. This suggests a paradoxical dynamic in which a retreat into solitude was related to a positive rebound on emotional well-being, possibly because it provides an occasion for coping and recentering. Moreover, in three separate studies we found a curvilinear relationship between the amount of time an adolescent spent alone and measures of adjustment, including depressive symptoms: Adolescents who spent an intermediate amount of time alone reported better average mood and adjustment than those who spent either little or a great deal of time alone. These patterns were not replicated for pre-adolescents or adults, so were adolescent-specific.

These findings suggest how hour-to-hour daily experiences in a particular context might contribute to both short- and long-term well-being. Under the right conditions, a period of time alone may serve as a resiliency mechanism and contribute to an adolescent's positive state. But under other conditions it does not; in fact spending large amounts of time alone is associated with depression. Data on other contexts suggests different dynamic relationships. For example there is evidence that depressed adolescents may reap fewer benefits from social interactions with friends and family than do their non-depressed peers (LaGreca *et al.*, see Chapter 17, this volume; Larson *et al.*, 1990; Tompson *et al.*, see Chapter 15, this volume). Individual differences may enter into these relationships by influencing not only how individuals experience a given context, but also which contexts they choose to enter (Caspi *et al.*, 2005).

Together, these two examples illustrate how daily emotions are part of dynamic processes. They suggest how depression may be manifest in the unfolding of adolescents' hour-to-hour experiences in response to stress and daily contexts. They suggest both vulnerability and resiliency processes that influence affective states; processes that may have consequences for development of depressive symptomatology. These daily processes, of course, are not the full explanation. There is substantial evidence that individuals' average patterns of daily affect, as well as their risk for depressive disorder, are influenced by stable underlying personality traits (Diener *et al.*, 2006; Klein *et al.*, see Chapter 13, this volume). However there is also evidence that the influences of these traits are at least partly mediated by how people respond to daily situations, and further that these responses can be influenced by development change (Caspi *et al.*, 2005; Diener *et al.*, 2006).

Adolescence, as we have seen, is a time of substantial change in daily emotions, so it may be an especially important period to understand this interplay of individual dispositions and daily experiences. It is essential to consider how these types of daily emotional dynamics might be both a cause and an effect of adolescents' longer-term patterns of depressive symptomatology.

Conclusion

To summarize, research with the ESM has provided both valuable information about normative patterns, and provocative hypotheses about what may lie behind these patterns. These studies present fairly strong evidence that, relative to adulthood, adolescence is a time of wide emotional swings, including not just negative but also strong positive emotions; indeed positive states are much more frequent than negative ones for most adolescents. Moreover, they have demonstrated that entry into adolescence is associated with the experience of more negative affect for many youth, at least within the socio-cultural groups covered by these studies. This research also has demonstrated correlational relationships between negative emotion and stress, and has suggested that stress may be a bigger factor than puberty in accounting for the increase in negative affect during this age period. Lastly, the data show robust relationships between this negative affect and depression, such that prolonged distress or despondency should not be dismissed as normal adolescence.

The major unanswered questions concern the processes and pathways that link individual differences, stress, negative emotion, and depression. Creative research designs will be required to capture these processes and pathways in the time frames in which they occur. The ESM addresses the time frame of hours and days, and, by itself may provide too granular a picture to detect dynamics that unfold in seconds and minutes, while being too fine-grained to capture longer-term change. Traditional longitudinal designs in which data are collected every 1–2 years may be suited to identifying this longer-term change, but miss the more proximate processes through which these changes occur. A strength of the ESM is that it obtains self-reports of emotional experiences in natural contexts, but clearly diverse methodologies, as represented in this volume, provide equally important pieces of this large and complex puzzle.

ENDNOTE

1 Analyses conducted by Larson on a data set described in Richards *et al.*, 2004.

REFERENCES

Barber, B.L., Jacobson, K.C., Miller, K.E., & Petersen, A.C. (1998). Ups and downs: daily cycles of adolescent moods. In A.C. Crouter & R. Larson (Eds.), *Temporal Rhythms in Adolescence: Clocks, Calendars, and the Coordination of Daily Life* (pp. 23–36). San Francisco, CA: Jossey-Bass.

Bradley, M.M., & Lang, P.J. (2000). Measuring emotion: behavior, feeling, and physiology. In R.D. Lane & L. Nagel (Eds.), *Cognitive Neuroscience of Emotion* (pp. 242–276). New York, NY: Oxford University Press.

Brooks-Gunn, J., & Warren, M.P. (1989). Biological and social contributions to negative affect in young adolescent girls. *Child Development*, 60, 40–55.

Caspi, A., Roberts, B., & Shiner, R. (2005). Personality development: stability and change. *Annual Review of Psychology*, 56, 453–484.

Chen, H., Mechanic, D., & Hansell, S. (1998). A longitudinal study of self-awareness and depressed mood in adolescence. *Journal of Youth and Adolescence*, 27(6), 719–734.

Cole, D.A., Nolen-Hoeksema, S., Girgus, J., & Paul, G. (2006). Stress exposure and stress generation in child and adolescent depression: a latent trait-state-error approach to longitudinal analyses. *Journal of Abnormal Psychology*, 115(1), 40–51.

Compas, B.E. (1987). Stress and life events during childhood and adolescence. *Clinical Psychology Review, 7*, 275–302.

Csikszentmihalyi, M., & Hunter, J. (2003). Happiness in everyday life: the uses of experience sampling. *Journal of Happiness Studies, 4*, 185–199.

Csikszentmihalyi, M., & Larson, R. (1984). *Being Adolescent.* New York: Basic Books.

Csikszentmihalyi, M., & Larson, R. (1987). Validity and reliability of experience-sampling method. *Journal of Nervous and Mental Disease, 175*, 526–536.

Diener, E., Lucas, R.E., & Scollon, C. (2006). Beyond the hedonic treadmill: revising the adaptation theory of well-being. *American Psychologist, 61*, 305–314.

Farkas, S., & Johnson, J. (1997). *Kids these Days: What Americans Really Think about the Next Generation.* New York, NY: Public Agenda.

Flament, M.F., Cohen, D., Choquet, M., Jeammet, P., & Ledoux, S. (2001). Phenom-enology, psychosocial correlates, and treatment seeking in major depression and dysthymia of adolescence. *Journal of the American Academy of Child and Adolescent Psychiatry, 40*, 1070–1078.

Fredrickson, B.L., & Losada, M.F. (2005). Positive affect and the complex dynamics of human flourishing. *American Psychologist, 60*, 678–686.

Fuligni, A.J., & Hardway, C. (2006). Daily variation in adolescents' sleep, activities, and psychological well-being. *Journal of Research on Adolescence, 16*, 353–378.

Graber, J.A., & Brooks-Gunn, J. (1996). Transitions and turning points: navigating the passage from childhood through adolescence. *Developmental Psychology, 32*, 768–776.

Greene, A.L., & Larson, R. (1991). Variations in stress reactivity during adolescence. In E.M. Cummings, A.L. Greene, & K.H. Karraker (Eds.), *Life Span Developmental Psychology: Perspectives on Stress and Coping* (pp. 195–209). Hillsdale, NJ: Lawrence Erlbaum.

Hektner, J.M., Schmidt, J.A., & Csikszentmihalyi, M. (2007). *Experience Sampling Method: Measuring the Quality of Everyday Life.* Thousand Oaks, CA: Sage.

Hess, R., & Goldblatt, I. (1957). The status of adolescence in American society: a problem in social identity. *Child Development, 28*, 459–468.

Hettema, J.M., Neale, M.C., Myers, J.M., Prescott, C.A., & Kendler, K.S. (2006). A population-based twin study of the relationship between neuroticism and intern-alizing disorders. *American Journal of Psychiatry, 163*, 857–864.

Holsen, I., Kraft, P., & Vittersø, J. (2000). Stability in depressed mood in adolescence: results from a 6-year longitudinal panel study. *Journal of Youth and Adolescence, 29*, 61–78.

Kahneman, D., & Riis, J. (2005). Living, and thinking about it: two perspectives on life. In F.A. Huppert, N. Baylis, & B. Keverne (Eds.), *The Science of Well-being* (pp. 284–304). Oxford, UK: Oxford University Press.

Keating, D. (2004). Cognitive and brain development. In R.M. Lerner & L. Steinberg (Eds.), *Handbook of Adolescent Psychology* (pp. 45–84). New York: Wiley.

Larson, R. (1989). Beeping children and adolescents: a method for studying time use and daily experience. *Journal of Youth and Adolescence, 18*, 511–530.

Larson, R. (1991). Adolescent moodiness. In R. Lerner, A. Peterson, & J. Brooks-Gunn (Eds.), *The Encyclopedia of Adolescence* (pp. 658–662). New York, NY: Garland.

Larson, R.W. (1990). The solitary side of life: an examination of the time people spend alone from childhood to old age. *Developmental Review, 10*, 155–183.

Larson, R.W. (1997). The emergence of solitude as a constructive domain of experience in early adolescence. *Child Development, 68*, 80–93.

Larson, R.W., & Asmussen, L. (1991). Anger, worry, and hurt in early adolescence: an enlarging world of negative emotions. In M.E. Colten & S. Gore (Eds.), *Adolescent Stress: Causes and Consequences* (pp. 21–41). New York: Adline de Gruyter.

Larson, R.W., & Csikszentmihalyi, M. (1978). Experiential correlates of time alone in adolescence. *Journal of Personality, 46*, 677–693.

Larson, R.W., & Ham, M. (1993). Stress and "storm and stress" in early adolescence: the relationship of negative events with dysphoric affect. *Developmental Psychology, 29*, 130–140.

Larson, R.W., & Lampman-Petraitis, C. (1989). Daily emotional states as reported by children and adolescents. *Child Development, 60*, 1250–1260.

Larson, R.W. & Pleck, J. (1999). Hidden feelings: emotionality in boys and men. In D. Bernstein (Ed.), *Nebraska Symposium on Motivation: Vol. 45. Gender and Motivation* (pp. 25–74). Lincoln, NE: University of Nebraska Press.

Larson, R.W., & Richards, M.H. (1991). Daily companionship in late childhood and early adolescence: changing developmental contexts. *Child Development, 62*(2), 284–300.

Larson, R.W., & Richards, M.H. (1994a). *Divergent realities: The Emotional Lives of Mothers, Fathers, and Adolescents.* New York, NY: Basic Books.

Larson, R.W., & Richards, M.H. (1994b). Family emotions: do young adolescents and their parents experience the same states? *Journal of Research on Adolescence, 4*, 567–583.

Larson, R.W., Csikszentmihalyi, M., & Graef, R. (1980). Mood variability and the psychosocial adjustment of adolescents. *Journal of Youth and Adolescence, 9*, 469–490.

Larson, R., Csikszentmihalyi, M., & Graef, R. (1982). Time alone in daily experience: loneliness or renewal? In L.A. Peplau & D. Perlman (Eds.), *Loneliness: A Sourcebook of Current Theory, Research, and Therapy* (pp. 41–53). New York, NY: Wiley-Interscience.

Larson, R.W., Raffaelli, M., Richards, M.H., Ham, M., & Jewell, L. (1990). Ecology of depression in late childhood and early adolescence: a profile of daily states and activities. *Journal of Abnormal Psychology, 99*(1), 92–102.

Larson, R.W., Moneta, G., Richards, M.H., & Wilson, S. (2002). Continuity, stability, and change in daily emotional experience across adolescence. *Child Development, 73*, 1151–1165.

Lewinsohn, P.M., Rohde, P., & Seeley, J.R. (1995). Adolescent psychopathology: III. The clinical consequences of comorbidity. *Journal of the American Academy of Child and Adolescent Psychiatry, 34*, 510–519.

Merrick, W.A. (1992). Dysphoric moods in depressed and non-depressed adolescents. In M.W. deVries (Ed.), *The Experience of Psychopathology: Investigating Mental Disorders in their Natural Settings* (pp. 148–156). New York: Cambridge University Press.

Moneta, G.B., Schneider, B., & Csikszentmihalyi, M. (2001). A longitudinal study of the self-concept and experiential components of self-worth and affect across adolescence. *Applied Developmental Science, 5*(3), 125–142.

Morris, N.M., & Udry, J.R. (1980). Validation of self-administered instrument to assess stage of adolescent development. *Journal of Youth and Adolescence, 9*, 271–280.

Richards, M.H., & Larson, R. (1993). Pubertal development and the daily subjective states of young adolescents. *Journal of Research on Adolescence*, **3**(2), 145–169.

Richards, M., Larson, R., Viegas Miller, B. *et al.* (2004). Risky and protective contexts and exposure to violence in urban African-American young adolescents. *Journal of Clinical Child and Adolescent Psychology*, **33**, 138–148.

Rosenblum, G.D., & Lewis, M. (2003). Emotional development in adolescence. In G.R. Adams & M.D. Berzonsky (Eds.), *Blackwell Handbook of Adolescence* (pp. 269–289). Malden, MA: Blackwell.

Rudolph, K.D., Hammen, C., Burge, D. *et al.* (2000). Toward an interpersonal life-stress model of depression: the developmental context of stress generation. *Development and Psychopathology*, **12**, 215–234.

Schneiders, J., Nicolson, N.A., Berkhof, J. *et al.* (2006). Mood reactivity to daily negative events in early adolescence: relationship to risk for psychopathology. *Developmental Psychology*, **42**, 543–554.

Selman, R.L. (2003). *The Promotion of Social Awareness: Powerful Lessons from the Partnership of Developmental Theory and Classroom Practice*. New York, NY: Russell Sage Foundation.

Sheeber, L.B., Allen, N., Davis, B., & Sorensen, E.D. (2000). Regulation of negative affect during mother-child problem-solving interactions: adolescent depressive status and family processes. *Journal of Abnormal Child Psychology*, **28**, 467–479.

Silk, J.S., Steinberg, L., & Morris, A.S. (2003). Adolescents' emotion regulation in daily life: links to depressive symptoms and problem behavior. *Child Development*, **74**, 1869–1880.

Simmons, R.G., Burgeson, R., Carlton-Ford, S., & Blyth, D.A. (1987). The impact of cumulative change in early adolescence. *Child Development*, **58**(5), 1220–1234.

Steinberg, L., Dahl, R., Keating, D. *et al.* (2006). The study of developmental psycho-pathology in adolescence: integrating affective neuroscience with the study of context. In D. Cicchetti & D.J. Cohen (Eds.), *Developmental Psychopathology, Vol 2. Developmental Neuroscience* (2nd edn, pp. 710–741). Hoboken, NJ: Wiley.

Verma, S., & Larson, R. (1999). Are adolescents more emotional? A study of the daily emotions of middle class Indian adolescents. *Psychology and Developing Societies*, **11**(2), 179–194.

Whalen, C.K., Jamner, L.D., Henker, B., & Delfino, R.J. (2001). Smoking and moods in adolescents with depressive and aggressive dispositions: evidence from surveys and electronic diaries. *Health Psychology*, **20**(2), 99–111.

Wilson-Shockley, S. (1995). *Gender Differences in Adolescent Depression: The Contribution of Negative Affect*. M.S. Thesis. University of Illinois at Urbana-Champaign.

3

Epidemiology of mood disorders during adolescence: implications for lifetime risk

John R. Seeley and Peter M. Lewinsohn

Prior to the 1970s, depression among adolescents received relatively little empirical attention. Indeed, some researchers maintained that depression did not exist in adolescents or that diagnostic criteria needed to be modified for use with adolescents (Glaser & Strauss, 1968; Toolan, 1962). Beginning in the 1970s, a number of researchers (Albert & Beck, 1975; Carlson & Cantwell, 1979; Cytryn & McKnew, 1972; Kashani & Simonds, 1979; Rutter *et al.*, 1986) began to focus on mood disorders in children and adolescents, concluding that depressive disorders clearly occur during this developmental period, are clinically debilitating, and are associated with numerous negative sequelae, including future psychopathology. Since the mid-1980s, our group at the Oregon Research Institute has been engaged in an extensive program of research on the epidemiology of adolescent psychopathology. The purpose of this chapter is to summarize our current understanding of mood disorders in adolescents based on this body of research and other epidemiological studies.

Although consensus regarding the number of depressive subtypes remains an unresolved issue, agreement is generally strong concerning (a) the importance of the distinction between unipolar and bipolar mood disorders; (b) the definition of major depressive disorder (MDD); and (c) the existence of dysthymia, a less severe but more chronic form of unipolar affective disorder. In addition, it is worth noting recent research highlighting the clinical importance of subthreshold depression and manic symptoms, and the arbitrary nature of the line between having a disorder and falling short of meeting criteria. Our research indicates that MDD is by far the most prevalent form of mood disorder among adolescents (Lewinsohn *et al.*, 1993); dysthymia has a lifetime occurrence of approximately 3% and bipolar disorders occur in less than

Adolescent Emotional Development and the Emergence of Depressive Disorders, ed. Nicholas B. Allen and Lisa B. Sheeber. Published by Cambridge University Press. © Cambridge University Press 2009.

1% of community adolescents. Given its greater prevalence, MDD will be the primary focus of this review, however, research findings regarding dysthymia, bipolar disorder, and subthreshold depression will also be presented.

The specific goals of this chapter are to provide information pertaining to the following issues regarding mood disorders during adolescence: (a) prevalence, incidence, recurrence, onset age, and duration; (b) comorbidity between depressive disorders and with other mental disorders; (c) symptomatic expression of depression; (d) psychosocial characteristics associated with being, becoming, and having been depressed; (e) continuity of depression from adolescence into early adulthood; (f) psychosocial functioning of young adults who experienced and recovered from MDD during adolescence; and (e) predictors of MDD recurrence in early adulthood. To begin, we describe our program of research on adolescent mood disorders.

The Oregon Adolescent Depression Project

Since 1985, we have been conducting a large, prospective, epidemiologic study on adolescent depression and other mental disorders, entitled the Oregon Adolescent Depression Project (OADP). Participants were randomly selected in three cohorts from nine senior high schools representative of urban and rural districts in western Oregon. Sampling was proportional to size of the school, grade within school, and gender within grade. A total of 1709 adolescents completed the initial assessment (T1) which included a diagnostic interview and a questionnaire assessment. Approximately one year later (T2), 1507 (88%) participants returned for a second wave of assessments. Participants were assessed on a comprehensive array of psychosocial constructs either known to be associated with depression in adults or hypothesized to be important with respect to depression in adolescents. We completed a third diagnostic assessment (T3) with a randomly selected subset of OADP participants ($n=941$) near the time of their 24th birthday and recently completed collecting a fourth diagnostic assessment (T4; $n=816$) from the participants around their 30th birthday.

Average age of the OADP sample at T1 was 16.6 (SD$=1.2$, range$=14–18$). Slightly over half of the participants (53%) were female; 91% were White; 12% had repeated a grade in school; 53% were living with both biological parents at the time of the T1 interview, and an additional 18% were living with a biological parent and step-parent. Most participants resided in households in which one or both parents worked as a minor professional or professional (for more detail, see Lewinsohn *et al.*, 1993).

Diagnostic information regarding current and past disorders as per the DSM (DSM–III–R; American Psychiatric Association, 1987; DSM–IV; American Psychiatric Association, 1994) was collected using adolescent report on the

Schedule for Affective Disorders and Schizophrenia for School-Age Children (K-SADS; Orvaschel *et al.*, 1982) at point of entry into study, and in conjunction with the Longitudinal Interval Follow-up Evaluation (LIFE; Keller *et al.*, 1987) at subsequent observation points. Inter-rater reliability of the interviews was high and comparable to what has been found in other studies.

Rates and course

Rates

Data from the OADP provide estimates of the basic epidemiologic parameters including *point prevalence* (i.e. percent in an episode of disorder at the time of the assessment), *lifetime prevalence* (i.e. percent who have experienced an episode during their lifetime), and *incidence* (i.e. percent who are not depressed at the beginning of an observation period but who develop an episode during a specified period of time). Incidence rates are customarily divided into *first incidence* (i.e. percent of the sample that develop an episode for the first time during the observation interval) and *recurrence* (i.e. percent with a previous episode that develop another episode during the interval). From a public health perspective, the total incidence rate is important for planning the delivery of mental health services because it indicates how many individuals in the population will become depressed during a certain time period.

Prevalence and incidence rates of unipolar depression are presented in Table 3.1. As can be seen, depression is common in adolescence. The lifetime prevalence rates of MDD for the OADP participants at T1 are especially high (19%). Conversely, the lifetime prevalence of dysthymia was only 3% during adolescence. The one-year first incidence rate for MDD was 7% for girls and 4% for boys; the rate of MDD recurrence for the T1–T2 interval of one year was 21% for girls and 9% for boys.

The OADP prevalence rates for adolescent MDD are comparable to the rates that have been reported for adults in more recent studies, such as the National Comorbidity Study Replication (NCS-R; Kessler *et al.*, 2003). Previous research reporting much lower rates of depression in younger children (e.g. Fleming *et al.*, 1989; Costello *et al.*, 1996) suggests a substantial increase in the prevalence of depression from childhood to adolescence. Indeed, the OADP rates of depression onset in childhood are low and sharply increase around the age of puberty (i.e. age 12 for girls and 14 for boys; see Figure 3.1).

The OADP lifetime prevalence of bipolar disorders at T2 (predominantly bipolar II and cyclothymia) was approximately 1% (Lewinsohn *et al.*, 2003); the lifetime prevalence of subthreshold bipolar disorder was approximately 4% during adolescence.

Table 3.1. Prevalence and incidence of major depressive disorder (MDD) and dysthymia in the Oregon Adolescent Depression Project

	Total		Female		Male	
	MDD	Dysthymia	MDD	Dysthymia	MDD	Dysthymia
Point prevalence						
T1	2.6	0.5	3.4	0.6	1.7	0.5
T2	3.1	0.1	3.6	0.3	2.6	0.0
Lifetime prevalence						
T1	18.5	3.2	24.8	4.0	11.6	2.3
T2	24.0	3.0	31.6	4.1	15.2	1.7
One-year incidence T1–T2[a]						
Total incidence	7.8	0.1	10.4	0.1	4.8	0.0
First incidence	5.7	0.1	7.1	0.1	4.4	0.0
Recurrence	17.9	0.0	21.1	0.0	9.1	0.0

Note:
[a] Total incidence = percentage who are not depressed at the beginning of an observation period but who develop an episode during a specified period of time; *first incidence* = percent of the sample that develop an episode for the first time during the observation interval; and *recurrence* = percent with a previous episode that develop another episode during the interval.

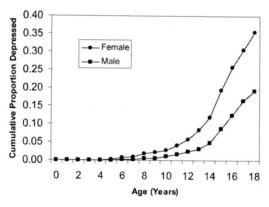

Figure 3.1. Cumulative proportion experiencing an onset of major depressive disorder as a function of age and gender.

Age at onset, episode duration, and time to recurrence

In a previous research report, we have summarized our research findings regarding the time course parameters of MDD (Lewinsohn *et al.*, 1994). The mean age of MDD onset was 14.9 years (SD = 2.8); median onset was 15.5. Earlier MDD onset was associated with being female, lower parental education, the presence of psychiatric comorbidity, and a history of suicide attempt. The mean duration of episodes of MDD was 26 weeks (range of 2 to 520 weeks). The duration was highly skewed with a median duration of 8.0 weeks. Longer MDD episodes were associated with earlier onset (i.e. age of 15 or younger), suicidal ideation, and seeking mental health treatment. Of the adolescents who recovered from the depressive episode, 5% experienced another episode within 6 months, 12% within 1 year, and approximately 33% within 4 years. Shorter time to MDD recurrence was associated with prior suicidal ideation and attempt and with later first onset. Formerly depressed females were more likely to have another episode between T1 and T2, although the mean time to recurrence for females and males who relapsed did not significantly differ. Among 26 adolescents who experienced three episodes of MDD by T2, the amount of well-time from second to third episode was significantly less than from first to second (13 vs. 27 weeks).

Comparing our findings with research with patient samples, depressive episodes in community adolescents appear to be shorter in duration and less likely to be recurrent. Kovacs (1996) reviewed findings from a number of studies of clinically referred adolescent patients, finding a median duration of MDD episodes of 7 to 9 months in child/adolescent patients (over three times as long as our findings). Approximately 70% of the depressed young patients experienced a recurrence of depression when followed for 5 or more years (approximately twice as high as our findings). One explanation for these discrepancies is that patient samples are more severely depressed. In our research (Lewinsohn *et al.*, 1998), as well as that of others (Coryell *et al.*, 1994; Kovacs, 1996), treatment utilization has been found to be associated with the severity of the episode.

We also can compare our results for adolescents to the duration and recurrence values for adults in the community (Lewinsohn *et al.*, 1986, 1989). The duration values of adult depressive episodes are approximately three times as long as adolescent episodes, while recurrence rates appear to be roughly comparable. Our analyses from the T3 diagnostic interviews indicate no significant increase in MDD durations between adolescence and early adulthood.

Impact of gender and age

Studies of gender differences in the rate of depression among adults have consistently reported a female-to-male ratio of 2:1 (Nolen-Hoeksema, 2002). Conversely, most studies of pre-adolescent children (i.e. 12 years of age or younger) find no gender difference in rates of depression or a slight elevation in boys compared to girls (Brooks-Gunn & Petersen, 1991; Garrison *et al.*, 1989; Nolen-Hoeksema *et al.*, 1991; Petersen *et al.*, 1991; Rutter, 1986). We found a significant gender difference, with females being twice as likely as males to be depressed. Comparing our results with other studies (Nolen-Hoeksema & Girgus, 1994; Petersen *et al.*, 1991) suggests that the gender difference in MDD levels probably emerges in the relatively small window between the ages of 12 and 14, as depicted in Figure 3.1.

Depression per self-report questionnaires

Adolescents have consistently been shown to report substantially higher scores on self-report depression questionnaires, such as the Center for Epidemiologic Studies Depression Scale (CES-D; Radloff, 1977), than adults. Using a standard self-report questionnaire criterion of depression "caseness" (i.e. CES-D scores of 16 or above), 40–50% of adolescents would be considered depressed at any point in time, in comparison with 16–20% of adults (Roberts *et al.*, 1990). Similar to the diagnostic rates, OADP girls scored significantly higher than boys on self-report depression questionnaires like the CES-D and the Beck Depression Inventory (BDI; Beck *et al.*, 1961). In addition, the gender difference in CES-D and BDI scores varied as a function of depression history. Currently depressed male and female adolescents did not differ on self-report scores; neither did males and females without a history of depression. Interestingly, the gender difference only appears to be between formerly depressed girls and boys.

Comorbidity

Interest in the co-occurrence, or comorbidity, of psychiatric disorders is a rather recent phenomenon. First introduced into the medical literature by Feinstein (1970), comorbidity refers to the fact that individuals with one disorder may be at elevated risk for a second disorder and this co-occurrence may affect the course of the two disorders. Comorbidity is said to exist either when persons with a current disorder have an elevated prevalence of other current disorders (concurrent comorbidity), or when persons with a history of a disorder have an elevated prevalence of other disorders (lifetime comorbidity). In addition, *homotypic comorbidity* refers to co-occurring disorders within disorder groups (e.g. within mood disorders); *heterotypic comorbidity* refers to co-occurring disorders across disorder groups (e.g. between mood and non-mood disorders). The study of comorbidity has been an active area of our research and some selected findings regarding lifetime comorbidity with depression are presented next.

Homotypic comorbidity

Among adolescents with unipolar depression, approximately 80% experienced MDD by itself or in conjunction with non-mood disorders, 10% experienced dysthymia without MDD, and the remaining 10% experienced MDD with lifetime comorbid dysthymia (Lewinsohn *et al.*, 1991), a condition that has been termed "double depression." Gender differences in the patterns of MDD-dysthymia comorbidity in the OADP sample were non-significant.

Heterotypic comorbidity

Almost half (43%) of adolescents with MDD also had a lifetime occurrence of a non-mood disorder at T1. The OADP rate of comorbidity of depression is comparable to the 53% reported by Angold & Costello (1993), but substantially lower than the 80–95% reported by Kovacs (1996). Depression during adolescence was significantly comorbid with eating disorders (odds ratio [OR] = 9.0), alcohol and drug abuse/dependence (OR = 4.5), anxiety disorders (OR = 4.4), and disruptive behavior disorders (OR = 2.2). Among comorbid cases, 80% of the youth developed the MDD episode *after* the other disorder.

Given the high degree of comorbidity, further study of the risk factors for "pure" and comorbid depressive episodes is needed. Many variables thought to be associated with depression may in fact only be risk factors for the comorbid disorder, as opposed to depression per se (Lewinsohn *et al.*, 1997). Although the occurrence of other disorders given an episode of MDD is much greater than expected by chance, the degree of comorbidity with depression appears to be lower than comorbidity of some other mental disorders (e.g. Lewinsohn *et al.*, 1993; Angold *et al.*, 1999). Given adolescent psychopathology, psychiatric comorbidity appears to be the rule rather than the exception.

Bipolar disorder

Adolescents with full-syndrome and subthreshold bipolar disorder had high rates of comorbidity (Lewinsohn *et al.*, 1995). Compared with adolescents without full-syndrome or subthreshold bipolar disorder, both groups had higher lifetime rates of anxiety (8% vs. 33%, 32%), disruptive behavior disorders (7% vs. 22%, 19%), and substance abuse/dependence (10% vs. 22%, 24%). It is important to note that while comorbidity with attention deficit hyperactivity disorder (ADHD) (3% vs. 11%, 8%) were significantly elevated in both groups, they are substantially below those reported by Biederman *et al.* (1997) and Geller *et al.* (2000) for prepubertal bipolar disorder cases.

Impact of comorbidity

Most combinations of mental disorders have serious negative consequences on functioning (Lewinsohn *et al.*, 1995; Seeley, 2001). Psychiatric comorbidity in adolescents is most strongly associated with academic problems and suicide attempts, followed by impaired role functioning and increased conflict with parents. Regarding specific patterns of comorbidity with depression, the co-occurrence of MDD and externalizing disorders (i.e. conduct disorder and alcohol or drug abuse/dependence) appears to be particularly deleterious, increasing the likelihood of treatment utilization, suicide attempt, impaired role functioning, and academic problems. The occurrence of a comorbid anxiety disorder has the smallest impact on MDD, increasing only the likelihood of treatment utilization. Furthermore, there is an interesting interaction between comorbidity and gender in that males who are only depressed had very low probability of being in treatment. The presence of a comorbid disorder, especially substance use disorder among boys, markedly increased treatment utilization. In girls, those with pure depression were more likely than those who had a comorbid disruptive behavior disorder to receive treatment.

Symptomatic expression of major depression

Researchers previously thought that children and adolescents, when depressed, would exhibit different symptoms than adults (e.g. "masked" depression; Welner, 1978). However, the trend over the past 25 years has been increasingly toward viewing MDD in children, adolescents, and adults as similar, as reflected in the DSM–III–R and DSM–IV criteria, which emphasize the commonalities in MDD across the age span. To examine the manifestation of an episode of MDD in adolescence, we calculated the relative frequency of DSM–III–R depressive symptoms for adolescents in an episode of MDD, for non-cases, and for the total sample at T1 (Roberts et al., 1995). As can be seen in Table 3.2, in addition to depressed mood, the most frequent symptoms are thinking difficulties and sleep and weight/appetite disturbances. The least frequent symptom is thoughts of death/suicide, which were reported by over half of the MDD cases. The relative rank ordering of depressive symptoms in the cases and non-cases was very similar (Spearman $r=0.83$). Of the adolescents who met criteria for MDD, the mean number of symptoms was 6.9 (SD$=1.2$). Of the two core symptoms of MDD, depressed mood is more prevalent than anhedonia in depressed adolescents (98% vs. 77%); anhedonia rarely exists in the absence of depressed mood (2% of MDD cases), and in 75% of MDD cases both core symptoms are present.

Age differences in symptom presentation

We also examined whether the phenomenology of MDD changes during childhood and adolescence. To accomplish this, symptom prevalence values were compared in MDD episodes that occurred before age 14 ($n=100$) with

Table 3.2. Rank order of DSM-III-R major depressive episode symptoms among adolescent cases, non-cases, and total sample at T1 in the Oregon Adolescent Depression Project

Symptom	Case %	Case Rank	Non-case %	Non-case Rank	Total %	Total Rank
Depressed mood	97.7	1	10.1	2	12.3	2
Anhedonia	77.3	5	3.7	8	5.6	8
Weight/appetite disturbance	79.5	4	8.6	4	10.5	4
Sleep disturbance	88.6	2	11.9	1	13.9	1
Motor disturbance	68.2	7	4.6	7	6.2	7
Loss of energy	68.2	7	8.6	4	10.2	5
Worthlessness/guilt	70.5	6	5.7	6	7.4	6
Thinking difficulties	81.8	3	9.7	3	11.5	3
Thoughts of death or suicide ideation	54.5	9	1.6	9	2.9	9

episodes that occurred after age 14 ($n=292$). None of the differences in symptom prevalence for the two age groups were significant.

A more important test of the age question would be to compare the symptom prevalence rates for MDD in adult samples. The pattern of symptoms in our depressed adolescents is generally similar to results from depressed adults identified in the Epidemiologic Catchment Area study (Robins & Regier, 1991). Depressed adolescents were more likely to report worthlessness/guilt than were depressed adults and were less likely to report weight/appetite changes and thoughts of death or suicide (Roberts et al., 1995). We also recently investigated the symptomatic expression of MDD among OADP participants as the progress into early adulthood (Lewinsohn et al., 2003). The analyses were based on 564 OADP participants who had experienced MDD in their lifetime. No systematic differences in the relative rate of occurrence of specific symptoms across episodes were found. In addition, age did not significantly influence the symptom picture. Consistent with other studies (Carlson & Kashani, 1988; Friedman et al., 1983), these findings suggest that there are relatively few differences in the MDD phenomenology between adolescent and young adult episodes. However, the concordance of specific symptoms and severity within individuals across episodes was low. Lack of consistency in symptom presentation across episodes is consistent with findings by Angst & Merikangas (1997), who found that the majority of their cases who displayed a particular depression subtype on one episode displayed a different subtype on a subsequent episode. Therefore, it should not be assumed that subsequent depressive episodes will resemble prior episodes with respect to symptom presentation and underscores the potential influence of environmental factors on symptom presentation.

Gender differences in symptom presentation

Among OADP participants with MDD, the prevalence rates of two of the nine symptoms were significantly different between genders. Compared with depressed boys, depressed girls reported higher symptom rates for weight/ appetite disturbance (77% vs. 59%) and worthlessness/guilt (83% vs. 68%). Among the non-cases, MDD symptom rates in girls were consistently higher than for boys, but the two patterns are quite similar and none of the gender differences were statistically significant.

Treatment utilization

Although 61% of the OADP adolescents with MDD reported receiving some type of treatment (Lewinsohn *et al.*, 1998), most of these treatments were relatively unsystematic and brief, and did not make use of recent research developments in the cognitive–behavioral treatment of depression (Hibbs & Jensen, 1996). Treatment in this population has typically been quite brief; we found that 22% of the treated adolescents received one or two sessions, and 27% received three to seven sessions. Unfortunately, those who received treatment were as likely to experience a subsequent episode of depression during early adulthood as those who had not received treatment (Lewinsohn *et al.*, 1998). We posit that this non-significant difference is probably due to greater depression severity in youth who sought treatment compared with depressed youth who did not, as well as the relatively unsystematic and brief treatments that were provided.

Psychosocial functioning during adolescence

Our research has allowed us to examine the psychosocial characteristics of adolescents before, during, and after an episode of MDD. Knowledge of each of these phases is important for informing on the design of preventive and treatment interventions.

Antecedents of MDD

The psychosocial characteristics which characterize adolescents before they become depressed enable us to identify those who are at elevated risk for *becoming* depressed and provide an opportunity for preventive interventions. The 19 variables marked in the "before" column of Table 3.3 are psychosocial risk/protective factors for becoming depressed in this age group. Variables that

Table 3.3. Variables associated with future, current, and past depression in adolescents

Variable	Before	During	After
Cognitive			
Pessimism	X	X	X
Depressotypic attributional style	X	X	X
Personality and other psychopathology			
Self-consciousness	X	X	X
Low self-esteem	X	X	X
Emotional reliance	X	X	X
Current depression	X	X	X
Internalizing problem behaviors	X	X	X
Externalizing problem behaviors	X	X	X
Past suicide attempt	X	X	X
Past depressive disorder	X	X	n/a
Past anxiety disorder	X	X	X
Stress			
Daily hassles	X	X	X
Major life events	X	X	X
Social and coping skills			
Low self-rated social competence		X	X
Poor coping skills	X	X	X
Interpersonal conflict with parents	X		X
Social support			
Low social support from family	X	X	X
Low social support from friends		X	X
Physical			
Physical illness	X	X	X
Poor self-rated health		X	X
Reduced level of activities		X	
Lifetime # of physical symptoms	X	X	
Current rate of tobacco use		X	X
Academic			
School absenteeism			X
Dissatisfaction with grades	X		

X indicates variable significant at $P < .001$.

are especially influential were internalizing problems (odds ratio [OR] = 2.8), subthreshold depressive symptomatology (OR = 1.8), past history of depressive disorder (OR = 3.6) or a suicide attempt (OR = 6.1), and the presence of a non-mood disorder (OR = 4.8).

Concomitants of MDD

The 22 variables in the "during" column of Table 3.3 highlight the types of psychosocial problems experienced by teenagers while they are depressed. The large number of correlates documents the pervasiveness of the psychosocial difficulties associated with being depressed. Being depressed clearly places youths at a disadvantage in situations requiring adaptive functioning. The psychosocial impairments associated with depression in adolescence are very similar to those that have been observed in adults (Gotlib & Hammen, 1992).

Characteristics of formerly depressed adolescents

The 21 variables on which formerly depressed adolescents differ from never-depressed controls are important for at least two reasons. First, they tell us that formerly depressed teenagers continue to manifest some of the depression-related psychosocial impairments. Hence, formerly depressed adolescents continue to experience some depressive symptoms, excessive interpersonal dependency, internalizing problems, pessimism, depressotypic attributions, and a greater number of major life stressors. Second, the characteristics of having been depressed are also important because they provide a possible explanation of why formerly depressed adolescents are at high risk for recurrence. This knowledge can guide the course of preventive interventions offered to formerly depressed youth and suggests that some degree of maintenance treatment needs to be offered after recovery from the acute phase of the episode.

Subthreshold depression

In recent years there has been considerable interest in the adult literature in what is being called "subthreshold," "subsyndromal," "mild," and "minor" depression with adults. A number of studies support the clinical significance of depressive symptoms including a 1-year study (Judd et al., 1997) in which patients with a core depression symptom were found to be elevated on multiple markers of adverse functioning, including excess healthcare utilization. In a previous paper, we report that adolescents with elevated CES-D scores who did not meet disorder criteria (labeled "false positive") resembled adolescents with depressive disorders on most measures of psychosocial dysfunction, including elevated risk of future depression (Gotlib et al., 1995). Adolescents who are false positive for depression manifest almost as much psychosocial dysfunction as those who met criteria for diagnosis, and that the level of psychosocial impairment increases as a direct function of the number of depressive symptoms (Lewinsohn et al., 2000). In fact, youth who are true positive (i.e. meet diagnostic criteria) only significantly differ from those that are false positive by having higher levels of suicidal ideation. Thus, contrary to implicit assumption, being false positive does not appear to be a benign condition, but rather warrants intervention efforts. Indeed, by intervening with youth who experience subthreshold depressive symptoms, escalation to full syndrome may be prevented (e.g. Clarke *et al.*, 1995, 2001).

Continuity from adolescence to early adulthood

Major depression

In Lewinsohn *et al.* (1999), we examined whether children and adolescents with a history of MDD were at increased risk for new episodes of MDD in adulthood, and whether they were also at increased risk for other mood and non-mood disorders during early adulthood. Participants with a history of MDD in childhood or adolescence ($n=261$) were compared with three groups: (a) participants with a history of adjustment disorder with depressed mood prior to age 19 ($n=73$); (b) participants with other non-mood disorders prior to age 19 ($n=133$; primarily anxiety, substance use and disruptive behavior disorders); and (c) participants with no history of psychiatric disorder prior to age 19 ($n=272$).

We included adjustment disorder with depressed mood as a comparison group for several reasons. First, as a "near-neighbor" category, it provided a good comparison for MDD, although its relationship to the mood disorders is unclear. Several studies have reported that most youths with adjustment disorder recover quickly, and that their risk of developing other psychiatric disorders is less than or does not differ from psychiatric controls, although it is perhaps greater than that of children without any psychiatric disorder (Kovacs *et al.*, 1984, 1994, 1995). Conversely, other studies have reported that the majority of children and adolescents with adjustment disorder have poor outcomes, and often develop more severe forms of psychopathology (Andreasen & Hoenk, 1982; Cantwell & Baker, 1989). Lastly, adjustment disorder is one of the most common psychiatric diagnoses in adolescents (Greenberg *et al.*, 1995; Newcorn & Strain, 1998).

Our data analytic strategy incorporated a hierarchical classification in which MDD took precedence over adjustment disorder, which in turn took precedence over non-mood disorder (e.g. participants with a lifetime history of MDD and adjustment disorder were included in the adolescent MDD group). As can be seen in Table 3.4, 45% of participants with adolescent MDD experienced another MDD episode between 19 and 23. This was significantly higher than MDD rates in the non-mood disorder group and the no-disorder control group. Whereas the MDD group had a very high rate of recurrence, the rate of MDD incidence in the adjustment disorder group

Table 3.4. Prevalence of DSM-IV disorder in young adulthood as a function of adolescent diagnostic group[a]

| Disorder 19–23 | Adolescent Diagnostic Group | | | | MDD contrasts |
	MDD	ADJUST	NON-MOOD	ND	
MDD	45	34	28	18	MDD > NON-MOOD and ND
ADJUST	8	4	10	8	ns
NON-MOOD	33	31	36	20	MDD > ND
Any Axis I	62	48	54	38	MDD > ADJUST and ND
Elevated antisocial PDE score	10	3	17	3	MDD > ADJUST and ND
Elevated borderline PDE score	10	3	5	1	MDD > ND

Note:
[a] MDD = major depressive disorder; ADJUST = adjustment disorder with depressed mood; NON-MOOD = non-mood disorder; ND = no disorder; ns = not significant.

was almost as high, and did not significantly differ from the MDD recurrence rate in the adolescent MDD group.

The adolescent MDD group also had an elevated rate of non-mood disorder compared to the no-disorder group. However, this difference appeared to be due to the presence of comorbid mental disorders in individuals with adolescent MDD. When rates of non-mood disorder between ages 19–24 were examined for the no-disorder group versus individuals with "pure" (non-comorbid) adolescent MDD, differences were non-significant (20% vs. 27%, respectively). Thus, it appears that having had an adolescent MDD resulted in a very substantial probability of MDD recurrence from age 19 to 24, and if the MDD was accompanied by another mental disorder, it was likely that the person would develop a non-mood disorder during early adulthood.

Being female increased the likelihood of future MDD (OR=1.7) and adjustment disorder (OR=2.1), whereas being male increased the likelihood of future non-mood disorder (OR=1.7), and elevated antisocial personality dimensional scores (OR=7.4). However, gender did not interact with adolescent diagnostic group in predicting young adult psychopathology, suggesting that the patterns of diagnostic continuity from adolescence to early adulthood were similar across gender.

To our knowledge, this is the largest community study addressing the continuity of MDD from childhood and adolescence to early adulthood currently in the literature. The results of this study document that adolescent

MDD confers a high degree of risk for MDD recurrence in early adulthood, as well as an increased probability of future non-mood disorders (predominantly substance use disorders) and Axis II pathology. These results have at least two compelling public health implications. First, given the negative consequences of early-onset MDD, the findings stress the importance of developing effective interventions to prevent the onset of depression during childhood and adolescence (Mrazek & Haggerty, 1994). Given that a few promising targeted preventive interventions with adolescents at risk for depression have shown encouraging results (for review, see Horowitz & Garber, 2006), a major public health priority should be to redouble these efforts. Second, children and adolescents who have experienced MDD need to be targeted for the prevention of future depressive episodes. Until efficacious depression prevention interventions are developed and validated, periodic clinical monitoring of at-risk adolescents to detect MDD recurrence is needed.

Bipolar disorder

There were six new cases of bipolar disorder (BD) from ages 19–23 (first incidence rate of 0.7%; Lewinsohn et al., 2000). Three of these cases had a history of MDD prior to age 19. However, they comprised only 1% of the adolescents with MDD in our sample, which is a much lower rate of "switching" than the 20–30% reported in previous studies of MDD in patient samples (Geller et al., 1994; Strober et al., 1993). Major depressive disorder before age 19 did not significantly predict the onset of BD during the age 19–23 period.

Young adult psychosocial functioning

The transition from adolescence to early adulthood represents one of the most demanding developmental stages in the life span. It is the time when individuals make important occupational and interpersonal choices that greatly influence the rest of their lives. Our primary aim in this next report (Lewinsohn et al., 2003) was to document the degree to which experiencing an episode of MDD during adolescence was associated with detectable differences in young adult functioning. Given the developmental demands required of adolescents as they enter early adulthood, our first objective was to document the degree to which experiencing an episode of MDD during adolescence was associated with detectable differences in young adult functioning. Our second objective was to test the specificity of associations between adolescent MDD and difficulties in young adult functioning. Lastly, our third objective was to examine the extent to which four categories of salient factors (i.e. psychiatric comorbidity, MDD recurrence, stability of functioning, current mood state) might account for any differences in young adult functioning that appear to be related to adolescent MDD.

Without adjusting for any of the relevant covariates, young adults who had experienced an episode of MDD during adolescence exhibited pervasive impairments across numerous domains of psychosocial functioning, including occupational performance, interpersonal functioning, quality of life, and physical well-being, although the effect sizes for each of these differences were generally small in magnitude. These findings replicate previous results indicating that young adults with a history of adolescent depression show numerous difficulties in psychosocial functioning (Brook *et al.*, 1996; Fergusson & Woodward, 2002; Geller *et al.*, 2001; Kandel & Davies, 1986; Rao *et al.*, 1999; Reinherz *et al.*, 1999).

When we examined the specificity of these associations, however, only one measure of young adult functioning emerged as uniquely associated with adolescent MDD: *reduced life satisfaction*. These results suggest that experiencing depression in adolescence may be associated with subsequent and enduring reductions in life satisfaction, although the causal nature of this association remains to be elucidated. For example, depression may lead to a longstanding decline in life satisfaction; dissatisfaction may precede, and perhaps play a causal role, in the development of depression; or both depression and low life satisfaction may be the result of a third factor, such as environmental stress, childhood abuse, or personality traits such as neuroticism. The remaining associations of adolescent MDD with young adult functioning were not stronger than comparable associations between adolescent non-mood disorders and future functioning. Thus, many of the impairments in early adulthood are associated with the occurrence of adolescent psychopathology more broadly.

To summarize the findings relevant to the third goal of the study, once we accounted for the effects of adolescent comorbidity, adolescent status on the outcome measures, young adult psychopathology, and current depressive symptomatology, the effects of adolescent MDD on young adult functioning disappeared. Thus, it appears that adolescent MDD, in and of itself, does not have significant effects on young adult psychosocial functioning. The pattern of findings suggests that these variables may mediate the associations between adolescent MDD and subsequent functioning. Future longitudinal studies designed to formally test mediational models would be particularly informative. The present findings are similar to a recent study by Fergusson & Woodward (2002), and taken together these results provide some reason for optimism regarding the long-term effects of adolescent MDD. However, it is important to bear in mind that we used a very conservative data analytic strategy, in which we included a number of covariates that are associated with both adolescent MDD and the young adult outcomes. Thus, the shared variance between adolescent MDD and the covariates in predicting young adult outcome was attributed to the covariates. Nevertheless, an optimistic interpretation of the results is applicable to the approximately 20% of formerly depressed adolescents whose adolescent MDD episode was non-recurrent and non-comorbid. Hence, an important area for future research is to identify the characteristics associated with depression that is adolescence-specific versus life-course persistent.

Predictors of MDD recurrence in early adulthood

Our primary goal in the next report (Lewinsohn *et al.*, 2000) was to identify the factors in formerly depressed adolescents (i.e. those who had recovered by age 19) that predicted MDD recurrence by early adulthood. The framework that guided our research is based on an integrative, multi-factorial model (Lewinsohn *et al.*, 1985), in which depression is conceptualized as the end result of environmentally initiated changes in behavior, affect, and cognition. The model distinguishes between antecedents (which occur before the onset of depression) and consequences (which are observable during and after an episode of depression). The model also recognizes individual vulnerabilities and protective factors which moderate the impact of antecedent events or consequences on depression incidence and recurrence. Vulnerabilities that were examined include the presence of psychopathology among family members, being female (which has often been shown to be a depression risk factor), elevated depressive symptomatology, depressotypic cognitions, excessive emotional reliance, academic problems, and poor physical health. Protective factors that were examined included self-rated social competence, adaptive coping skills, and social support from family and friends.

Based on the often-observed finding that the experience of having an episode of depression increases the likelihood of another episode (Amenson & Lewinsohn, 1981), clinical aspects of the adolescent MDD episode (e.g. early onset, longer duration, recurrence during adolescence, greater severity, treatment utilization, and suicide attempts) also were hypothesized to lead to recurrence. Comorbid adolescent psychopathology was also hypothesized to be a vulnerability for recurrence. Lastly, traits measuring selected young adult personality disorders (i.e. antisocial and borderline personality disorders) were posited to reflect stable characteristics of the person which act as vulnerabilities for MDD recurrence.

Variables that specifically predicted MDD recurrence included multiple depressive episodes in adolescence, a family history of recurrent MDD, borderline personality disorder symptomatology, and for females only, increased conflict with parents. These findings suggest that clinical characteristics, both of the proband and of the first-degree relatives, are among the strongest predictors of MDD recurrence and are consistent with previous research indicating that the presence of MDD in family members significantly increases the likelihood of MDD recurrence in adults (Merikangas *et al.*, 1994; Weissman *et al.*, 1987). The results of this study extend previous research by indicating that recurrent depression breeds true across generations.

The clinical implications of this study are straightforward. Clinicians are routinely faced with decisions about what to do with young people who have a history of MDD. We found that roughly one quarter of formerly depressed adolescents experienced subsequent non-comorbid MDD in early adulthood, one quarter experienced comorbid MDD, one quarter remained free from depression recurrence but experienced a non-mood disorder, and only one quarter remained free of disorder during the assessment period. Earlier and better identification of the most salient risk factors is the first step in avoiding a protracted course of disorder. Our study indicates that depressed female adolescents (especially those who experience high conflict with parents), adolescents with multiple MDD episodes, and those with a family history of recurrent depression are at particularly high risk for depression recurrence. These individuals should be closely monitored or receive continued prophylactic treatment. Future studies need to examine the effects of Axis II psychopathology on the course of depression and determine whether treatments specifically addressing the personality disorder symptomatology are necessary in impacting the course of depression.

Future directions

Epidemiological research conducted over the past few decades has clearly established that mood disorders frequently occur during childhood and adolescence, co-occur with other mental disorders at a high rate, have a profound impact on psychosocial functioning, and have a high likelihood of recurrence in adulthood. Indeed, as a result of the increased understanding of the nature and course of mood disorders, efficacious treatment and preventive interventions are being developed and empirically validated. However, as previously discussed in this chapter, there are many unresolved issues that remain to be addressed in future research.

Based on longitudinal studies such as the OADP, the putative early risk and protective factors for youth depression need to be clearly established in order to refine models of etiology and guide further treatment and prevention efforts. Factors that contribute to the onset of depression need to be distinguished from those that maintain depression or predict depression recurrence. Furthermore, risk and protective mechanisms that are specific to certain developmental periods, or that are gender- or culturally specific, should be identified. As presented earlier in Figure 3.1, the risk for major depressive disorder begins to sharply increase at age 12 for girls and age 14 for boys. Thus, early adolescence represents an important developmental period in which to target preventive interventions for reducing the lifetime risk for depression and the associated negative sequelae.

REFERENCES

Albert, N., & Beck, A.T. (1975). Incidence of depression in early adolescence: a preliminary study. *Journal of Youth and Adolescence*, **4**, 301–306.

Amenson, C.S., & Lewinsohn, P.M. (1981). An investigation into the observed sex difference in prevalence of unipolar depression. *Journal of Abnormal Psychology*, **90**, 1–13.

American Psychiatric Association (1987). *Diagnostic and Statistical Manual of Mental Disorders* (3rd edn). Washington, DC: American Psychiatric Association.

American Psychiatric Association (1994). *Diagnostic and Statistical Manual of Mental Disorders* (4th edn). Washington, DC: American Psychiatric Association.

Andreasen, N.C., & Hoenk, P.R. (1982). The predictive value of adjustment disorders: a follow-up study. *American Journal of Psychiatry*, **139**, 584–590.

Angold, A., & Costello, E.J. (1993). Depressive comorbidity in children and adolescents: empirical, theoretical, and methodological issues. *American Journal of Psychiatry*, **150**, 1779–1791.

Angold, A., Costello, E.J., & Erkanli, A. (1999). Comorbidity. *Journal of Child Psychology and Psychiatry and Allied Disciplines*, **40**, 57–87.

Angst, J., & Merikangas, K. (1997). The depressive spectrum: diagnostic classification and course. *Journal of Affective Disorders*, **45**, 31–40.

Beck, A.T., Ward, C.H., Mendelson, M., Mock, J., & Erbaugh, J. (1961). An inventory for measuring depression. *Archives of General Psychiatry*, **4**, 561–571.

Biederman, J., Faraone, S.V., Hatch, M. *et al.* (1997). Conduct disorder with and without mania in a referred sample of ADHD children. *Journal of Affective Disorders*, **44**, 177–188.

Brook, J.S., Whiteman, M., Finch, S.J., & Cohen, P. (1996). Young adult drug use and delinquency: childhood antecedents and adolescent mediators. *Journal of the American Academy of Child and Adolescent Psychiatry*, **35**, 1584–1592.

Brooks-Gunn, J., & Petersen, A. (1991). Studying the emergence of depression and depressive symptoms during adolescence. *Journal of Youth and Adolescence*, **20**, 115–119.

Cantwell, D.P., & Baker, L. (1989). Stability and natural history of DSM-III childhood diagnoses. *Journal of the American Academy of Child and Adolescent Psychiatry*, **28**, 691–700.

Carlson, G.A., & Cantwell, D.P. (1979). A survey of depressive symptoms in a child and adolescent psychiatric population. *Journal of the American Academy of Child Psychiatry*, **18**, 587–599.

Carlson, G.A., & Kashani, J.H. (1988). Phenomenology of major depression from childhood through adulthood: analysis of three studies. *American Journal of Psychiatry*, **145**, 1222–1225.

Clarke, G.N., Hawkins, W., Murphy, M. *et al.* (1995). Targeted prevention of unipolar depressive disorder in an at-risk sample of high school adolescents: a randomized trial of a group cognitive intervention. *Journal of the American Academy of Child and Adolescent Psychiatry*, **34**, 312–321.

Clarke, G.N., Hornbrook, M., Lynch, F. *et al.* (2001). Offspring of depressed parents in an HMO: a randomized trial of a group cognitive intervention for preventing depression in adolescent offspring of depressed parents. *Archives of General Psychiatry*, **58**, 1127–1134.

Coryell, W., Akiskal, H.S., Leon, A.C. *et al.* (1994). The time course of nonchronic major depressive disorder. *Archives of General Psychiatry*, **51**, 405–410.

Costello, E.J., Angold, A., Burns, B.J. *et al.* (1996). The Great Smoky Mountains Study of Youth: goals, design, methods, and the prevalence of DSM-III-R disorders. *Archives of General Psychiatry*, **53**, 1129–1136.

Cytryn, L., & McKnew, D.H., Jr. (1972). Proposed classification of childhood depression. *American Journal of Psychiatry*, **129**, 149–155.

Feinstein, A.R. (1970). The pretherapeutic classification of comorbidity in chronic disease. *Journal of Chronic Diseases*, **23**, 455–468.

Fergusson, D.M., & Woodward, L.J. (2002). Mental health, educational and social role outcomes of adolescents with depression. *Archives of General Psychiatry*, **59**, 225–231.

Fleming, J.E., Offord, D.R., & Boyle, M.H. (1989). Prevalence of childhood and adolescent depression in the community: Ontario child health study. *British Journal of Psychiatry*, **155**, 647–654.

Friedman, R.C., Hurt, S.W., Clarkin, J.F., Corn, R., & Aronoff, M.S. (1983). Symptoms of depression among adolescents and young adults. *Journal of Affective Disorders*, **5**, 37–43.

Garrison, C.Z., Schluchter, M.D., Schoenbach, V.J., & Kaplan, B.K. (1989). Epidemiology of depressive symptoms in young adolescents. *Journal of the American Academy of Child and Adolescent Psychiatry*, **28**, 343–351.

Geller, B., Fox, L.W., & Clark, K.A. (1994). Rate and predictors of prepubertal bipolarity during follow-up of 6- to 12-year old depressed children. *Journal of the American Academy of Child and Adolescent Psychiatry*, **33**, 461–468.

Geller, B., Zimerman, B., Williams, M. *et al.* (2000). Diagnostic characteristics of 93 cases of a prepubertal and early adolescent bipolar disorder phenotype by gender, puberty and comorbid attention deficit hyperactivity disorder. *Journal of Child and Adolescent Psychopharmacology*, **10**, 157–164.

Geller, B., Zimerman, B., Williams, M., Bolhofner, K., & Craney, J.L. (2001). Adult psychosocial outcome of prepubertal major depressive disorder. *Journal of the American Academy of Child and Adolescent Psychiatry*, **40**, 673–677.

Glaser, B.G., & Strauss, A.I. (1968). *A Time for Dying*. Chicago, IL: Aldine.

Gotlib, I.H., & Hammen, C. (1992). *Psychological Aspects of Depression: Toward an Interpersonal Integration*. New York, NY: John Wiley & Sons.

Gotlib, I.H., Lewinsohn, P.M., & Seeley, J.R. (1995). Symptoms versus a diagnosis of depression: differences in psychosocial functioning. *Journal of Consulting and Clinical Psychology*, **63**, 90–100.

Greenberg, W.M., Rosenfeld, D.N., & Ortega, E.A. (1995). Adjustment disorder as an admission diagnosis. *American Journal of Psychiatry*, **152**(3), 459–461.

Hibbs, E.D., & Jensen, P.S.E. (1996). *Psychosocial Treatments for Child and Adolescent Disorders: Empirically Based Strategies for Clinical Practice*. Washington, DC: American Psychological Association.

Horowitz, J.L., & Garber, J. (2006). The prevention of depressive symptoms in children and adolescents: a meta-analytic review. *Journal of Consulting and Clinical Psychology*, **74**, 401–415.

Judd, L.L., Paulus, M.P., Wells, K.B., & Rapaport, M.H. (1997). Socioeconomic burden of subsyndromal depressive symptoms and major depression in a sample of the general population. *American Journal of Psychiatry*, **153**, 1411–1417.

Kandel, D.B. & Davies, M. (1986). Adult sequelae of adolescent depressive symptoms. *Archives of General Psychiatry*, **43**, 255–262.

Kashani, J., & Simonds, J.F. (1979). The incidence of depression in children. *American Journal of Psychiatry*, **136**, 1203–1205.

Keller, M.B., Lavori, P.W., Friedman, B. *et al.* (1987). The longitudinal interval follow-up evaluation. *Archives of General Psychiatry*, **44**, 540–548.

Kessler, R.C., Berglund, P., Demler, O. *et al.* (2003). The epidemiology of major depressive disorder: results from the National Comorbidity Survey Replication (NCS-R). *Journal of the American Medical Association*, **289**, 3095–3105.

Kovacs, M. (1996). Presentation and course of major depressive disorder during childhood and later years of the life span. *Journal of the American Academy of Child and Adolescent Psychiatry*, **35**, 705–715.

Kovacs, M., Feinberg, T.L., Crouse-Novack, M.A., Paulauskas, S.L., & Finkelstein, R. (1984). Depressive disorders in childhood I: a longitudinal prospective study of characteristics and recovery. *Archives of General Psychiatry*, **41**, 229–237.

Kovacs, M., Gatsonis, C., Pollock, M., & Parrone, P.L. (1994). A controlled prospective study of DSM-III adjustment disorder in childhood: short-term prognosis and long-term predictive validity. *Archives of General Psychiatry*, **51**(7), 535–541.

Kovacs, M., Ho, V., & Pollock, M.H. (1995). Criterion and predictive validity of the diagnosis of adjustment disorder: a prospective study of youths with new-onset insulin-dependent diabetes mellitus. *American Journal of Psychiatry*, **152**(4), 523–528.

Lewinsohn, P.M., Hoberman, H., Teri, L., & Hautzinger, M. (1985). An integrative theory of depression. In S. Reiss & R. Bootzin (Eds.), *Theoretical Issues in Behavior Therapy* (pp. 331–359). San Diego, CA: Academic Press.

Lewinsohn, P.M., Fenn, D.S., Stanton, A.K., & Franklin, J. (1986). Relation of age at onset to duration of episode in unipolar depression. *Journal of Psychology and Aging*, **1**, 63–68.

Lewinsohn, P.M., Zeiss, A., & Duncan, E.M. (1989). Probability of relapse after recovery from an episode of depression. *Journal of Abnormal Psychology*, **98**, 107–116.

Lewinsohn, P.M., Rohde, P., Seeley, J.R., & Hops, H. (1991). Comorbidity of unipolar depression: I. Major depression with dysthymia. *Journal of Abnormal Psychology*, **100**, 205–213.

Lewinsohn, P.M., Hops, H., Roberts, R.E., Seeley, J.R., & Andrews, J.A. (1993). Adolescent psychopathology: I. Prevalence and incidence of depression and other DSM-III-R disorders in high school students. *Journal of Abnormal Psychology*, **102**, 133–144.

Lewinsohn, P.M., Clarke, G.N., Seeley, J.R., & Rohde, P. (1994). Major depression in community adolescents – age at onset, episode duration, and time to recurrence. *Journal of the American Academy of Child and Adolescent Psychiatry*, **33**, 809–818.

Lewinsohn, P.M., Klein, D.N., & Seeley, J.R. (1995). Bipolar disorders in a community sample of older adolescents: prevalence, phenomenology, comorbidity, and course. *Journal of the American Academy of Child and Adolescent Psychiatry,* **34**, 454–463.

Lewinsohn, P.M., Rohde, P., & Seeley, J.R. (1995). Adolescent psychopathology: III. The clinical consequences of comorbidity. *Journal of the American Academy of Child and Adolescent Psychiatry,* **34**, 510–519.

Lewinsohn, P.M., Gotlib, I.H., & Seeley, J.R. (1997). Depression-related psychosocial variables in adolescence: are they specific to depression? *Journal of Abnormal Psychology,* **106**, 365–375.

Lewinsohn, P.M., Rohde, P., & Seeley, J.R. (1998). Treatment of adolescent depression: frequency of services and impact on functioning in young adulthood. *Depression and Anxiety,* **7**, 47–52.

Lewinsohn, P.M., Rohde, P., Klein, D.N., & Seeley, J.R. (1999). Natural course of adolescent major depressive disorder: I. Continuity into young adulthood. *Journal of the American Academy of Child and Adolescent Psychiatry,* **38**, 56–63.

Lewinsohn, P.M., Klein, D.N., & Seeley, J.R. (2000). Bipolar disorder during adolescence and young adulthood in a community sample. *Bipolar Disorders,* **2**, 281–293.

Lewinsohn, P.M., Rohde, P., Seeley, J.R., Klein, D.N., & Gotlib, I.H. (2000). Natural course of adolescent major depressive disorder in a community sample: predictors of recurrence in young adults. *American Journal of Psychiatry,* **157**, 1584–1591.

Lewinsohn, P.M., Solomon, A., Seeley, J.R., & Zeiss, A. (2000). The clinical implications of "subthreshold" depressive symptoms. *Journal of Abnormal Psychology,* **109**, 345–351.

Lewinsohn, P.M., Pettit, J., Joiner, T.E., Jr., & Seeley, J.R. (2003). The symptomatic expression of major depressive disorder in adolescents and young adults. *Journal of Abnormal Psychology,* **112**, 244–252.

Lewinsohn, P.M., Rohde, P., Seeley, J.R., Klein, D.N., & Gotlib, I. (2003). Psychosocial functioning of young adults who have experienced and recovered from major depressive disorder during adolescence. *Journal of Abnormal Psychology,* **112**, 353–363.

Lewinsohn, P.M., Seeley, J.R., & Klein, D.N. (2003). Epidemiology and suicidal behavior of juvenile bipolar disorder. In B. Geller & M. Delbello (Eds.), *Child and Early Adolescent Bipolar Disorder* (pp. 7–24). New York: Guilford Publications.

Merikangas, K.R., Wicki, W., & Angst, J. (1994). Heterogeneity of depression: classification of depressive subtypes by longitudinal course. *British Journal of Psychiatry,* **164**, 342–348.

Mrazek, P.J., & Haggerty, R.J. (1994). *Reducing Risks for Mental Disorders: Frontiers for Preventive Intervention Research.* Washington, DC: National Academy Press.

Newcorn, J.H., & Strain, J. (1998). Adjustment disorder in children and adolescents. *Journal of the American Academy of Child and Adolescent Psychiatry,* **31**(2), 318–326.

Nolen-Hoeksema, S. (2002). Gender differences in depression. In I.H. Gotlib & C.L. Hammen (Eds.), *Handbook of Depression* (pp. 492–509). New York, NY: Guilford Press.

Nolen-Hoeksema, S., & Girgus, J.S. (1994). The emergence of gender differences in depression during adolescence. *Psychological Bulletin,* **115**, 424–443.

Nolen-Hoeksema, S., Girgus, J.S., & Seligman, M.E.P. (1991). Sex differences in depression and explanatory style in children. *Journal of Youth and Adolescence,* **20**, 233–245.

Orvaschel, H., Puig-Antich, J., Chambers, W.J., Tabrizi, M.A., & Johnson, R. (1982). Retrospective assessment of prepubertal major depression with the Kiddie-SADS-E. *Journal of the American Academy of Child Psychiatry*, **21**, 392–397.

Petersen, A.C., Sarigiani, P.A., & Kennedy, R.E. (1991). Adolescent depression: why more girls? *Journal of Youth and Adolescence*, **20**, 247–271.

Radloff, L.S. (1977). The CES-D Scale: a self-report depression scale for research in the general population. *Applied Psychological Measurement*, **1**, 385–401.

Rao, U., Hammen, C., & Daley, S.E. (1999). Continuity of depression during the transition to adulthood: a 5-year longitudinal study of young women. *Journal of the American Academy of Child and Adolescent Psychiatry*, **38**, 908–915.

Reinherz, H., Giaconia, R.M., Carmola, A.M., Wasserman, M.W., & Silverman, A.B. (1999). Major depression in young adulthood: risks and impairments. *Journal of Abnormal Psychology*, **108**, 500–510.

Roberts, R.E., Andrews, J.A., Lewinsohn, P.M., & Hops, H. (1990). Assessment of depression in adolescents using the Center for Epidemiologic Studies Depression Scale. *Psychological Assessment: A Journal of Consulting and Clinical Psychology*, **2**, 122–128.

Roberts, R.E., Lewinsohn, P.M., & Seeley, J.R. (1995). Symptoms of DSM-III-R major depression in adolescence: evidence from an epidemiological survey. *Journal of the American Academy of Child and Adolescent Psychiatry*, **34**, 1608–1617.

Robins, L., & Regier, D. (1991). *Psychiatric Disorders in America*. New York, NY: Free Press.

Rutter, M. (1986). The developmental psychopathology of depression: issues and perspectives. In M. Rutter, C. Izard, & P. Read (Eds.), *Depression in Young People: Developmental and Clinical Perspectives* (pp. 3–30). New York, NY: Guilford Press.

Rutter, M., Izard, C.E., & Read, P.B. (1986). *Depression in Young People: Developmental and Clinical Perspectives*. New York, NY: Guilford Press.

Seeley, J.R. (2001). *Comorbidity between Conduct Disorder and Major Depression: Phenomenology, Correlates, Course, and Familial Aggregation.* (Doctoral Dissertation, University of Oregon.)

Strober, M., Lampert, C., Schmidt, S., & Morrell, W. (1993). The course of major depressive disorder in adolescents: I. Recovery and risk of manic switching in a follow-up of psychotic and nonpsychotic subtypes. *Journal of the American Academy of Child and Adolescent Psychiatry*, **32**, 34–42.

Toolan, J.M. (1962). Depression in children and adolescents. *American Journal of Orthopsychiatry*, **32**, 404.

Weissman, M.M., Gammon, G.D., John, K. *et al.* (1987). Children of depressed parents: increased psychopathology and early onset of major depression. *Archives of General Psychiatry*, **44**, 847–853.

Welner, Z. (1978). Childhood depression: an overview. *Journal of Nervous and Mental Disease*, **166**, 588–593.

4

Pubertal development in early adolescence: implications for affective processes

Laura M. DeRose and Jeanne Brooks-Gunn

Introduction

Puberty is considered to be the most significant developmental event during early adolescence. The multitude of changes that characterize the pubertal transition have significant implications for understanding affective processes during this time period. In addition to the drastic physical changes that occur, pubertal development coincides with the restructuring of social roles, expectations, and relationships within the family, peer group, and school environment (Feldman & Elliott, 1990; Graber & Brooks-Gunn, 1996). New emotions related to these multiple changes are emerging for the early adolescent (Graber & Brooks-Gunn, 2002). Additionally, the physiological changes of puberty, such as hormonal increases, have been associated with some variation in affect (Brooks-Gunn *et al.*, 1994; Buchanan *et al.*, 1992; Susman *et al.*, 1991). Affective processes during early adolescence may be associated directly with physiological and physical changes, or may be linked via timing of the transition (Brooks-Gunn & Reiter, 1990).

Affect is an important outcome to study because the emergence of the gender differential in depressive disorder coincides with pubertal development. Rates of depression in girls and boys are nearly indistinguishable up until the pubertal transition (Nolen-Hoeksema & Girgus, 1994). By mid-adolescence, the gender difference in both subclinical levels of depressive symptoms and diagnosable unipolar depression is at the rate of about 2:1 for girls to boys; this rate persists through adulthood (Nolen-Hoeksema, 2001). An evaluation of potential gender differences in affective processes during the pubertal transition may help elucidate why the gender differential in depressive disorder emerges during this time period.

Adolescent Emotional Development and the Emergence of Depressive Disorders, ed. Nicholas B. Allen and Lisa B. Sheeber. Published by Cambridge University Press. © Cambridge University Press 2009.

The current chapter will begin with a brief description of the biological aspects of pubertal development as well as methods of measuring puberty. The second section is a description of the empirical research linking pubertal development to affective processes, with an emphasis on pubertal timing models. In the final section, proposed mechanisms for the association between pubertal timing and affect are presented.

Biological aspects of pubertal development

Pubertal development is a series of inter-related processes resulting in maturation and adult reproductive functioning. Pubertal development begins in middle childhood and takes 5 to 6 years for most adolescents to complete (Brooks-Gunn & Reiter, 1990; Marshall & Tanner, 1969, 1970; Petersen, 1987). A wide range of individual differences exists in the timing of onset and rate of puberty. The following sections describe both the physiological and physical changes of pubertal development, as well as an explanation of how the different aspects of pubertal development are measured. The studies linking pubertal development with affective processes have used a range of pubertal indicators as well as different ways of measuring them (Dorn et al., 2006).

Physiological changes of puberty

The physiological changes of puberty primarily involve the hypothalamic-pituitary-adrenal (HPA) axis and to a larger extent the hypothalamic-pituitary-gonadal (HPG) axis. The HPA axis is responsible for adrenarche, the initial increases in the adrenal androgen hormones dehydroepiandrosterone (DHEA) and DHEAS (the sulfated form of DHEA). Adrenarche begins around age 6 or 7 in girls and possibly later for boys. Adrenal androgens are responsible for the appearance of axillary (i.e. armpit) hair and, in part, pubic hair.

Hormones of the HPG axis play a main role in the initiation of puberty. The hypothalamic gonadotropin releasing hormone (GnRH) pulse generator, or "gonadostat" is active prenatally and during early infancy, suppressed during childhood, then reactivated at the onset of puberty (Fechner, 2003). In order for puberty to begin, the brain's sensitivity to the negative feedback of gonadal sex steroids (testosterone in males and estrogen in females) decreases, which then releases the HPA axis from inhibition. Puberty begins with the release of GnRH pulses, which activates pulsatile bursts of gonadotropins, luteinizing hormone (LH), and follicle stimulating hormone (FSH), from the pituitary gland.

The LH and FSH pulses secreted in response to the GnRH occur first at night and then during the day. Increases in LH and FSH are some of the earliest measurable hormonal indications of pubertal development, and both

LH and FSH rise progressively during puberty (Grumbach & Styne, 2003; Reiter & Grumbach, 1982). In females, the function of LH and FSH is to initiate follicular development in the ovaries, which stimulates them to produce estrogen. Estrogen sensitive tissues, such as the breasts and uterus, then respond to the increase. In males, increased LH stimulates the testes to secrete testosterone, resulting in an increase in testicular size, and FSH stimulates spermatogenesis (Fechner, 2003).

Physical changes of puberty

The physical indicators of puberty most commonly measured in studies include breast development in girls and testicular growth in boys, as well as pubic hair development in both sexes. These physical indicators are most commonly classified by Marshall & Tanner's (1969) five stages of development, ranging from no development ("1") to fully developed ("5"), even though development is continuous. The mean ages of onset for the secondary sex characteristics described below are based on a study of girls only (Herman-Giddens *et al.*, 1997) that used Marshall & Tanner's developmental stages to classify levels of physical development.

Girls

In females, secondary sex characteristic development is a result of estrogen from the ovaries. Breast development begins in the USA between ages 8 and 13, with a mean age of 9.96 for White girls and a mean age of 8.87 for Black girls (Herman-Giddens *et al.*, 1997). The process of developing mature breasts from breast budding takes approximately 4.5 years, regardless of whether or not girls enter puberty earlier or later than average (Brooks-Gunn & Reiter, 1990). Pubic hair development typically begins shortly after breast budding; however, approximately 20% of girls experience pubic hair development prior to breast budding. Pubic hair development begins in the USA between the ages of 8 and 13 years, with a mean age of 10.5 years in White girls and 8.8 years for Black girls (Herman-Giddens *et al.*, 1997). Menarche is a late sign of pubertal development in girls and occurs following the peak in height velocity and during the rapid increase in weight and body fat (Tanner, 1978). The mean age of menarche in North America is 12.88 years for White girls and 12.16 years for Black girls (Herman-Giddens *et al.*, 1997).

Boys

In males, secondary sexual characteristic development is a result of testosterone from the testes. The onset of testicular growth is the initial sign of pubertal development, which occurs on average between ages 11 and 11.5, but can begin as early as age 9.5 (Brooks-Gunn & Reiter, 1990). Pubic hair growth begins on average at about age 12; however, 41% of boys are in Tanner Stage 4 of testicular growth when initial pubic hair growth begins. The average length of time between initial genital growth and the development of mature genitalia in boys is 3 years (Brooks-Gunn & Reiter, 1990). Spermarche, or first ejaculation, usually occurs between 13 and 14 years of age. More noticeable physical changes in boys include voice changing and the development of facial hair (Brooks-Gunn & Reiter, 1990).

Measuring pubertal development

Self- and parent-report measures

The majority of studies that assess secondary sex characteristic development include self- or parent-report ratings of the above-mentioned Tanner stages, since they are easier to obtain than assessments by health professionals. Correlations between parent and health examiner ratings of Tanner stages range from 0.75 to 0.87 (Brooks-Gunn et al., 1987; Dorn et al., 1990). Correlations between self- and physician-reports have been reported as ranging between 0.77 and 0.91, which were slightly more accurate than parent ratings in the same study (Dorn et al., 1990).

The Pubertal Development Scale (PDS) is another commonly used measure that includes questions about growth spurt, body hair (not specifically pubic hair) and skin change in boys and girls, facial hair growth and voice change in boys, and breast development and menarche in girls, rated on 4-point scales, from "no development" to "development already completed" (Petersen et al., 1988). Correlations between physician Tanner ratings and self-reports of the PDS were between 0.61 and 0.67 (Brooks-Gunn et al., 1987). A study that assessed the reliability and validity of four pubertal assessment measures including the PDS and Tanner concluded that the measures showed both predictive and discriminate validity (Schmitz et al., 2004).

Hormone measures

Due to the difficulty in measuring GnRH caused by its short half life (Rockett et al., 2004), the hormones regulated directly or indirectly by GnRH are measured. These hormones include the gonadotropins (LH, FSH) and sex steroid hormones (testosterone and estrogen). Methods for measuring these hormones include blood draws and blood spots, salivary collection, and urinary collection. Although more invasive, the assays for blood are more sensitive than the assays for urine and saliva (Worthman & Stallings, 1997).

Important issues in measurement

Indicators of puberty are correlated, but not equivalent, as each indicator captures a different aspect of the pubertal process (Brooks-Gunn & Warren, 1985; Graber et al., 1996). In a comprehensive review of 447 articles that include assessments of puberty, there were considerable inconsistencies across studies in methods, definitions, and conceptualizations of puberty and its stages (Dorn *et al.*, 2006). One of the conclusions from this review article was that the selection of methods to measure pubertal status and timing needs to be aligned with the framework of the specific study and its research questions. A key issue is to determine which aspect of puberty may be most relevant to the main questions of the research study (Dorn *et al.*, 2006).

Empirical studies examining associations between pubertal processes and affect

In most studies examining the association between pubertal development and affect, affect has been measured via self- or parent-report measures. More often negative affect has been assessed in studies, via measures of depressive and/or aggressive symptoms. Measures of internalizing and externalizing problems have also been used to assess affect. In general studies have not included questionnaires that measure positive affect specifically. Also, many studies have focused on girls only. The following sections will present empirical research from studies that examine links between pubertal status and pubertal timing on the one hand, and affective outcomes on the other.

Pubertal status

Pubertal status models refer to adolescents' degree of physical maturation as well as their levels of hormones. Models that examine hormone levels directly are considered direct effect models, and those that measure physical change secondary to hormone levels are considered indirect effect models.

Hormonal change and affect

Across studies that include hormone measures, effects vary by gender, hormone, and outcome under investigation. Compared to examinations of pubertal status and timing, studies that include hormonal indicators are few, due to the cost of hormone collection and assays, and the more invasive nature of the process for research participants.

The National Institute of Mental Health (NIMH) study of puberty and psychopathology examined direct links between hormone concentrations and affect (Nottelmann *et al.*, 1987a, 1987b; Susman *et al.*, 1987a, 1987b). In general, results of this study ($n = 108$) indicated stronger effects of hormones on affect in boys compared with girls. For boys, negative associations were found between pubertal status measures (testosterone:estradiol ratio, sex hormone binding globulin, androstenedione concentration) and negative emotional tone. Adrenal androgen concentrations were correlated with negative emotional tone in boys, while FSH was linked with negative emotional tone in girls (Susman *et al.*, 1985). As hormone levels were age-adjusted, these results indicate effects of both status and timing.

A study on hormone-affect links in girls only was conducted by Brooks-Gunn and colleagues with 100 White girls ranging in age from 10 to 14 (Brooks-Gunn & Warren, 1989; Warren & Brooks-Gunn, 1989). Five hormonal indicators were included in the study – FSH, LH, estradiol, testosterone, and DHEAS. Outcomes included depressive and aggressive affect. The major finding to emerge was a significant quadratic effect of estradiol on depressive affect. Based on this finding, girls were categorized into four hormonal stages based on the range of their estradiol levels; each range affects reproductive organs and functioning of the reproductive system differently. Stage I girls were considered prepubertal, stage II girls were experiencing the beginning of pubertal development, stage III girls were considered to be in mid- or late-puberty, and stage IV girls were experiencing cyclic menstrual function. Estradiol levels were 0–25, 26–50, 51–74, and greater than 75 pg/ml, respectively, for each stage.

Highest levels of depressive affect were found in the groups (stages II and III) that demonstrated initial increases in estradiol (Brooks-Gunn & Warren, 1989; Warren & Brooks-Gunn, 1989). In follow-up analysis ($n=72$), this hormone-affect association was found to persist over the course of 1 year (Paikoff *et al.*, 1991). The curvilinear nature of the hormone-affect association fits the premise that activational effects may be greatest when the endocrine system is being turned on. However, the magnitude of the hormone effect was small, accounting for only 4% of the variance in negative affect. Other studies have also indicated that when hormone-affect associations are found, they generally account for a small portion of variance in outcome (Buchanan *et al.*, 1992). These findings imply that puberty likely has more indirect effects on affective outcomes, as the percent of variance accounted for by hormones is generally small.

Secondary sex characteristic status and affects

The assumption underlying potential associations between secondary sex characteristic development and affect is that adolescents experience negative reactions or receive negative feedback from others about their development when they reach certain stages, or that they may feel that certain behaviors are expected with increasing physical development. The physical changes of puberty may also change how adolescents view themselves. Since hormonal changes are the cause of the changes in physical growth and development, it is often difficult to disentangle hormonal and status effects on adjustment. For example, a study of diagnosed depression found that only after reaching Tanner stage III were girls more likely than boys to experience higher rates of depressive disorder (Angold *et al.*, 1998). However, subsequent analyses showed that effects of elevated estradiol and testosterone levels eliminated effects due to secondary sex characteristics (Angold *et al.*, 1999). In sum, direct effects of secondary sex characteristics on affect are not evident. Rather, effects may be moderated via variables such as how others perceive girls who are nearly fully developed and the social pressures that accompany looking more like an adult (Stattin & Magnusson, 1990).

Pubertal timing

A large body of literature examines links between pubertal timing and affect in adolescents, mainly because there is a substantial degree of variation among individuals regarding when puberty begins and how it progresses (Tanner, 1970). Classifications of maturational timing may differ by study, even when the same pubertal status measure is used, such as the Tanner (for a review, see Dorn *et al.*, 2006). The varied methods result in cross-study variation in the maturational and chronological ages of adolescents classified in the same timing group. In the cases where the same classification system is used, different samples, having different distributions, may exhibit various percentages of off-time and on-time girls (even if same definition of timing is used).

A few hypotheses have emerged to explain links between pubertal timing and psychological development. The "off-time" hypothesis is the most general one; it predicts that both earlier and later development in girls and boys compared to one's same-age, same-gender peers is a risk factor for problem behaviors (Caspi & Moffitt, 1991). A more specific hypothesis is the gendered "deviation" pattern of pubertal timing effects, where early maturation is a risk factor for females but late maturation is a risk factor for males. This hypothesis is based on the developmental pattern that girls, on average, mature earlier than boys. Girls who mature earlier than their peers or boys who mature later than their peers are considered to be in the "deviant" categories (Brooks-Gunn *et al.*, 1985; Petersen & Taylor, 1980).

The "early maturation" hypothesis is also referred to as the "stage-termination" hypothesis (Petersen & Taylor, 1980). This hypothesis posits that early maturation is a risk factor for adjustment problems among both females and males across a range of outcomes (Brooks-Gunn *et al.*, 1985; Caspi & Moffitt, 1991; Ge *et al.*, 1996; Tschann *et al.*, 1994). Early maturation may be disadvantageous because early maturers experience social pressure to adopt more adult norms and engage in adult behaviors, even though they may not be socially, emotionally, or cognitively prepared (Brooks-Gunn *et al.*, 1985; Caspi & Moffitt, 1991; Magnusson *et al.*, 1985) for the new experiences. This hypothesis involves the notion of stage termination (Petersen & Taylor, 1980), which means that early maturation disrupts the normal course of development such that early maturers have less time and are less experienced to handle adult behaviors.

Early maturation has been repeatedly associated with more internalizing symptoms and psychological distress in girls, compared with on-time or later maturing peers (Brooks-Gunn *et al.*, 1985; Ge *et al.*, 1996; Graber *et al.*, 1997,

2004; Hayward *et al.*, 1997; Stattin & Magnusson, 1990). In a longitudinal study investigating links between pubertal transition and depressive symptoms in rural White youth living in Iowa, girls began to experience more symptoms than boys in the 8th grade and this difference persisted through mid- and late adolescence (Ge *et al.*, 2001a). Girls who experienced menarche at a younger age subsequently experienced a higher level of depressive symptoms than their on-time and late-maturing peers, at each annual assessment during the 6-year study. Additionally, the interaction between early menarche and recent life events predicted subsequent depressive symptoms for girls. Interestingly, the significant main effect of gender on depressive symptoms disappeared when pubertal timing, recent life events, and their interaction were included in models, suggesting that pubertal timing may explain a significant part of the observed gender differences in depressive symptoms during adolescence.

Findings on links between pubertal timing and negative affect in boys are more inconsistent. Many of the earlier studies on pubertal timing in boys found that early-maturing boys were better off than their later-maturing counterparts, on measures of social, psychological, and behavioral outcomes (Jones, 1957, 1965; Mussen & Jones, 1957). Studies since the 1950s and 1960s have found more mixed effects. In the NIMH study of puberty and psychopathology, a higher rate of negative emotional tone has been found in late maturing boys during mid- and late adolescence as compared with their age-mates (Nottelmann *et al.*, 1987a). However, studies have also found that early-maturing boys experience more internalizing symptoms (Petersen & Crockett, 1985; Susman *et al.*, 1991, 1985) or that both early- and late maturing boys show more depressive tendencies (Alsaker, 1992). Another study found that late maturing boys experienced more internalizing symptoms than their on-time peers, and that both early- and late maturing boys showed significantly higher rates of depression than on-time maturing boys (Graber *et al.*, 1997). In a longitudinal study with White boys living in a rural area, early-maturing boys, compared with their on-time and late-maturing peers, exhibited more internalized distress (Ge *et al.*, 2001b). Results from a large-scale study of Black boys also indicated that early-maturers reported higher levels of internalizing symptoms (Ge *et al.*, in press). In sum, a trend emerges for both early- and late-maturing boys to experience more internalizing symptoms than their on-time peers.

According to the early maturation, or stage-termination, hypothesis, if Black girls are experiencing pubertal onset earlier than their White counterparts (they are the earliest to mature across ethnic groups), it is expected that they would experience the most stress. Few studies have tested links between pubertal timing and affect across ethnic groups. While one study found associations between early menarche and depressive symptoms in White girls but not Black or Hispanic girls (Hayward *et al.*, 1999), another study including only Black children, results showed that early maturing girls had higher rates of depressive symptoms than their non-early peers (Ge *et al.*, 2003). In the National Study of Adolescent Health (Add Health), adolescents who reported being overweight were more likely to be distressed by pubertal growth if they were Anglo– or Hispanic–American girls than boys or African–Americans (Ge *et al.*, 2001c).

A study that examined pubertal timing across Latina, Black, and White children from economically diverse Chicago neighborhoods found that Latina girls reached menarche earlier than Black and White girls (Obeidallah *et al.*, 2000). The difference between Latina and White girls was accounted for by socioeconomic factors. Interestingly, *perceptions* of pubertal timing did not vary across ethnic groups, which may have been because girls were comparing themselves to their friends, who were similar demographically. These results suggest that pubertal timing may be most relevant when comparing girls within racial groups rather than across groups (Obeidallah *et al.*, 2000). Another study using the same sample (Project on Human Development in Chicago Neighborhoods) found that girls in each ethnic group who matured "off-time," that is, earlier or later than their same-age, same-gender peers, experienced more clinical levels of depression/anxiety, with strongest effects found in White girls (Foster & Brooks-Gunn, manuscript under review). Research needs to better address associations between pubertal timing and affect across different ethnic groups. It is possible that perceptions of pubertal change by families and peers differ by ethnicity, as well as by the extent of preparation for pubertal change that adolescents experience (e.g. how much it is discussed in social contexts).

Mechanisms for associations between pubertal timing and affect

As stated earlier, pubertal development is marked by a multitude of physiological, psychological, and social changes for the adolescent. How well the adolescent copes with these changes may depend on how well the adolescent copes with stress in general as well as the psychological vulnerability of the adolescent before puberty begins. Several pathways have been proposed that may explain how the stress that the adolescent experiences during the pubertal transition is linked with their affective states. One such pathway is the individual diathesis-stress model, in which puberty is thought to accentuate the effects of psychosocial factors that exist prior to the onset of puberty. Another is the transition stress model, which focuses on the emotional and physiological arousal linked with pubertal change. A third pathway focuses on the frequency and types of stressors during the transition. Fourth, weight changes that accompany puberty, for girls in particular, may mediate puberty-affect associations.

Individual diathesis-stress model

The individual diathesis-stress model posits that psychosocial vulnerability factors that exist prior to adolescence accentuate the probability of increases in emotional distress during pubertal development (Caspi & Moffitt, 1991; Dorn & Chrousos, 1997; Nolen-Hoeksema & Girgus, 1994; Susman et al., 2003). Results of a longitudinal study of 501 girls who were assessed every 2 years from age 3 through 15 indicated that the early onset of menarche magnified and accentuated behavioral problems among girls who were predisposed to behavior problems earlier in childhood (Caspi & Moffitt, 1991). As studies on puberty have rarely explored the full range of adolescence, including the transition from childhood and the transition into adulthood, we have few examples from other studies.

Transitional stress model

Reproductive transitions are periods of development that involve reorganization of biological and behavioral systems, as the transitional stress model indicates (Susman, 1997, 1998). This reorganization may increase emotional arousal and vulnerability to the onset of psychiatric disorders (Dorn & Chrousos, 1997). For example, aroused physiological states may trigger increased moodiness, sudden mood changes, feelings of self-consciousness, or elevated intensity of moods, all of which, if interpreted negatively, could lead to affective problems.

Graber et al. (2006) illustrate the use of the transitional stress model in a study of potential mediated pathways from pubertal development to changes in depressive affect and aggression in girls between the ages of 10 to 14. Pubertal development was measured in three ways: (a) estradiol categories to tap gonadal maturation, (b) dehydroepiandrosterone sulfate (DHEAS) to indicate adrenal maturation, and (c) pubertal timing (early maturation versus other). The three potential mediators included emotional arousal, attention difficulties, and negative life events. Findings indicated that early pubertal timing predicted higher emotional arousal which subsequently predicted increased depressive affect. A mediated association with aggression via negative life events was found for both estradiol category and DHEAS. The authors concluded that there is a need for more intensive investigation of gonadal and adrenal processes in explaining affective changes associated with early maturation (Graber et al., 2006).

Frequency and type of stressors

Evidence from longitudinal studies suggests that adolescents experience more life events, both negative and positive, in early adolescence than in later adolescence, with the number of events peaking around age 14 (Brooks-Gunn,

1991; Ge *et al.*, 1994). Findings indicate that girls face more stressful life events than boys in adolescence (Compas & Wagner, 1991; Ge *et al.*, 1994; Larson & Ham, 1993). Adolescent females have also been found to report significantly more negative interpersonal events than adolescent males, to perceive these events as more stressful (Wagner & Compas, 1990), and to be more vulnerable to stress in peer and family contexts (Greene & Larson, 1991; Rudolph, 2002). For example, girls have been found to be more aware of threat of conflict to friendships, which intensifies with age (Laursen, 1996).

The experience of several simultaneous (or in close proximity) stressful events can overtax the coping resources of adolescents (Simmons & Blyth, 1987). Because girls tend to transition through puberty earlier than boys, the stressful events that co-occur with this transition are different for them, especially early-maturing girls. For example, going through a school change at the same time as going through peak pubertal development, as early-maturing girls are likely to do, has been identified as an experience that sets adolescents on course for poorer adjustment across adolescence (Petersen *et al.*, 1991). Boys most often transition schools before the onset of puberty, making this cumulative stress situation more frequent for girls.

Puberty-related weight and body-image change

In a review of the literature on puberty-related weight and body-image change in girls, Stice (2003) concluded that the association between puberty and affect is mediated by body dissatisfaction. It is likely that girls more often experience increased body size negatively due to the media images in Western cultures that value the thin physique of a prepubertal body over the mature body for girls (Attie & Brooks-Gunn, 1989). Stice (2003) highlights studies in which early-puberty induced body dissatisfaction predicted subsequent onset of depressive pathology (Rierdan *et al.*, 1989; Stice *et al.*, 2000) and increases in depressive symptoms (Stice & Bearman, 2001). Interestingly, when body satisfaction is statistically controlled, the sex difference in depression is substantially reduced (Allgood-Merten *et al.*, 1990; Rierdan *et al.*, 1989; Siegel *et al.*, 1999; Stice, 2003; Wichstrom, 1999). This research demonstrates that body dissatisfaction plays a role in mediating links between pubertal change and negative affect in girls. Studies have not focused on boys' responses to increases in height and weight during puberty. However, these are most likely positive changes for boys, due to their increase in lean muscle mass and decrease in body fat.

Conclusions

As pubertal development is considered to be the most significant developmental event in early adolescence and as this is the period where the gender differential in depression emerges, it is particularly important to study puberty–affect associations. The past few decades have witnessed a proliferation in research on pubertal development and its implications. Studies have examined how puberty-related biological, psychological, and social changes are linked to adolescent outcomes, including affective states. Many of the studies have included samples of girls only, with the assumption that pubertal change has a more significant impact on girls than boys. However, studies that include girls and boys have found effects for both.

A few key findings have emerged from the research. One is that when direct effects of pubertal hormones are found on affect (e.g. Brooks-Gunn & Warren, 1989), they generally account for a small portion of the variance in outcome, with social factors having a stronger effect. Rapid increases in hormones during pubertal development seem to be the factor that is associated with affect, particularly depressive symptoms. With regard to timing of puberty, one of the most consistent findings has been that early-maturing girls tend to experience more negative affect than their on-time and late-maturing peers. For boys, findings are more mixed, although early- and late-maturers, compared to their on-time peers, seem to be at some risk for more negative affect. In examining mechanisms for the association between pubertal timing and affect, stress may exacerbate existing psychological vulnerability or result in increased physiological or emotional arousal for the adolescent. The frequency and types of stressors that coincide with an early pubertal transition may impact affective processes. Additionally, for girls, increased body dissatisfaction has been found to mediate the association between early maturation and depressive symptoms.

Although the past few decades have been marked by many pioneering studies examining associations between pubertal development and affect, there are a few key areas for future research. First, while many studies do find significant effects of pubertal development on affect, most adolescents progress through puberty without experiencing significant psychopathology. In order to identify the adolescents who develop more significant and long-lasting problems, studies need to be designed to examine the full span of pubertal development, as well as development into young adulthood. Most studies begin assessment of puberty once the process has already begun, and do not follow participants beyond mid- or late-adolescence. Additionally, more research needs to be conducted on antecedents of pubertal timing, which may also influence consequences of timing. Second, the measurement of affective processes in the studies of pubertal development has been limited. Most studies include self- or parent-report measures of affective states, namely, depressive and aggressive symptoms. A recommendation would be for studies to include more diverse measures of affective processes, such as measurements of emotion regulation, and physiological measures of emotion (i.e. heart rate, skin conductance, etc.), as well as specific measures of positive affect. The third suggestion, as emphasized in the comprehensive review by Dorn and colleagues (2006), would be to better standardize methods of assessing pubertal status and timing. Inconsistencies in measurement make it difficult to compare results across studies.

Fourth, studies need to include more non-white adolescents, especially since variations in pubertal onset have been identified between Black and White girls (e.g. Herman-Giddens *et al.*, 1997). Also, not much research has examined effects of neighborhood during the pubertal transition (Obeidallah *et al.*, 2004). In most past studies, samples have not been representative; exceptions include the Dunedin (New Zealand) Multidisciplinary Health and Development Study, the Great Smoky Mountains Study of Youth, the National Longitudinal Study of Adolescent Health, and the Project on Human Development in Chicago Neighborhoods. It is particularly important to include representative samples in the research due to the differences found in pubertal timing across various ethnic and socioeconomic groups. Finally, a piece that is missing in the literature is how preparation for pubertal onset, via education and interactive discussion in family, school, or community settings, may influence how adolescents affectively experience the transition.

REFERENCES

Allgood-Merten, B., Lewinsohn, P.M., & Hops, H. (1990). Sex differences in adolescent depression. *Journal of Abnormal Psychology*, **99**, 55–63.

Alsaker, F.D. (1992). Pubertal timing, overweight, and psychological adjustment. *Journal of Early Adolescence*, **12**, 396–419.

Angold, A., Costello, E.J., & Worthman, C.W. (1998). Puberty and depression: the roles of age, pubertal status and pubertal timing. *Psychological Medicine*, **28**, 51–61.

Angold, A., Costello, E.J., Erkanli, A., & Worthman, C.W. (1999). Pubertal changes in hormone levels and depression in girls. *Psychological Medicine*, **29**, 1043–1053.

Attie, I., & Brooks-Gunn, J. (1989). Development of eating problems in adolescent girls: a longitudinal study. *Developmental Psychology*, **25**, 70–79.

Brooks-Gunn, J. (1991). How stressful is the transition to adolescence for girls? In M.E. Colton & S. Gore (Eds.), *Adolescent Stress: Causes and Consequences* (pp. 131–149). New York, NY: Aldine de Gruyter.

Brooks-Gunn, J., & Reiter, E.O. (1990). The role of pubertal processes. In S.S. Feldman & G.R. Elliott (Eds.), *At the Threshold: The Developing Adolescent* (pp. 16–53). Cambridge, MA: Harvard University Press.

Brooks-Gunn, J., & Warren, M.P. (1985). Measuring physical status and timing in early adolescence: a developmental perspective. *Journal of Youth and Adolescence*, **14**, 163–189.

Brooks-Gunn, J., & Warren, M.P. (1989). Biological and social contributions to negative affect in young adolescent girls. *Child Development*, **60**, 40–55.

Brooks-Gunn, J., Petersen, A.C., & Eichorn, D. (1985). The study of maturational timing effects in adolescence. *Journal of Youth and Adolescence*, **14**, 149–161.

Brooks-Gunn, J., Warren, M.P., Rosso, J., & Gargiulo, J. (1987). Validity of self-report measures of girls' pubertal status. *Child Development*, **58**, 829–841.

Brooks-Gunn, J., Graber, J., & Paikoff, R.L. (1994). Studying links between hormones and negative affect: models and measures. *Journal of Research on Adolescence*, **4**, 469–486.

Buchanan, C.M., Eccles, J.S., & Becker, J.B. (1992). Are adolescents the victims of raging hormones: evidence for activational effects of hormones on moods and behavior at adolescence. *Psychological Bulletin*, **111**, 62–107.

Caspi, A., & Moffitt, T.E. (1991). Individual differences are accentuated during periods of social change: the sample case of girls at puberty. *Journal of Personality and Social Psychology*, **61**, 157–168.

Compas, B., & Wagner, B.M. (1991). Psychosocial stress during adolescence: intrapersonal and interpersonal processes. In M.E. Colton & S. Gore (Eds.), *Adolescent Stress: Causes and Consequences* (pp. 67–85). New York, NY: Aldine de Gruyter.

Dorn, L.D., & Chrousos, G.P. (1997). The neurobiology of stress: understanding regulation of affect during female biological transitions. *Seminars in Reproductive Endocrinology*, **15**, 19–35.

Dorn, L.D., Susman, E.J., Nottelmann, E.D., Inoff-Germain, G., & Chrousos, G.P. (1990). Perceptions of puberty: adolescent, parent, and health care personnel. *Developmental Psychology*, **26**, 322–329.

Dorn, L.D., Dahl, R.E., Woodward, H.R., & Biro, F. (2006). Defining the boundaries of early adolescence: a user's guide to assessing pubertal status and pubertal timing in research with adolescents. *Applied Developmental Science*, **10**, 30–56.

Fechner, P.Y. (2003). The biology of puberty: new developments in sex differences. In C. Hayward (Ed.), *Gender Differences at Puberty* (pp. 17–28). New York, NY: Cambridge University Press.

Feldman, S., & Elliott, G. (1990). *At the Threshold: The Developing Adolescent.* Cambridge, MA: Harvard University Press.

Ge, X., Conger, R.D., Lorenz, F.O., & Simons, R.L. (1994). Parents' stressful life events and adolescent depressed mood. *Journal of Health and Social Behavior*, **35**, 28–44.

Ge, X., Conger, R.D., & Elder, G.H., Jr. (1996). Coming of age too early: pubertal influences on girls' vulnerability to psychological distress. *Child Development*, **67**, 3386–3400.

Ge, X., Conger, R.D., & Elder, G.H., Jr. (2001a). Pubertal transition, stressful life events, and the emergence of gender differences in adolescent depressive symptoms. *Developmental Psychology*, **37**, 404–417.

Ge, X., Conger, R.D., & Elder, G.H., Jr. (2001b). The relationship between puberty and psychological distress in adolescent boys. *Journal of Research on Adolescence*, **11**, 49–70.

Ge, X., Elder, G.H., Jr., Regnerus, M., & Cox, C. (2001c). Pubertal transitions, perceptions of being overweight, and adolescents' psychological maladjustment: gender and ethnic differences. *Social Psychology Quarterly*, **64**, 363–375.

Ge, X., Kim, I.J., Brody, G.H., *et al.* (2003). It's about timing and change: pubertal transition effects on symptoms of major depression among African American youths. *Developmental Psychology*, **39**, 430–439.

Ge, X., Brody, G.H., Conger, R.D., & Simons, R.L. (in press). Pubertal transition and African American children's internalizing and externalizing symptoms. *Journal of Youth and Adolescence*.

Graber, J.A., & Brooks-Gunn, J. (1996). Transitions and turning points: navigating the passage from childhood through adolescence. *Developmental Psychology*, **32**, 768–776.

Graber, J.A., & Brooks-Gunn, J. (2002). Adolescent girls' sexual development. In G.M. Wingood & R.J. DiClemente (Eds.), *Handbook of Women's Sexual and Reproductive Health* (pp. 21–42). New York, NY: Kluwer Academic/Plenum.

Graber, J.A., Petersen, A.C., & Brooks-Gunn, J. (1996). Pubertal processes: methods, measures, and models. In J.A. Graber, J. Brooks-Gunn & A.C. Petersen (Eds.), *Transitions through Adolescence: Interpersonal Domains and Context* (pp. 23–53). Mahwah, NJ: Lawrence Erlbaum.

Graber, J.A., Lewinsohn, P.M., Seeley, J.R., & Brooks-Gunn, J. (1997). Is psychopathology associated with the timing of pubertal development? *Journal of the American Academy of Adolescent Psychiatry*, **36**, 1768–1776.

Graber, J.A., Seeley, J.R., Brooks-Gunn, J., & Lewinsohn, P.M. (2004). Is pubertal timing associated with psychopathology in young adulthood? *Journal of the American Academy of Child and Adolescent Psychiatry*, **43**, 718–726.

Graber, J.A., Brooks-Gunn, J., & Warren, M.P. (2006). Pubertal effects on adjustment in girls: moving from demonstrating effects to identifying pathways. *Journal of Youth and Adolescence*, **35**, 413–423.

Greene, A.L., & Larson, R.W. (1991). Variation in stress reactivity during adolescence. In E.M. Cummings, A.L. Greene, & K.H. Karraker (Eds.), *Life-span Developmental Psychology: Perspectives on Stress and Coping* (pp. 195–209). Hillsdale, NJ: Lawrence Erlbaum.

Grumbach, M.M., & Styne, D.M. (2003). Puberty: ontogeny, neuroendocrinology, physiology, and disorders. In P.R. Larsen, H.M. Kronenberg, S. Melmed, & K.S. Polonsky (Eds.), *Williams Textbook of Endocrinology* (pp. 1115–1286). Philadelphia, PA: W.B. Saunders.

Hayward, C., Killen, J.D., Wilson, D.M. *et al.* (1997). Psychiatric risk associated with early puberty in adolescent girls. *Journal of the American Academy of Child and Adolescent Psychiatry*, **36**, 255–262.

Hayward, C., Gotlib, I., Schraedley, P.K., & Litt, I.F. (1999). Ethnic differences in the association between pubertal status and symptoms of depression in adolescent girls. *Journal of Adolescent Health*, **25**, 143–149.

Herman-Giddens, M.E., Slora, E.J., Wasserman, R.C. *et al.* (1997). Secondary sexual characteristics and menses in young girls seen in office practice: a study from the pediatric research in office settings network. *Pediatrics*, **99**, 505–512.

Jones, M.C. (1957). The later careers of boys who were early- or late-maturing. *Child Development*, **28**, 113–128.

Jones, M.C. (1965). Psychological correlates of somatic development. *Child Development*, **36**, 899–911.

Larson, R., & Ham, M. (1993). Stress and "storm and stress" in early adolescence: the relationship of negative events with dysphoric affect. *Developmental Psychology*, **29**, 130–140.

Laursen, B. (1996). Closeness and conflict in adolescent peer relationships: interdependence with friends and romantic partners. In W.M. Bukowski, A.F. Newcomb, & W.W. Hartup (Eds.), *The Company they Keep: Friendship in Childhood and Adolescence* (pp. 186–210). New York, NY: Cambridge University Press.

Magnusson, D., Stattin, H., & Allen, V. (1985). Biological maturation and social development: a longitudinal study of some adjustment processes from mid-adolescence to adulthood. *Journal of Youth and Adolescence*, **14**, 267–283.

Marshall, W.A., & Tanner, J.M. (1969). Variations in the pattern of pubertal changes in girls. *Archives of Disease in Childhood*, **44**, 291–303.

Marshall, W.A., & Tanner, J.M. (1970). Variations in the pattern of pubertal changes in boys. *Archives of Disease in Childhood*, **45**, 13–23.

Mussen, P.H., & Jones, M.C. (1957). Self-conceptions, motivations, and interpersonal attitudes of late- and early-maturing boys. *Child Development*, **28**, 243–256.

Nolen-Hoeksema, S. (2001). Gender differences in depression. *Current Directions in Psychological Science*, **10**, 173–176.

Nolen-Hoeksema, S., & Girgus, J.S. (1994). The emergence of gender differences in depression during adolescence. *Psychological Bulletin*, **115**, 424–443.

Nottelmann, E.D., Susman, E.J., Dorn, L.D. *et al.* (1987a). Developmental processes in early adolescence: relations among chronologic age, pubertal stage, height, weight, and serum levels of gonadotropins, sex steroids, and adrenal androgens. *Journal of Adolescent Health*, **8**, 246–260.

Nottelmann, E.D., Susman, E.J., Inoff-Germain, G. *et al.* (1987b). Developmental processes in American early adolescence: relations between adolescent adjustment problems and chronologic age, pubertal stage and puberty-related serum hormone levels. *Journal of Pediatrics*, **110**, 473–480.

Obeidallah, D.A., Brennan, R.T., Brooks-Gunn, J., Kindlon, D., & Earls, F. (2000). Socioeconomic status, race, and girls' pubertal maturation: results from the Project on Human Development in Chicago Neighborhoods. *Journal of Research on Adolescence*, **10**, 443–488.

Obeidallah, D.A., Brennan, R.T., Brooks-Gunn, J., & Earls, F. (2004). Links between puberty timing, neighborhood contexts, and girls' violent behavior. *Journal of the American Academy of Child and Adolescent Psychiatry*, **43**, 1460–1468.

Paikoff, R., Brooks-Gunn, J., & Warren, M.P. (1991). Predictive effects of hormonal change on affective expression in adolescent females over the course of one year. *Journal of Youth and Adolescence*, **20**, 191–214.

Petersen, A.C. (1987). The nature of biological-psychosocial interactions: the sample case of early adolescence. In R.M. Lerner & T.T. Foch (Eds.), *Biological-Psychosocial Interactions in Early Adolescence: A Life-span Perspective* (pp. 35–61). Hillsdale, NJ: Lawrence Erlbaum.

Petersen, A.C., & Crockett, L.J. (1985). Pubertal timing and grade effects on adjustment. *Journal of Youth and Adolescence*, **14**, 191–206.

Petersen, A.C., & Taylor, B. (1980). The biological approach to adolescence: biological change and psychological adaptation. In J. Adelson (Ed.), *Handbook of Adolescent Psychology* (pp. 117–155). New York: John Wiley & Sons.

Petersen, A.C., Crockett, L., Richards, M., & Boxer, A. (1988). A self-report measure of pubertal status: reliability, validity, and initial norms. *Journal of Youth and Adolescence*, **17**, 117–133.

Petersen, A.C., Sargiani, P.A., & Kennedy, R.E. (1991). Adolescent depression: why more girls? *Journal of Youth and Adolescence*, **20**, 247–271.

Reiter, E.O., & Grumbach, M.M. (1982). Neuroendocrine control mechanisms and the onset of puberty. *Annual Review of Physiology*, **44**, 595–613.

Rierdan, J., Koff, E., & Stubbs, M.L. (1989). A longitudinal analysis of body image as a predictor of the onset and persistence of adolescent girls' depression. *Journal of Early Adolescence*, **9**, 454–466.

Rockett, J.C., Lynch, C.D., & Buck, G.M. (2004). Biomarkers for assessing reproductive development and health: Part 1-pubertal development. *Environmental Health Perspectives*, **112**, 105–112.

Rudolph, K.D. (2002). Gender differences in emotional responses to interpersonal stress during adolescence. *Journal of Adolescent Health*, **30**, 3–13.

Schmitz, K.E., Hovell, M.F., Nichols, J.F. *et al.* (2004). A validation study of early adolescents' pubertal self-assessments. *Journal of Early Adolescence*, **24**, 357–384.

Siegel, J.M., Yancey, A.K., Aneshensel, C.S., & Schuler, R. (1999). Body image, perceived pubertal timing, and adolescent mental health. *Journal of Adolescent Health*, **25**, 155–165.

Simmons, R.G., & Blyth, D.A. (1987). *Moving into Adolescence: The Impact of Pubertal Change and School Context*. New York, NY: Aldine de Gruyter.

Stattin, H., & Magnusson, D. (1990). *Pubertal Maturation in Female Development*. Hillsdale, NJ: Lawrence Erlbaum.

Stice, E. (2003). Puberty and body image. In C. Hayward (Ed.), *Gender Differences at Puberty* (pp. 61–76). New York, NY: Cambridge University Press.

Stice, E., & Bearman, S.K. (2001). Body image and eating disturbances prospectively predict growth in depressive symptoms in adolescent girls: a growth curve analysis. *Developmental Psychology*, **37**, 597–607.

Stice, E., Hayward, C., Cameron, R.P., Killen, J.D., & Taylor, C.B. (2000). Body image and eating disturbances predict onset of depression among female adolescents: a longitudinal study. *Journal of Abnormal Psychology*, **109**, 438–444.

Susman, E.J. (1997). Modeling developmental complexity in adolescence: hormones and behavior in context. *Journal of Research on Adolescence*, **7**, 283–306.

Susman, E.J. (1998). Biobehavioural development: an integrative perspective. *International Journal of Behavioral Development*, **22**, 671–679.

Susman, E.J., Nottelmann, E.D., Inoff-Germain, G. *et al.* (1985). The relation of relative hormonal levels and physical development and social-emotional behavior in young adolescents. *Journal of Youth and Adolescence*, **14**, 245–264.

Susman, E.J., Inoff-Germain, G., Nottelmann, E.D. *et al.* (1987a). Hormones, emotional dispositions, and aggressive attributes in young adolescents. *Child Development*, **58**, 1114–1134.

Susman, E.J., Nottelmann, E.D., Inoff-Germain, G., Dorn, L.D., & Chrousos, G.P. (1987b). Hormonal influences on aspects of psychological development during adolescence. *Journal of Adolescent Health Care*, **8**, 492–504.

Susman, E.J., Dorn, L.D., & Chrousos, G.P. (1991). Negative affect and hormone levels in young adolescents: concurrent and predictive perspectives. *Journal of Youth and Adolescence*, **20**, 167–189.

Susman, E.J., Dorn, L.D., & Schiefelbein, V. (2003). Puberty, sexuality, and health. In M. Lerner, M.A. Easterbrooks, & J. Mistry (Eds.), *The Comprehensive Handbook of Psychology: Vol. 6* (pp. 295–324). New York, NY: Wiley.

Tanner, J.M. (1962). *Growth at Adolescence*. Oxford: Blackwell Scientific.

Tanner, J.M. (1970). Physical growth. In P.H. Mussen (Ed.), *Carmichael's Manual of Child Psychology* (pp. 77–155). New York, NY: John Wiley & Sons.

Tanner, J.M. (1978). *Fetus into Man: Physical Growth from Conception to Maturity.* Cambridge, MA: Harvard University Press.

Tschann, J.M., Adler, N.E., Irwin, C.E. *et al.* (1994). Initiation of substance use in early adolescence: the roles of pubertal timing and emotional distress. *Health Psychology,* 13, 326–333.

Wagner, B.M., & Compas, B.E. (1990). Gender, instrumentality, and expressivity: moderators of the relation between stress and psychological symptoms during adolescence. *American Journal of Community Psychology,* 18, 383–406.

Warren, M.P., & Brooks-Gunn, J. (1989). Mood and behavior at adolescence: evidence for hormonal factors. *Journal of Clinical Endocrinology and Metabolism,* 69, 77–83.

Wichstrom, L. (1999). The emergence of gender difference in depressed mood during adolescence: the role of intensified gender socialization. *Developmental Psychology,* 35, 232–245.

Worthman, C.M., & Stallings, J.F. (1997). Hormone measures in finger-prick blood spot samples: new field methods for reproductive endocrinology. *American Journal of Physical Anthropology,* 104, 1–21.

5

Pubertal and neuroendocrine development and risk for depression

Julia A. Graber

Puberty has often been identified as an important marker, if not a causal factor, of changes in adjustment from childhood to adolescence. Although most discussions of adolescent development cite puberty as an important, defining, or critical process, the evidence that behavior demonstrates meaningful changes in connection with puberty is less voluminous than our beliefs would indicate. At the same time, the circumstantial evidence has been quite compelling. Rates of subclinical symptoms and depressive disorders begin to increase in the early adolescent period (Seeley & Lewinsohn, see Chapter 3, this volume). Furthermore, the 2:1 gender difference of females to males in rates of depressive disorder also emerges in this time period (Costello *et al.*, 2006; Seeley & Lewinsohn, see Chapter 3, this volume). Given the extent of physical, neurological, and physiological processes that are subsumed under puberty, as well as the commensurate psychological and social changes that occur either because of or along with puberty, the logical assumption is that puberty plays an important role in increases in rates of depression and the gender difference in rates. Yet, puberty is, in fact, a normative developmental process, or rather set of processes, that everyone experiences (with the exception of individuals with relatively rare genetic and endocrine disorders). Thus, this chapter considers the question: how or why does something that happens to everyone lead to disorder for some individuals?

Before considering this question, some general points about the literature are worth noting. First, the literature on puberty and disorder is relatively small, with a few studies of neuroendocrine processes and a few additional studies on links between depressive disorders and pubertal timing, that is, going through puberty early, at the same time, or later than one's peers. Second, much of this work has not had sufficient power to examine different

Adolescent Emotional Development and the Emergence of Depressive Disorders, ed. Nicholas B. Allen and Lisa B. Sheeber. Published by Cambridge University Press. © Cambridge University Press 2009.

depressive disorders separately in connection with puberty. As such, the literature is mostly limited to major depressive disorder (MDD) or dysthymia with no studies to date on connections between puberty and bipolar mood disorders. Third, as others have discussed in detail (Dorn *et al.*, 2003; DeRose & Brooks-Gunn, see Chapter 4, this volume), which aspects of puberty are assessed and how each is measured has an impact on interpretation of findings and identification of consistent themes in the literature. Fourth, in addition to the impact of assessment of puberty on understanding findings, assessment of disorder also influences the interpretation of findings (Kessler *et al.*, 2001). Hence, methodological overlap in the studies that have examined both pubertal processes and depressive disorders is limited. Initial studies of puberty typically examined normative developmental process rather than disorder. Studies of disorder tended to focus on only a few aspects of puberty (see Ryan & Dahl, 1993, and Angold *et al.*, 1999, as notable exceptions). Several researchers have called for nationally representative studies of the epidemiology and etiology of depressive disorders, or child and adolescent disorders more generally, taking a developmental epidemiology approach and including comprehensive assessment of pubertal development (Costello *et al.*, 2006; Kessler *et al.*, 2001). As yet, no such study exists. Finally, as noted, a major challenge to the field is understanding the role that puberty plays in the development of depressive disorders for some individuals. Whereas several models have been delineated to explain the role of puberty in affective changes during adolescence, and presumably subsequent onset of disorder (e.g. Buchanan *et al.*, 1992), the literature on depressive disorders and puberty has mainly focused on demonstrating a puberty-adjustment association with only limited consideration of how or why the effect occurs.

Given these issues, the present chapter first discusses the findings of studies that have examined links between puberty and depressive disorders. Then, explanatory models are examined. Implications of the literature for prevention or intervention as well as future research are also presented.

Are the changes of puberty linked to depressive disorders?

The L-HPA and HPG endocrine systems

The limbic-hypothalamus-pituitary-adrenal (L-HPA) and the hypothalamus-pituitary-gonadal (HPG) systems control the hormonal changes of puberty and subsequent morphological changes to the body and reproductive functioning. Moreover, these systems are linked to increases in subclinical depressive symptoms and depressive disorders. In particular, studies of L-HPA functioning and the stress system have identified biological markers that differentiate disordered from non-disordered individuals. As well, critical developmental research demonstrates gene–environment interactions in the development of L-HPA functioning (Caspi *et al.*, 2003; Francis *et al.*, 1999). The following provides a brief review of how changes in each system at puberty may be linked to depression.

The L-HPA stress system

Activation of the L-HPA occurs in response to novelty and stress, especially social stressors. Briefly, hormones in the brain stimulate the pituitary to secrete adrenocorticotropin hormone (ACTH) which in turn stimulates the adrenal gland to secrete cortisol (see McEwen, 2000; Meyer *et al.*, 2001, for a detailed discussion). As the individual assesses the threat level or copes with the challenge, cortisol levels decrease. Normative diurnal cycles in cortisol occur with peak levels observed just before waking, followed by a rapid decline, and then relatively stable, low levels in the late afternoon and evening, with increases during sleeping. Interestingly, acute elevations of cortisol in response to stressful situations may promote cognitive processing of emotions; that is, humans and animals remember experiences that activate stress responses (McEwen, 2000). However, chronic production of cortisol appears to damage brain structures. Some individuals do not show the typical adaptation to the situation either due to behavioral failures to cope with the challenge or longer-term adaptations of the physiological system that maintain elevated levels of cortisol to frequently occurring stressors. Hence, over time, some individuals are exposed to elevated levels of cortisol that impact emotional, cognitive, and immune systems (McEwen, 2000).

Changes in L-HPA at puberty and depression

Discussion of L-HPA changes at puberty which might be linked to depression has focused on adrenarche, or maturation of the adrenal glands. Adrenarche involves the production of dehydroepiandrosterone (DHEA) and its sulfate (DHEAS) as well as other hormones, including testosterone. A different area of the adrenal gland is responsible for the secretion of cortisol. Walker *et al.* (2001) have found that the adrenal-cortisol areas mature linearly and continue to mature in the post-pubertal period. They have also suggested that this maturation may be linked to expression of symptoms and disorder, most likely among individuals with vulnerabilities to these problems.

Depression in adulthood is often characterized by dysregulation in the stress system (see Meyer *et al.*, 2001, for a review). Much of the initial research on puberty and depression has consisted of clinical studies designed to determine if depression in pre-pubertal children was different from depression in post-pubertal adolescents and adults (Ryan & Dahl, 1993). Initial studies reported that physiological dysregulation observed in adult patients, such as elevated morning cortisol levels (i.e. hypersecretion), was not observed in depressed children and adolescents (Birmaher *et al.*, 1996). More recently, several studies have identified alterations in diurnal patterns of cortisol secretion among children with anxiety disorders and adolescents with depression (Forbes *et al.*, 2006; Forbes *et al.*, see Chapter 7, this volume). An emerging literature indicates that the neuroendocrine dysregulation observed with MDD in adulthood is not fully present in children with MDD. Diurnal alterations in cortisol may be seen in adolescents with MDD and hence, it is hypothesized that pubertal maturation involving the L-HPA is necessary before adult-type neuroendocrine concomitants of depression are observed. Notably, studies often find few differences in the experience of symptoms of depression in childhood versus adolescence despite these differences in physiology (Birmaher *et al.*, 1996, 2004).

Levels of DHEA and DHEAS

Hormonal changes in DHEA and DHEAS have also been associated with affective changes including internalizing and externalizing symptoms during puberty (see DeRose & Brooks-Gunn, Chapter 4, this volume; Susman & Rogol, 2004, for recent reviews). In studies with adolescents at high risk for depression, Goodyer *et al.* (2000a, 2000b) initially reported that hypersecretion of DHEA in the evening or high morning cortisol were predictive of MDD onset. However, in subsequent work following this sample, Goodyer *et al.* (2003) reported that higher morning cortisol/DHEA ratios distinguished those adolescents who experienced persistent depression from those whose episodes remitted or who were never depressed. As Goodyer and his colleagues (2000b) noted, they did not directly assess puberty. The initial finding that MDD was preceded by high DHEA levels could be indicative of a link between MDD and either more advanced pubertal development or hormone levels that are high for pubertal stage. In contrast, the finding that persistent MDD was linked with low DHEA relative to cortisol might suggest an association with less advanced pubertal development.

The work by Goodyer and his colleagues indicates that additional research is needed in order to clarify associations between DHEA and DHEAS and depression in adolescents. Research with adults and on adolescent symptoms may shed light on the expected direction of effects. Wolf & Kirschbaum (1999) suggest that high DHEAS levels are consistently associated with depression in adults but that findings among adolescents are more mixed. It is important to note that the adult studies were often not prospective but rather examined hormonal correlates of depression. In the adolescence literature, low DHEAS is often associated with aggressive symptoms (see Susman & Rogol, 2004 for a review). In addition, my colleagues and I have found that high DHEAS in combination with earlier age at menarche was associated with higher emotional arousal and depressive symptoms in early adolescent girls (Graber *et al.*, 2006). Given the interconnections among L-HPA and HPG systems, Angold (2003) recommends considering neuroendocrine processes of both systems before drawing conclusions about effects of adrenal or gonadal hormones. In fact, Angold and his colleagues have taken this approach in their own work.

Hypothalamus-pituitary-gonadal hormonal effects

In examinations of HPG hormones such as estradiol or testosterone, Angold and colleagues (1999) have found that hormone levels predicted the onset of depression in girls, and accounted for the effects of secondary sexual characteristics on depression. Note that the Great Smoky Mountain Study (GSM) used a representative sampling approach and followed three age cohorts (9-, 11-, and 13-year-olds) over time; as such, it is one of the few studies of puberty and depression to use an epidemiologic approach. Angold (2003) has since reported that DHEAS was also positively associated with rates of depression but that inclusion of estradiol and testosterone in the models accounted for the effect of DHEAS. Because rates of depression were highest in the upper part of the hormone distributions, these findings suggest that depression starts to occur at higher rates once more adult-like levels of gonadal hormones are reached but does not explain why some girls become depressed and others do not.

Pubertal timing

Whereas studies of pubertal hormone-depression links are limited, more attention has been given to the social-contextual aspects of puberty such as pubertal timing. The timing of when a transition occurs may be an important factor in how the individual navigates that transition. For example, an adolescent's development (neural, cognitive, emotional) at the time of the transition may be salient to the outcome of the transition; earlier maturation may result in the individual entering puberty prior to developing competencies needed to adapt to the changes (Graber & Brooks-Gunn, 1996). Also, social context often defines the transition – what it means to have an adult body, whether being off-time is deviant in the peer group, and so forth. Over the past 15 years, a literature has emerged linking pubertal timing, especially early maturation, to a range of affective and behavioral problems (see DeRose & Brooks-Gunn, Chapter 4, this volume; Graber, 2003, for recent reviews). While the literature on disorder is much smaller, it is also quite compelling.

In a community sample of girls followed longitudinally from early adolescence into young adulthood, my colleagues and I have found that earlier age at menarche was associated with several inter-correlated subclinical problems. These studies used established screeners for disorders and compared patterns (e.g. persistent problems versus transient or no problems) during adolescence and young adulthood. Earlier maturation was associated with persistent eating problems during adolescence (Graber *et al.*, 1994) and co-occurring eating and depressive problems during mid-adolescence, the time period when rates of depressive scores over the cut-off peaked for this sample (Graber & Brooks-Gunn, 2001).

In 1997, two articles were published that examined early maturation in connection with internalizing disorders using stringent diagnostic criteria. In the first, Hayward and colleagues (1997) found that earlier maturation was associated with higher levels of internalizing symptoms during early adolescence in a community sample of girls. Furthermore, girls who had internalizing problems in early adolescence and who were early maturers were more likely to have internalizing disorders (e.g. MDD, any anxiety disorder, or eating disorder) at follow-up in mid adolescence. Interestingly, Caspi & Moffitt (1991) reported quite similar findings in a large, epidemiological study of a birth-cohort in New Zealand. In that study, girls with childhood behavior problems and early maturation had the highest rates of behavior problems by age 16.

In the other study from 1997, my colleagues and I conducted a comprehensive examination of off-time puberty (both early and late) in connection with a range of subclinical and diagnostic outcomes for girls and boys using the Oregon Adolescent Depression Project (OADP), a large epidemiological study of depression in the high-school years (Graber *et al.*, 1997). For girls, early and late maturation were associated with higher lifetime rates of MDD. Early maturing girls also reported higher rates of suicide attempts than other youth. For boys, timing was not associated with lifetime or current experience of disorder. Although the focus of the present discussion is on depression, we also found that early maturation in girls was associated with higher lifetime rates of substance use disorder, eating disorders, and disruptive behavior disorder, as well as higher current rates of disruptive behavior disorder.

A subsequent community study of girls, ages 11–15, has replicated links between earlier ages at menarche and diagnosis of depression (with some modifications to criteria) and substance use disorder over a 2-year period (Stice *et al.*, 2001); effects for eating disorders were not replicated. In addition, Stice and his colleagues examined comorbidity among the three disorders of interest – depression, substance use, and eating disorders – and found that early menarche in girls was associated with greater risk for comorbid depression and substance use.

In a follow-up analysis of the OADP when participants were 24 years of age, my colleagues and I examined whether pubertal timing effects demonstrated in the mid adolescent period (ages 14–18) persisted into adulthood (Graber *et al.*, 2004). In young adulthood, late maturation was no longer associated with higher prevalence of MDD. In contrast, early maturation effects were maintained into young adulthood in that these women continued to have higher lifetime prevalence rates of MDD than on-time maturers. Furthermore, early maturation was not predictive of age of onset in a survival analysis, indicating that early maturation was associated with higher rates of onset of MDD across adolescence. As with our prior findings, young women who had been early maturers also had higher lifetime prevalence rates of other disorders including anxiety and disruptive behavior disorders, as well as higher lifetime rates of attempted suicide and Antisocial Personality traits in comparison other young women. The follow-up analyses of the OADP (Graber *et al.*, 2004), again, found no association between pubertal timing and lifetime or current rates of MDD in young adult men. Timing effects, which were found in late maturing males for other disorders and behaviors, are not discussed here.

One exception to the emerging consistency in this literature is analysis of pubertal timing in the GSM project. Angold *et al.* (1998) found no association between early maturation and MDD. In their analyses, they defined early maturation as reaching Tanner stage III prior to age 12. However, this approach necessitated that most of their oldest age cohort was excluded from some analyses. Additional analyses based on age at menarche were only conducted for those girls who had reached Tanner stage III or higher resulting in an unusual truncation of range in that more of the sample who had reached this stage of development was comprised of early maturers. Also, under this approach potential effects of late maturation were not examined. Subsequent examination of the GSM when all youth are post-pubertal may be informative.

Interestingly, the emerging consistency in the literature has occurred despite differences in protocols for assessing puberty. Hayward and colleagues (1997) assessed pubertal timing via differences in stage of development, the OADP analyses were based on perceived timing (Graber *et al.*, 1997, 2004), and Stice and his colleagues (2001) examined age at menarche and all found that earlier pubertal maturation in girls was linked to depressive disorders. Notably, the GSM study, in which timing-depression links were not found, also used age at menarche and stage of pubertal development (Angold *et al.*, 1998); hence, it does not appear that the discrepant findings were attributable to method.

In part, one reason that findings have become more consistent, especially for girls, is that recent studies have used more comprehensive assessments of psychopathology, both subclinical and disorder. This approach is quite useful in longitudinal assessments, as the critical challenge for studies of adjustment is to predict more accurately who will develop disorders over time. For example, Ge *et al.* (2006) have described pubertal status and timing effects on internalizing and externalizing symptoms using diagnostic interviews. In this study of 10–12-year-old African–American children, advanced pubertal status and pubertal timing were associated with more symptoms of general anxiety disorder and MDD in girls and boys. Within the restricted age range of 10–12, more advanced pubertal status may be confounded with early timing so it will be interesting to see if these early adolescent associations translate into timing effects for disorder over time. Also, Ge and his colleagues are one of the few groups to examine pubertal effects on internalizing symptoms in an African–American sample. Recent studies have found comparable effects of early maturation on externalizing behaviors in African–American and Latino youth (e.g. Lynne *et al.* in press).

In general, consistent findings for early timing effects on depression in girls are found in the mid-adolescent, and most recently young adulthood, periods rather than during puberty. Hence, increases in rates of disorder occur in the advanced to postpubertal period for girls. Girls who mature earlier than their peers are likely to reach menarche earlier than age 12, well before rates of disorder rise. Hence, timing does not confer immediate risk at the entry to puberty, but rather appears to be the beginning, or part of, a pathway for social or biological experiences that result in disorder over time.

Conclusions regarding puberty and depression

The answer to the original question, "Are the changes of puberty linked to depressive disorders?", appears to be yes. However, putting aside the studies of subclinical symptoms, it is alarming to see how few studies have actually assessed this question; the paucity of studies stands in contrast to the number of times that puberty is mentioned in the literature as an important transition that is likely linked to changes in affect, behavior, and adjustment. In terms of depressive disorders, adult-like levels of estrogen were associated with increases in rates of depression seen in the advanced to post-pubertal period for girls in one study. A comparable "level-of-maturation" effect may also exist for adrenal androgens (i.e. DHEA and DHEAS), but two groups report different findings. Early pubertal timing is associated with depressive disorders in girls in several studies. Late maturation in girls may also be linked to depressive disorders but this is based on only one study. Overall, the literature reviewed is small and has not directly tested mechanisms underlying the effects.

Explanations for puberty-depression associations

Puberty is a "necessary" but not sufficient condition for depression

One interpretation of the hormone-depression associations is that being either in the advanced stages of puberty or post-pubertal is "necessary" for the experience of depression. Of course, pre-pubertal children can become depressed; yet, as noted, the change in rates of disorder by the post-pubertal period is marked. Once the neuroendocrine system is mature, it may be more likely to respond to the factors that lead to depression via dysregulation and affective and physical symptoms of disorder. The following sections highlight findings regarding mechanisms for the emergence of depression in the post-pubertal period, and also identify some assumptions about these processes that may not be fully supported.

Maturation of the HPG system

Links between maturation of the HPG system, specifically estradiol levels, and depression are particularly intriguing. Whereas substantial evidence has confirmed that the L-HPA system is central to stress responses and psycho-pathology, the HPG system also interacts with neural functioning with effects beyond regulation of puberty and reproductive functioning. Estrogen receptors are found not only in the hypothalamus but also in the hippocampus where cortisol impacts memory (McEwen, 1994). Recently, Taylor and her colleagues (2000) have suggested that for women, physiological stress responses may involve estrogen and oxytocin, the latter being a hormone that is often associated with maternal caregiving behaviors and pair bonding in other species.

Exposure to estrogen across the life span has also been linked to health problems such as breast cancer (e.g. Apter *et al.*, 1989). Specifically, women who were early maturers have higher rates of breast cancer than other women. This link is not strictly due to longer exposure to estrogen because of longer periods of fertility but early maturers may also have higher estrogen levels during adulthood (Lai *et al.*, 2001). Overall, estrogen studies seem to speak to the negative effect of elevated hormone levels on women's health and that early maturers may be at risk for poor mental and physical health. Hence, the assertion that depression is more likely in a "mature" system is incomplete as individual differences are found in how the HPG system functions.

At the same time, several studies have examined the positive effect of hormone replacement therapy on depression in peri-menopausal women (e.g. de Novaes Soares *et al.*, 2001). Of course, hormone replacement is not intended to create high estrogen levels but rather to prevent low levels. Although the literature on HPG hormones and depression is sparse, the nature of the findings and related research using animal models suggests that further investigation is merited.

Puberty and gene–environment interactions

Other evidence for "maturation" as a factor comes from recent studies of gene–environment interactions. Though an extensive review of the genetics of depression is beyond the purview of this chapter, studies have reported that pubertal status may influence the expression of gene–environment interactions.

Silberg and her colleagues (1999) observed that the influence of genetic factors or genetic similarity in twins for depressive symptoms (from diagnostic interviews) was evident among post-pubertal adolescents but not for pre-pubertal children. Furthermore, although negative life events were predictive of depressive symptoms in both boys and girls, depressive symptoms increased with age even for girls who did not experience negative life events. Furthermore, genetic similarity was associated with the reporting of negative life events. Hence, girls may experience greater heritability for depression that is mediated by the heritability of another factor (e.g. personality) that leads to the experience of negative life events (Moffitt et al., 2006). Synthesizing estrogen findings with genetics and life-event findings suggests that both HPG maturation and emergence of a genetic vulnerability occur at about the same time.

Caspi and his colleagues (2003) have identified a specific gene polymorphism that moderates whether the experience of stressful life events will result in having a depressive disorder. In particular, they examined the influence of maltreatment during childhood (e.g. consistently harsh discipline, sexual abuse, severe physical punishment, and disruptive caregiver changes), on the experience of depression in young adulthood. The 5-HTTLPR gene, which is hypothesized to moderate serotonergic responses to stress, moderated the link between childhood maltreatment and young adult depression; childhood experience was only salient to onset of depression in individuals with the short allele of the gene. Again, it is possible that maturation of the endocrine system and brain maturation may be necessary before outcomes, such as MDD, of gene–environment interactions such as that described by Caspi and colleagues (2003) are experienced.

Diathesis stress models and puberty

Maturation, in and of itself, is not a particularly explanatory process. The "maturation" of the endocrine system is based on continual gene–environment interactions that occur through puberty and beyond. Caspi and his colleagues (2003) suggested that these types of gene–environment interactions fit a diathesis-stress model of depressive disorders. It is well documented that diathesis, propensity, or vulnerability for disorders can develop over time. In rodents, Meaney and his colleagues (e.g. Francis et al., 1999) have delineated an animal model involving genetics, maternal care behaviors, and subsequent alternations in the L-HPA that result in consistent individual differences in behavioral and physiological responses to stress and subsequent health outcomes. Work by Suomi and his colleagues (see Suomi, 1999, for a review) has demonstrated similar processes in the development of individual differences in vulnerability to depressive behaviors in non-human primates.

The advances in articulating explanatory models for diathesis-stress interactions and the subsequent prediction of disorder (or disease, more broadly) do not, however, tend to explain why things change at puberty. In part, the notion is that puberty is an additional stressor, and those with vulnerabilities for disorders have the most difficulty with this transition either socially or physiologically. Notably, early maturing girls with prior problems showed an accentuation of these problems over time in two studies (Caspi & Moffitt, 1991; Hayward *et al.*, 1997). Prior symptoms may not constitute vulnerability per se, but rather may be markers for vulnerabilities that put children on pathways to disorder. Hence, it would be useful to know more about specific vulnerabilities, such as affect regulation difficulties that develop in response to childhood maltreatment, and why some vulnerabilities seem to interact with puberty, in particular, pubertal timing in girls.

Alternately, returning to the findings for adrenal androgens, hormone levels that increase in childhood such as DHEA and DHEAS may already demonstrate individual differences in levels that are indicative of vulnerability or altered physiological functioning; that is, the propensity to have consistently high-for-age estrogen or DHEAS levels could be vulnerability. In this case, it would be a vulnerability that does not emerge until puberty. Of course, given the limited literature on estrogen and depression, as well as the inconsistent findings for adrenal androgens, more evidence would be needed to move beyond conjecture.

Puberty is interconnected with other adolescent challenges

Another explanatory model of puberty–depression links focuses on puberty as one of several changes occurring during early adolescence. When listing the changes that young adolescents experience, it is difficult to find a domain that has not been linked to puberty (e.g. parent–child interactions, sexually based experiences among peers, school changes, etc.). These cumulative or simultaneous changes result in increases in depressive symptoms (see Graber & Brooks-Gunn, 1996, for a review). In discussions of pubertal timing, it is often suggested that early maturation leads to disorder because youth face challenges prior to having the skills needed to cope with these experiences (see DeRose and Brooks-Gunn, Chapter 4). Or, off-time maturation confers risks due to feeling different or out-of-synch with peers. In particular, early maturing girls have peer and dating relationships that may put them at risk for problem behaviors and emotional challenges associated with managing intimate relationships (see Graber & Sontag, 2006, for a discussion of these issues), and are more likely to have extended periods of parent–child conflict than other adolescents (Steinberg, 2001). Rudolf (2002) has suggested that girls, in general, have higher risk for depression because girls place more importance on their social interactions and experience more stress in comparison to boys in these interactions.

In the OADP, early maturation in females was not only associated with higher rates of MDD in adolescence and adulthood but also with less social support from family and friends at both assessments (Graber *et al.*, 1997, 2004). Impaired social interactions may have been a result of their history of disorder, or may be one of the factors that led to disorder. Moreover, in the OADP, early maturation was linked to serious externalizing problems (conduct disorder in adolescence) and higher rates of antisocial personality disorder in young adulthood. A defining feature of antisocial personality disorder is impaired social relationships.

Though the existing literature does not fully explain why early maturing girls have higher rates of depression, there are clues from the subclinical literature and studies of normative development that speak to factors that put some girls at risk. Specifically, changes in social relationships during adolescence occur in existing relationships (e.g. with parents and peers), and in many cases occur in new relationships (e.g. navigating romantic and sexual feelings). Early maturing girls often have less healthy experiences with these relationship changes (Graber & Sontag, 2006).

Puberty is not meaningfully associated with disorder but is a marker for other processes

A final explanation is that puberty is a marker for other processes that predict depression. Studies of predictors of the onset of puberty have focused on a range of genetic, behavioral, and environmental factors. Belsky *et al.* (1991) delineated an evolutionary model of socialization in which stressful family environments lead to behavioral problems, and earlier onset of pubertal development as well as other life outcomes. Prospective studies have identified the quality of family relations, specifically, warmth and conflict in family relations, as important to timing of maturation in girls, such that lower warmth and more conflict were associated with earlier maturation (see Graber, 2003, for a review). Consistent with these initial studies, Ellis *et al.* (1999) reported that affection in parent–child interactions when girls were in preschool (ages 4–5) predicted pubertal timing differences in early adolescence. Ellis & Garber (2000) subsequently reported that maternal mood disorders were associated with earlier maturation in girls but the association was mediated by poor quality of family relationships and father absence; both factors seemed to be independent pathways to earlier maturation in girls. In addition, research on girls who experience maltreatment has found that sexual abuse prior to the onset of puberty is associated with earlier ages of menarche (Trickett & Putnam, 1993; Zabin *et al.*, 2005). Because Zabin and her colleagues (2005) could differentiate whether abuse happened prior to external signs of puberty, they were able to conclude that the effect was more likely accounted for by stress processes than by abusers choosing victims who were beginning puberty. Childhood sexual abuse has been identified as a predictor of several disorders, including depression (Trickett & Putnam, 1993).

Although none of these studies have investigated physiological mechanisms, in studies of adult women and in animal models, psychosocial or environmental stress influences the estrogen system and a range of health outcomes (e.g. McEwen, 1994). Hence, a gender-specific mechanism may exist for these findings.

One point to consider in this discussion is how much of early timing effects on disorder in girls may, in fact, be accounted for by unhealthy family relationships. The types of family interactions that predict earlier puberty are potentially also the types of family interactions associated with the development of vulnerabilities for depression (see Tompson, McKowen, and Asarnow, Chapter 15). Furthermore, youth who enter adolescence with poor quality family relationships are likely to continue to have low warmth and high conflict, and higher risk for psychopathology during adolescence (Steinberg, 2001). As yet, no studies have fully examined the interconnection of these factors in childhood in order to determine if early timing effects on depression are mediated by family relationships or other factors. It may be that both pubertal timing and family relationships have unique contributions as well as a combined contribution to the development of depression. Prospective research would be beneficial not just from a scientific standpoint but would also provide insight for prevention and intervention efforts.

Is puberty relevant to depressive disorders or adolescent psychopathology more generally?

The extent to which pubertal changes and timing are uniquely connected to the affective or neuroendocrine dysregulations that characterize MDD is relevant more broadly to discussions of classification of disorder. In particular, individual differences in pubertal development are associated with several disorders, not just depression. Adrenal and gonadal hormone changes have more often been associated with externalizing behaviors such as aggression rather than depression (see Susman & Rogol, 2004, for a review). In the timing literature, studies examining multiple diagnostic categories typically reported early maturation effects on externalizing disorders (e.g. substance use, conduct disorder; Graber et al., 1997, 2004; Stice et al., 2001). Hence, the existing, albeit limited, literature suggests that early maturation in girls is a risk for both internalizing and externalizing problems and may not be specific to one disorder.

At the same time, internalizing and externalizing problems are often highly correlated during adolescence (e.g. Krueger et al., 1998) and nearly half, or even two-thirds, of all adolescents who meet diagnostic criteria for depression have a comorbid condition (Rohde *et al.*, 1991). Often, the other disorder precedes the development of depression (Rohde *et al.*, 1991). Hence, it is not surprising that pubertal processes may not represent a unique pathway to depressive disorders. Only one study discussed here, investigated comorbidity; in that project, Stice and his colleagues (2001) found that earlier age of menarche was associated with comorbid depression and substance use.

As indicated previously, no study has yet considered puberty and the development of bipolar disorders. It has been suggested that symptoms consistent with bipolar disorders in children may be mistaken for externalizing symptoms or behaviors (Birmaher *et al.*, 1996). Moreover, among adolescents who had a MDD episode, comorbid substance use problems and high rates of psychosocial problems have been linked to subsequent development of a bipolar disorder (for bipolar II; Birmaher *et al.*, 1996). Hence, these symptom patterns share similarities with the early maturation-disorder literature in girls. Clearly, future studies need to account not only for comorbidity but also for the full range of diagnostic possibilities over sufficient time for disorders to emerge – a daunting task for research.

Implications for prevention

If puberty is associated with depression or disorder, in general, a logical question arises: Are there targets of intervention when studying puberty? An initial response is to say "no;" if the biological changes of puberty are occurring within the normal developmental range then it seems illogical to suggest that intervention be directed at altering puberty itself. In actuality, pediatricians and other health practitioners, as well as parents, have undertaken direct "treatment" of puberty via drugs that halt or slow the progression of puberty even in cases of normative development (Paterson *et al.*, 1998). In addition, cancer prevention researchers have found that a low-fat diet resulted in lower estradiol levels in young adolescent girls (Dorgan *et al.*, 2003); they concluded that regular exercise during early adolescence combines with diet to lower estradiol, and hence, may impact long-term risk for breast cancer. Of course, simply recommending that girls keep their weight down and in so doing keep estrogen levels lower may have unintended consequences (i.e. eating disorders) if there is not a focus on healthy practices.

In contrast to direct intervention on puberty, using puberty or timing as a marker for identifying individuals at increased risk for disorder may be helpful to parents and health practitioners. In part, recommending more or better information to parents does not necessarily make them more adept at dealing with problems that may emerge, it only tells them to keep an eye out for them. The difficulty here is that parent–child relationship problems are one reason girls may mature earlier than peers. Parents having problems before their children enter adolescence may be least able to help their children navigate the transition. Early family intervention or prevention efforts as described by others (see Tompson, McKowen, and Asarnow, Chapter 15) may be particularly salient to puberty-disorder pathways.

Given that puberty is hypothesized to confer risk via interaction with social-contextual factors, focus on those factors (parents, healthy peer relationships, coping skills for managing stressful events) would likely be the most fruitful approach to prevention efforts. For example, if genetic factors impact the tendency to experience stressful life events post-pubertally, then the ability to cope with these events is critical and a target for intervention. It may be particularly important to identify or create gender-specific programming that focuses on the unique stressors faced by young adolescent girls (e.g. social stressors) and effective strategies for regulating their emotions and developing competence in dealing with these experiences (Graber & Sontag, 2006).

Throughout this discussion, I have identified gaps in the literature. As noted initially, there is an alarming absence of comprehensive examinations of puberty-disorder links, and testing of mechanisms for these effects. The fact is that comprehensive examinations of most issues are expensive, and this is particularly true for puberty. At the same time, although several large, national studies of development that include pubertal measures are in progress, most of these do not include diagnostic protocols. Some new, smaller studies of puberty with diagnostic protocols have been undertaken. It is hoped that these studies will be able to follow their samples for sufficient time to identify pathways to disorder. Another approach to filling this gap is to encourage greater inclusion of pubertal measures into prevention and intervention trials focusing on depressive disorders. Prevention studies can be particularly useful for understanding mechanisms for etiology of behaviors and disorders through examination of mechanisms of change and via examination of normative developmental process in the control group. Overall, puberty is definitely a component of multiple pathways to depressive disorder, as well as other disorders. Better identification of these pathways is likely the best approach for identifying prevention and treatment strategies for youth and families.

REFERENCES

Apter, D., Reinila, M., & Vihko, R. (1989). Some endocrine characteristics of early menarche, a risk factor for breast cancer, are preserved into adulthood. *International Journal of Cancer*, **44**, 783–787.

Angold, A. (2003). Adolescent depression, cortisol, and DHEA [Editorial]. *Psychological Medicine*, **33**, 573–581.

Angold, A., Costello, E.J., & Worthman, C.M. (1998). Puberty and depression: the roles of age, pubertal status and pubertal timing. *Psychological Medicine*, **28**, 51–61.

Angold, A., Costello, E.J., Erkanli, A., & Worthman, C.M. (1999). Pubertal changes in hormone levels and depression in girls. *Psychological Medicine*, **29**, 1043–1053.

Belsky, J., Steinberg, L., & Draper, P. (1991). Further reflections on an evolutionary theory of socialization. *Child Development*, **62**, 682–685.

Birmaher, B., Ryan, N.D., Williamson, D.E. *et al.* (1996). Childhood and adolescent depression: a review of the past 10 years. Part I. *Journal of the American Academy of Child and Adolescent Psychiatry*, **35**, 1427–1439.

Birmaher, B., Williamson, D.E., Dahl, R.E. *et al.* (2004). Clinical presentation and course of depression in youth: does onset in childhood differ from onset in adolescence? *Journal of the American Academy of Child and Adolescent Psychiatry*, **43**, 63–70.

Buchanan, C.M., Eccles, J.S., & Becker, J.B. (1992). Are adolescents the victims of raging hormones: evidence for activational effects of hormones on moods and behavior at adolescence. *Psychological Bulletin*, **111**, 62–107.

Caspi, A., & Moffitt, T.E. (1991). Individual differences are accentuated during periods of social change: the sample case of girls at puberty. *Journal of Personality and Social Psychology*, **61**, 157–168.

Caspi, A., Sugden, K., Moffitt, T.E. *et al.* (2003). Influence of life stress on depression: moderation by a polymorphism in the 5-HTT gene. *Science*, **301**, 386–389.

Costello, E.J., Foley, D.L., & Angold, A. (2006). Ten-year research update review: The epidemiology of child and adolescent psychiatric disorders. II. Developmental epidemiology. *Journal of the American Academy of Child and Adolescent Psychiatry*, **45**, 8–25.

de Novaes Soares, C., Almeida, O.P., Joffe, H., & Cohen, L.S. (2001). Efficacy of estradiol for the treatment of depressive disorders in perimenopausal women. *Archives of General Psychiatry*, **58**, 529–534.

Dorn, L.D., Dahl, R.D., Williamson, D.E. *et al.* (2003). Developmental markers in adolescence: implications for studies of pubertal processes. *Journal of Youth and Adolescence*, **32**, 315–324.

Dorgan, J.F., Hunsberger, S.A., McMahon, R.P. *et al.* (2003). Diet and sex hormones in girls: findings from a randomized controlled clinical trial. *Journal of the National Cancer Institute*, **95**, 132–141.

Ellis, B.J., & Garber, J. (2000). Psychosocial antecedents of variation in girls' pubertal timing: maternal depression, stepfather presence, and marital and family stress. *Child Development*, **71**, 485–501.

Ellis, B.J., McFadyen-Ketchum, S., Dodge, K.A., Pettit, G.S., & Bates, J.E. (1999). Quality of early family relationships and individual differences in the timing of pubertal maturation in girls: a longitudinal test of an evolutionary model. *Journal of Personality and Social Psychology*, **77**, 387–401.

Forbes, E.E., Williamson, D.E., Ryan, N.D., Birmaher, B., Axelson, D.A., & Dahl, R.E. (2006). Peri-sleep-onset cortisol levels in children and adolescents with affective disorders. *Biological Psychiatry*, **59**, 24–30.

Francis, D.D., Champagne, F.A., Liu, D., & Meaney, M.J. (1999). Maternal care, gender expression, and the development of individual differences in stress reactivity. *Annals of the New York Academy of Sciences*, **896**, 66–84.

Ge, X., Brody, G.H., Conger, R.D., & Simons, R.L. (2006). Pubertal maturation and African American children's internalizing and externalizing symptoms. *Journal of Youth and Adolescence*, **35**, 531–540.

Goodyer, I.M., Herbert, J., Tamplin, A., & Altham, P.M.E. (2000a). First-episode major depression in adolescents: affective, cognitive, and endocrine characteristics of risk status and predictors of onset. *British Journal of Psychiatry*, **176**, 142–149.

Goodyer, I.M., Herbert, J., Tamplin, A., & Altham, P.M.E. (2000b). Recent life events, cortisol, dehydroepiandrosterone and the onset of major depression in high-risk adolescents. *British Journal of Psychiatry*, **177**, 499–504.

Goodyer, I.M., Herbert, J., & Tamplin, A. (2003). Psychoendocrine antecedents of persistent first-episode major depression in adolescents: a community-based longitudinal inquiry. *Psychological Medicine*, **33**, 601–610.

Graber, J.A. (2003). Puberty in context. In C. Hayward (Ed.), *Gender Differences at Puberty* (pp. 307–325). New York: Cambridge University Press.

Graber, J.A., & Brooks-Gunn, J. (1996). Transitions and turning points: navigating the passage from childhood through adolescence. *Developmental Psychology*, **32**, 768–776.

Graber, J.A., & Brooks-Gunn, J. (2001). Co-occurring eating and depressive problems: an 8-year study of adolescent girls. *International Journal of Eating Disorders*, **30**, 37–47.

Graber, J.A., & Sontag, L.M. (2006). Puberty and girls' sexuality: why hormones aren't the complete answer. In L.M. Diamond (Vol. Ed.), *New Directions for Child and Adolescent Development: Vol. 112. Rethinking Positive Adolescent Female Sexual Development* (pp. 23–38). San Francisco, CA: Jossey-Bass.

Graber, J.A., Brooks-Gunn, J., Paikoff, R.L., & Warren, M.P. (1994). Prediction of eating problems: an eight year study of adolescent girls. *Developmental Psychology*, **30**, 823–834.

Graber, J.A., Lewinsohn, P.M., Seeley, J.R., & Brooks-Gunn, J. (1997). Is psychopathology associated with the timing of pubertal development? *Journal of the American Academy of Child and Adolescent Psychiatry*, **36**, 1768–1776.

Graber, J.A., Seeley, J.R., Brooks-Gunn, J., & Lewinsohn, P.M. (2004). Is pubertal timing associated with psychopathology in young adulthood? *Journal of the American Academy of Child and Adolescent Psychiatry*, **43**, 718–726.

Graber, J.A., Brooks-Gunn, J., & Warren, M.P. (2006). Pubertal effects on adjustment in girls: moving from demonstrating effects to identifying pathways. *Journal of Youth and Adolescence*, **35**, 413–423.

Hayward, C., Killen, J.D., Wilson, D.M. *et al.* (1997). Psychiatric risk associated with early puberty in adolescent girls. *Journal of the American Academy of Child and Adolescent Psychiatry*, **36**, 255–262.

Kessler, R.C., Avenevoli, S., & Merikangas, K.R. (2001). Mood disorders in children and adolescents: an epidemiologic perspective. *Biological Psychiatry*, **49**, 1002–1014.

Krueger, R.F., Caspi, A., Moffitt, T.E., & Silva, P.A. (1998). The structure and stability of common mental disorders (DSM-III-R): a longitudinal-epidemiological study. *Journal of Abnormal Psychology*, **107**, 216–227.

Lai, J., Vesprini, D., Chu, W., Jernström, H., & Narod, S.A. (2001). CYP gene polymorphisms and early menarche. *Molecular Genetics and Metabolism*, **74**, 449–457.

Lynne, S.D., Graber, J.A., Nichols, T.R., Brooks-Gunn, J., & Botvin, G.J. (in press). Links between pubertal timing, peer influences, and externalizing behaviors among urban students followed through middle school. *Journal of Adolescent Health*.

McEwen, B.S. (1994). How do sex and stress hormones affect nerve cells? *Annals of the New York Academy of Sciences*, **743**, 1–18.

McEwen, B.S. (2000). The neurobiology of stress: from serendipity to clinical relevance. *Brain Research*, **886**, 172–189.

Meyer, S.E., Chrousos, G.P., & Gold, P.W. (2001). Major depression and the stress system: a life span perspective. *Development and Psychopathology*, **13**, 565–580.

Moffitt, T.E., Caspi, A., & Rutter, M. (2006). Measured gene-environmental interactions in psychopathology: concepts, research strategies, and implications for research, intervention, and public understanding of genetics. *Perspectives on Psychological Science*, **1**, 5–27.

Paterson, W.F., McNeill, E., Reid, S., Hollman, A.S., & Donaldson, M.D.C. (1998). Efficacy of Zoladex LA (goserelin) in the treatment of girls with central precocious or early puberty. *Archives of Disease in Childhood*, **79**, 323–327.

Rohde, P., Lewinsohn, P.M., & Seeley, J.R. (1991). The comorbidity of unipolar depression: II. Comorbidity with other mental disorders in adolescents and adults. *Journal of Abnormal Psychology*, **100**, 214–222.

Rudolf, K.D. (2002). Gender differences in emotional responses to interpersonal stress during adolescence. *Journal of Adolescent Health*, **30** (Suppl.), 3–13.

Ryan, N.D., & Dahl, R.E. (1993). The biology of depression in children and adolescents. In J.J. Mann & D.J. Kupfer (Eds.), *The Biology of Depressive Disorders, Part B: Subtypes of Depression and Comorbid Disorders* (pp. 37–58). New York: Plenum Press.

Silberg, J., Pickles, A., Rutter, M. *et al.* (1999). The influence of genetic factors and life stress on depression among adolescent girls. *Archives of General Psychiatry*, **56**, 225–232.

Steinberg, L. (2001). We know some things: parent-adolescent relationships in retrospect and prospect. *Journal of Research on Adolescence*, **11**, 1–19.

Stice, E., Presnell, K., & Bearman, S.K. (2001). Relation of early menarche to depression, eating disorders, substance abuse, and comorbid psychopathology among adolescent girls. *Developmental Psychology*, **37**, 608–619.

Suomi, S.J. (1999). Attachment in Rhesus monkeys. In J. Cassidy & P.R. Shaver (Eds.), *Handbook of Attachment: Theory, Research, and Clinical Applications* (pp. 181–197). New York: Guilford Press.

Susman, E.J., & Rogol, A. (2004). Puberty and psychological development. In R.M. Lerner & L. Steinberg (Eds.), *Handbook of Adolescent Psychology* (2nd edn, pp. 15–44). Hoboken, NJ: John Wiley & Sons.

Taylor, S.E., Klein, L.C., Lewis, B.P. *et al.* (2000). Biobehavioral responses to stress in females: tend-and-befriend, not fight-or-flight. *Psychological Review*, **107**, 411–429.

Trickett, P.K., & Putnam, F.W. (1993). Impact of child sexual abuse on females: toward a developmental, psychobiological integration. *Psychological Science*, **4**, 81–87.

Walker, E.F., Walder, D.J., & Reynolds, F. (2001). Developmental changes in cortisol secretion in normal and at-risk youth. *Development and Psychopathology*, **13**, 721–732.

Wolf, O.T., & Kirschbaum, C. (1999). Actions of dehydroepiandrosterone and its sulfate in the central nervous system: effects on cognition and emotion in animals and humans. *Brain Research Reviews*, **30**, 264–288.

Zabin, L.S., Emerson, M.R., & Rowland, D.L. (2005). Childhood sexual abuse and early menarche: the direction of their relationship and its implications. *Journal of Adolescent Health*, **36**, 393–400.

6

Mapping brain maturation and sexual dimorphism in adolescence

Tomáš Paus

Introduction

Adolescence represents a major transition that takes place over most of the second decade of human life. In the shift from a caregiver-dependent child to a fully autonomous adult, adolescents undergo multiple changes in their physical growth and physiology, as well as in their cognitive and emotional skills. The timing of some of these changes, such as the onset of sexual maturation, can be readily determined. On the other hand, defining the moment of becoming an adult member of the society, especially in the legal sense, varies widely (Poythress *et al.*, 2006). Recognizing that "gonadal maturation" and "behavioral maturation" are two distinct, albeit interacting, processes with separate timing is essential (Sisk & Foster, 2004).

It can be argued that, during adolescence, "behavioral maturation" is attained by acquiring a well-balanced interface between emotion, reasoning and decision-making, and action. How does brain maturation during this period of human development influence the attainment of such an interface? Furthermore, given the presence of sex differences in cognitive abilities (Kimura, 1999) and affect-related processes (Herba & Phillips, 2004), as well as in the incidence of depression and other psychopathology (Angold *et al.*, 1998, 1999; see Seeley and Lewinsohn, Chapter 3), do girls and boys show different trajectories in their brain maturation? Finally, are the age and sex differences in brain structure a product of nature or nurture?

In order to answer some of the above questions and to provide a conceptual framework for designing and interpreting new studies of brain–behavior relationships during adolescence, this chapter focuses on the current trends in the use of magnetic resonance imaging (MRI) in quantifying subtle

Adolescent Emotional Development and the Emergence of Depressive Disorders, ed. Nicholas B. Allen and Lisa B. Sheeber. Published by Cambridge University Press. © Cambridge University Press 2009.

differences in brain structure, and for measuring brain activity during task performance using functional MRI (fMRI). The chapter begins with a brief overview of the techniques used for the analysis of structural MR images aimed at deriving brain features such as regional volumes of gray and white matter, cortical thickness, and structural properties of white-matter fiber tracts.

To aid the reader's understanding of fMRI studies, I also discuss current views regarding the physiological basis of the fMRI signal. The chapter continues with an overview of the maturation of various morphological features and functional processes during childhood and adolescence, and with the review of the known sex differences in the structure of the adolescent and adult brain. The chapter finishes with a discussion of the role of genes and experience in shaping the human brain; it will highlight the possibility that some of the differences in brain structure may be the consequence of experience associated with, for example, depressive behavior.

Principles of structural MRI: analysis

Over the past decade, a large number of computational tools have been developed that allow us to extract various brain features from MR images, such as the volume of various gray-matter (GM) structure, regional tissue "density," or cortical thickness (for details, see legend to Figure 6.1). When interpreting morphometric findings, it is important to bear in mind that changes extracted by computational analysis of structural MR images reflect the uneven and largely unknown contribution of the different cellular components constituting a given sample of brain tissue (Figure 6.2b).

Principles of functional MRI: what do we measure?

The most common parameter measured with fMRI in studies of brain–behavior relationships is the blood oxygenation-level dependent (BOLD) signal. As its name suggests, BOLD signal is based on our ability to detect, with MRI, changes in blood concentration of deoxyhemoglobin. Upon neural activation, the disproportionate increase in regional cerebral blood flow (CBF) "dilutes" the amount of deoxyhemoglobin in the small veins leaving the "activated" region ("red veins" phenomenon). This leads to a positive signal on images that we use, in turn, to infer regional changes in brain activity. Although there is no dispute about the existence of a relationship between local hemodynamics and brain activity, there is still little agreement about the role of various neural events in driving the hemodynamic signal. It is likely that changes in local hemodynamics reflect a sum of excitatory

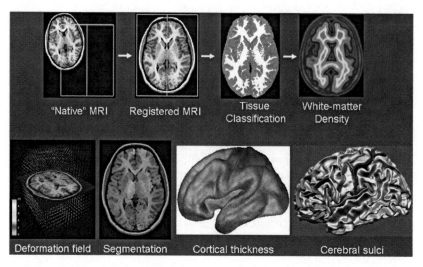

Figure 6.1. This figure is also reproduced in color between pages 144 and 145. A typical image-processing "pipeline" begins with a *linear transformation* of a T1W image from the acquisition ("native") space to standardized stereotaxic space, namely that of the average MNI-305 atlas (Collins *et al.*, 1994; Evans *et al.*, 1993), aligned with Talairach & Tournoux (1988) space, note that there is a negligible difference in the overall brain size between adolescent brains and those of young adults (23.4±4.1 years) who constitute the MNI-305 atlas. The next step involves *brain-tissue classification* into gray matter (GM), white matter (WM), and cerebrospinal fluid (CSF); an automatic classification is achieved by combining information from different types of MR images, namely T1W, T2W, and PDW acquisitions (Zijdenbos *et al.*, 2002; Cocosco *et al.*, 2003). The tissue-classification step yields three sets of binary 3-D images (i.e. GM, WM, and CSF). Each of the binary images can be smoothed to generate *probabilistic "density" images*. These maps are used in voxel-wise analyses of age- or group-related differences in GM or WM density (see Ashburner & Friston, 2000 for methodological overview). Another important processing step is a non-linear registration of the subject's image to a template brain; local differences between the subject and the template are captured in a *deformation field*. The template brain contains information about anatomical boundaries; this anatomical information can be "projected" onto each subject's brain using the corresponding deformation field and fine-tuned by combining it with the tissue-classification map (Collins *et al.*, 1994, 1995). In this way, the pipeline provides automatic estimates of *regional volumes of GM and WM*, such as those constituting the major lobes. Another voxel-wise approach has been developed to quantify individual differences in the 3-D anatomy of the cerebral cortex. These include estimates of the *cortical thickness* (Fischl & Dale, 2000; Han *et al.*, 2006; Lerch & Evans, 2005) and the quantification of individual differences in the position, depth and length of the *cerebral sulci* (Mangin *et al.*, 2004). Voxel-wise analysis can also be employed when analyzing diffusion tensor-imaging datasets (Smith *et al.*, 2006). Figure reprinted with permission from Paus, 2005.

(a)

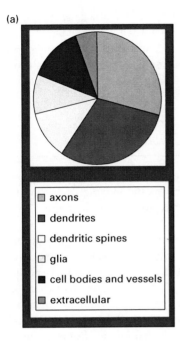

(b)

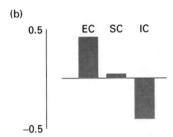

Factor 1: EC > SC > IC
 • Dendrite/Neuron
 • Mitochondria/Neuron
 • Axon/Neuron
 • Dendrite volume
 • Neuronal density
 • Density of Neurons/Glia
 • Capillary volume/Neuron
 • Mitochondrial volume

Figure 6.2. (a) Proportion of various cellular elements that make up 1 mm³ of the cerebral cortex in mice (data from Braitenberg, 2001). Please see color plate section. (b) Cellular elements affected by rearing environment: EC, enriched complex environment; SC, socially complex environment; IC, individually caged animals (data from Sirevaag & Greenough, 1988).

postsynaptic inputs in the sample of scanned tissue (Logothetis *et al.*, 2001). The firing rate of "output" neurons may be related to local blood flow (Heeger *et al.*, 2000; Rees *et al.*, 2000) but only inasmuch as it is linked in linear fashion to excitatory postsynaptic input. Inhibitory neurotransmission may lead to decreases in CBF indirectly, through its presynaptic effects on postsynaptic excitation (Mathiessen *et al.*, 1998).

Brain maturation

Over the past decade, a number of investigators have used structural MRI and described age-related changes in white and gray matter in typically developing children and adolescents. We have recently reviewed this literature (Paus, 2005) and noted the following findings.

The overall volume of *white matter* (WM) increases in a linear way during childhood and adolescence, with several interesting regional variations. These include age-related increases in WM density in the internal capsule and the putative arcuate fasciculus (Paus *et al.*, 1999), regional variations in the growth of the corpus callosum where the splenium continues to increase, whereas the genu does not (Giedd *et al.*, 1996a, 1999b; Pujol *et al.*, 1993), and an age-related increase in the WM volume of the left inferior frontal gyrus in boys but not girls (Blanton *et al.*, 2004). More recently, diffusion tensor imaging (DTI) has been employed to assess age-related changes in magnitude (apparent diffusion coefficient, ADC) and directionality (fractional aniso-tropy, FA) of the diffusion of water in the human brain during childhood and adolescence. Overall, DTI-based studies reveal age-related decreases in ADC and increases in FA in a number of WM regions, many of which are identical to those revealed by the above MRI studies (Klingberg *et al.*, 1999; Schmithorst *et al.*, 2002; Snook *et al.*, 2005); changes in FA are interpreted as reflecting an increase in density of fibers and/or increase in myelination.

The monotonic nature of the developmental changes in brain maturation observed for WM does not appear to hold in the case of *gray matter* (GM). Gray matter volume in the frontal and parietal lobes appears to peak at between 10 and 12 years, and decreases slightly afterwards; in the temporal lobes the peak occurs around the age of 16 years (Giedd *et al.*, 1999b). Other investigators found similar age-related GM "loss" in the frontal, parietal, and temporal lobes; it appears to start around puberty in the sensori-motor areas and spreads rostrally over the frontal cortex and caudally over the parietal and then temporal cortex (Gogtay *et al.*, 2004; Sowell *et al.*, 2001). The dorsolat-eral prefrontal cortex and the posterior part of the superior temporal gyrus appear to "lose" GM last of all (Gogtay *et al.*, 2004). More recently, similar age-related "loss" of the cortical gray-matter has been observed using cortical thickness as the parameter of interest (Shaw *et al.*, 2006). But as I (Paus, 2005) and others (Sowell *et al.*, 2001) have argued, such an apparent loss of cortical GM may be a partial-volume artifact: increased intra-cortical myelination could "dilute" the GM signal and result in an apparent decrease in GM volume.

Knowledge of the functional organization of the human brain, gleaned from previous lesion and functional imaging work, provides a foundation for the initial functional interpretations of the above structural observations. For example, changes in WM volume along the arcuate fasciculus and in the left inferior frontal gyrus are likely to correlate with language, while the late maturational changes in GM of the prefrontal cortex and the superior temporal gyrus/sulcus may be related, respectively, to executive functions and processing of biological motion (see below). The latter may be important for non-verbal interactions between peers. Only a handful of studies have acquired structural (MRI) and functional (e.g. neuropsychological assessment) datasets in the same group of individuals. In these studies, significant correlations were found between IQ and GM volume of the prefrontal cortex (Reiss *et al.*, 1996), IQ and FA in the white matter of the frontal lobes (Schmithorst *et al.*, 2005), IQ and cortical thickness (Shaw *et al.*, 2006), and between reading skills and FA in the left temporo-parietal WM (Beaulieu *et al.*, 2005; Deutsch *et al.*, 2005).

Functional MRI (fMRI) provides yet another avenue for exploring brain–behavior relationships in the maturing human brain. Before discussing some of the findings obtained with this technique, we should point out a few challenges facing investigators using fMRI in children and adolescents (see also Davidson *et al.*, 2003). Head motion during acquisition of fMRI datasets compromises the quality of data; in our experience, for example, up to 25% of scans must be excluded from further analyses for this reason (e.g. in 10-year-old healthy volunteers). Arguably, this number can be reduced with the use of a mock scanner (Rosenberg *et al.*, 1997). Putting aside such technical issues and the complexity of interpreting the BOLD signal (see above), the most difficult conceptual problem is the confounding interaction between age and performance. In other words, when studying age-related changes in brain activity during the performance of a given task, how do we interpret fMRI findings on the background of concomitant age-related differences in the task performance? Note that for many of the "executive" abilities (see Kesek, Zelazo and Lewis, Chapter 8), 10-year-old children appear to differ significantly from their younger peers but less so from the older ones (Figure 6.3). Is the brain activity different because the behavior (performance) is different, or vice versa?

One of the approaches used to overcome this issue is matching subjects either by age or by performance, and examining the differences in fMRI response in these matched groups. This approach has been used extensively in studies of *verb generation* (Brown *et al.*, 2004; Schlaggar *et al.*, 2002). In the executive

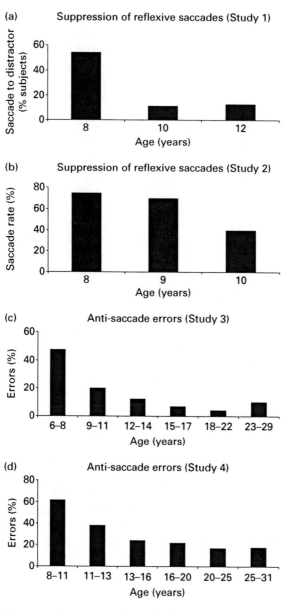

Figure 6.3. Performance of typically developing children, adolescents and adults in a number of cognitive tasks requiring behavioral inhibition and/or resistance to interference. Reprinted with permission from Paus, 2005.

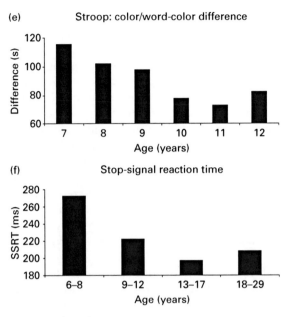

(e) Stroop: color/word-color difference

(f) Stop-signal reaction time

Figure 6.3. (*cont.*)

domain, Kwon *et al.* (2002) used this approach in a study of *visuo-spatial working memory* and found age-related (age 7 to 22 years) increases in the BOLD signal in the prefrontal and parietal cortex even after factoring out inter-individual differences in performance. Similar BOLD increases were also observed in these regions during the performance of a variety of tasks involving some form of response inhibition, including the *Stroop task* (Adleman *et al.*, 2002), *anti-saccade task* (Luna *et al.*, 2001), the *stop task* (Rubia *et al.*, 2000), and, to a certain extent, during the performance of a *Go/No-Go task* (Tamm *et al.*, 2002) and the Eriksen flanker task (Bunge, 2002).

During adolescence, high demands are placed not only on the executive systems but also on the interplay between cognitive and affect-related processes. Such cognition-emotion interactions are particularly crucial in the context of peer-peer interactions and the processing of verbal and non-verbal cues. It is therefore of interest to note that the cortex of the superior temporal sulcus (STS) contains a set of regions engaged during the processing of non-verbal cues such as those carried by eye and mouth movements (Puce *et al.*, 1998), hand movements/actions (Beauchamp *et al.*, 2002; Decety *et al.*, 1997; Grezes *et al.*, 1999), or body movements (Bonda *et al.*, 1996). As suggested by Allison *et al.* (2000), feedforward and feedback interactions between the STS and amygdala may be critical for the discrimination of various facial expressions and for the attentional enhancement of the neural response to socially salient stimuli.

Consistent with such an "amplification" mechanism, Kilts and colleagues (2003) observed significantly stronger neural response to dynamic, as compared with static, facial expressions of anger in both the STS and amygdala. We have also observed a strong BOLD response in amygdala, not only while adult subjects viewed video clips of angry hand movements or angry faces, but also during viewing of (dynamic) neutral facial expressions (Grosbras & Paus, 2006). Although the basic aspects of face perception are in place shortly after birth (Goren *et al.*, 1975), both the quantity and quality of face processing continues to increase all the way through adolescence (Carey *et al.*, 1992; McGivern *et al.*, 2002; Taylor *et al.*, 1999). Developmental fMRI studies of the processing of facial expressions are consistent with this pattern. For example, *happy, but not sad, faces* elicit significant BOLD response in the amygdala in adolescent subjects (Yang *et al.*, 2003). Studies of *fearful facial expressions* suggest that an increase in the BOLD signal in amygdala can be detected in adolescents (Baird *et al.*, 1999), but it is relatively weak (Thomas *et al.*, 2001).

In summary, significant changes in brain structure and function take place during childhood and adolescence. These changes occur both in white matter and cortical gray matter. It seems that structures showing the most robust age-related changes overlap with regions involved in language, executive functions and non-verbal communication. The presence of maturational changes in white matter underscores the importance of inter-regional communication in cognitive development, and suggests that neural connectivity might mediate the attainment of a well-balanced interface between emotion, reasoning and decision-making, and action during adolescence.

Sex differences

This section will review the current literature with regard to whether girls and boys show different trajectories in their brain maturation. We shall start by describing sex differences in the adult brain and, with this background, we will then evaluate the current knowledge of the presence or absence of such differences at different stages of brain development and maturation. Right from the outset, it should be pointed out that – in most instances – the relative contributions of genetic (nature) and environmental (nurture) factors in gender differences are unclear. To what extent "function" can shape the "structure" is the topic of the last section.

In biology, sexual dimorphism typically refers to apparent sex differences in external features such as the body size, color of the feathers, or presence of horns. In humans, there are few qualitative differences between men and women other than the genitalia and secondary sexual characteristics. Most of the sex differences are quantitative and show a considerable overlap between men and women (e.g. height and weight). In a broad sense, the latter is also true about sex differences in the structure of the human brain.

Overall, the male brain is larger (by ~10%) than the female brain; it contains larger absolute volume of both gray and white matter (Carne *et al.*, 2006; Good *et al.*, 2001; Gur *et al.*, 2002; Luders *et al.*, 2002). This difference remains after co-varying body height or weight (Ankney, 1992; Jerison, 1987; Peters *et al.*, 1998; Skullerud, 1985). When expressed as a percentage of total brain (or cranial) volume, sex differences in the volume of white matter disappear (Gur *et al.*, 2002; Luders *et al.*, 2002), while those in gray matter remain (Good *et al.*, 2001), disappear (Gur *et al.*, 2002) or even reverse (i.e. female > male; Luders *et al.*, 2002).

Moving beyond global volumes of gray and white matter, only a handful of regions are *relatively* (i.e. after removing the effect of brain size) larger in the male vs. the female brain, including the amygdala and the hippocampus (Good *et al.*, 2001; Gur *et al.*, 2002), and the paracingulate sulcus (Paus *et al.*, 1996a, 1996b; Yucel *et al.*, 2001). There are many more brain structures that are *relatively* larger in the female vs. the male brain, including the lateral orbitofrontal cortex (Good *et al.*, 2001; Gur *et al.*, 2002), anterior (Paus *et al.*, 1996a; Good *et al.*, 2001) and posterior (Good *et al.*, 2001) cingulate cortex, and the inferior frontal gyrus (Good *et al.*, 2001). Compared with the male brain, the female brain also appears to contain more white matter constituting the corpus callosum (Bermudez & Zatorre, 2001; Steinmetz *et al.*, 1992; Cowell *et al.*, 1992), internal and external capsule and optic radiation (Good *et al.*, 2001), and shows greater extent of inter-hemispheric connections between the posterior temporal regions (Hagmann *et al.*, 2006).

Finally, there are striking sex differences in the extent of hemispheric asymmetries in brain structure. Overall, it seems that the male brains are more asymmetric than female brains (Kovalev *et al.*, 2003). This is especially true for left-larger-than-right (L > R) structural asymmetries of language-related structures, such as the planum temporale (Good *et al.*, 2001; Kulynych *et al.*, 1994; Sequeira Sdos *et al.*, 2006) and planum parietale (Jancke *et al.*, 1994). It is of interest to note that left-handed, but not right-handed, females show the same L > R hemispheric asymmetry for both the planum temporale (Sequeira Sdos *et al.*, 2006) and parietale (Jancke *et al.*, 1994). The presence of larger language-related structures in the left vs. right hemispheres in the male brain appears to include hemispheric asymmetries in major fiber tracts. Two recent reports observed strong L > R asymmetry in males, but not in females, in the structural organization of the arcuate fasciculus, as derived from DTI-based tractography (Hagmann *et al.*, 2006; Catani, pers. comm.). This fiber tract most likely contains axons connecting the posterior and anterior speech regions; it continues to mature throughout childhood and adolescence (Paus *et al.*, 1999). Finally, the male brain also shows a clear L > R asymmetry vis-à-vis the depth of the central sulcus in a region of cortical hand representation; this asymmetry was present in right-handed males, it reversed (R>L) to some extent in left-handed males, and was absent in all females (Amunts et al., 2000). One exception from the above preponderance of hemispheric asymmetries in the male brains is the R>L asymmetry in the size of the anterior cingulate gyrus that is present in females but not in males (Pujol et al., 2002). It is also of note that the size of the anterior cingulate gyrus correlates with harm avoidance and that sex differences in this personality trait are substantially reduced when the area of the anterior cingulate gyrus is used as a covariate (Pujol et al., 2002).

When do the above gender differences emerge? Answering this question would further our understanding of the mechanisms underlying sexual dimorphism in the human brain and may help us in distinguishing between genetic and environmental influences. Sex differences in the overall brain size appear to be present even before birth. Using head circumference as a proxy of brain size, male infants showed slightly higher (2%) values than female infants with comparable femur length both prenatally and during the first year of life (Joffe et al., 2005). Using autopsy material, sex differences in brain weight are seen as early as in infancy (Dekaban, 1978). On the other hand, Matsuzawa and colleagues (2001) found no sex differences in MRI-derived measures of the total brain volume; but as noted by the authors, their study was underpowered and hampered by the fact that girls were slightly older than boys. Regarding regional sex differences after birth, an ultrasound-based study examined the total area and subdivisions of the corpus callosum in neonates (Hwang et al., 2004) and observed sex differences (Female>Male) in the thickness of the splenium. Overall, the brain weight is about 90% of the adult brain by about the age of 5 years (Dekaban, 1978) and it reaches the adult size by about the age of 10 years (Dekaban, 1978; Pfefferbaum et al., 1994). The rather sparse amount of in vivo data available regarding the brain growth during the first 5 years of life does not allow us, however, to make any conclusions regarding sex differences in the rate of the growth during this period.

Much richer literature exists on sex differences during childhood and adolescence. On a global level, it appears that males compared with females show larger age-related increases in the total volume of white matter (De Bellis et al., 2001; Giedd et al., 1999a). This sexual dimorphism is particularly striking during adolescence, as was recently observed in one of our studies (Perrin et al., 2006; Figure 6.4). Are such sex differences in age-related global increases in white matter seen also regionally? This question has been asked in several morphometric studies of the corpus callosum. Two studies reported no sex differences in the rate of age-related increases in the area of the corpus callosum (Giedd et al., 1999a; Rauch & Jinkins, 1994). Two other studies found sex differences in the rate of growth over a 2-year period during late adolescence and early adulthood (M>F; Pujol et al., 1993), and in the time when the maximum width of certain parts of the corpus callosum is

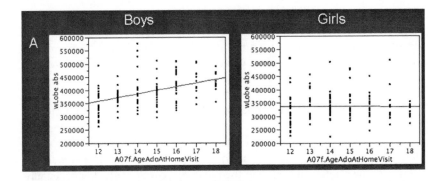

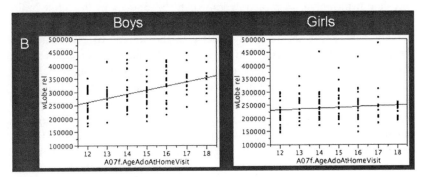

Figure 6.4. Age-related changes in the volume of white matter in the cerebral lobes during adolescence. Note that the significant age-related increases in both absolute (A) and relative (B) volumes are present in boys ($n=131$) but absent in girls ($n=143$). Relative volumes were calculated by dividing the absolute volumes by a brain-size index.

attained during adulthood (Cowell *et al.*, 1992). It thus seems that, in the case of the corpus callosum, maturation of white matter continues through early and middle adulthood, with sex differences emerging during these later periods of maturation.

Changes in gray matter also seem to follow different timetables in girls and boys. Between the ages of 5–21 years, the volume of gray matter in all but the occipital lobe increases with age and then declines. The peak of these changes occurs, however, at different ages in different lobes and, for a given lobe, at different ages in boys and girls (Frontal female: 11.0 yr, Frontal male: 12.1 yr; Parietal female: 10.2 yr, Parietal male: 11.8 yr; Temporal female: 16.7 yr, Temporal male: 16.5 yr; Giedd *et al.*, 1999a). This timetable suggests that girls are ahead of boys during the early (10–12 yr) stages of the cortical maturation during adolescence and that this sex difference evens out at the later (~16 yr) stage. Obviously, one needs to keep in mind that this statement only applies to those biological processes that could be captured by the rather gross MRI-based estimates of gray-matter volume available at the time of this particular study. As described above, adult females and males differ in the size of several gray-matter structures, including amygdala and hippocampus (M > F), and the different regions of the frontal cortex (F > M). The available data suggest that the amygdala volume does increase more with age in males, as compared with females (Giedd *et al.*, 1996c).

This is also the case for the hippocampus (Suzuki *et al.*, 2005); but note that the opposite trend was reported in another study, namely age-related increase in the hippocampal volume found in females but not males (Giedd *et al.*, 1996c). Boys but not girls also seem to show age-related increase in the volume of the caudate nucleus and the putamen (Giedd *et al.*, 1996b). Finally, very few hemispheric asymmetries known to be present in the adult brain (see above) have been examined in the maturing brain. It appears that males but not females present L > R asymmetry in the volume of gray matter in the inferior frontal gyrus (Blanton *et al.*, 2004). Unlike the adult brain, L > R hemispheric asymmetry in the planum temporale and planum parietale appears to be more developed in females than in males, with no changes with age (Preis *et al.*, 1999). Given the overwhelming evidence of larger hemispheric asymmetries in these regions in adult males (see above), this observation is puzzling, especially in light of the reports of the presence of the L > R planum temporale in newborns and infants (Witelson & Pallie, 1973; Wada *et al.*, 1975).

Overall, the female and male brains differ in several respects. Most of the differences are quantitative in nature and rather subtle. These include, for example, differences in the brain size, volume of the white matter, and the size of brain regions such as the amygdala and hippocampus (M > F), or the orbitofrontal and anterior cingulate cortices, and the corpus callosum (F > M). The most striking and, perhaps, qualitative differences between male and female brains lie in the degree of hemispheric asymmetries involving, but not limited to, language-related areas. The available data suggest that some of the above sex differences continue to develop during childhood and adolescence. Most notably, this is the case for age-related increase in global and local (i.e. corpus callosum, inferior frontal gyrus) white matter, as well as the size of some brain regions, such as the amygdala and the hippocampus. It is also clear that the timing of cellular processes influencing the overall cortical volume in the different lobes varies not only as a function of location (e.g. frontal vs. temporal lobes) but also as a function of sex.

Effects of genes and experience on brain structure

If we are to understand neural mechanisms underlying affect, its expression and regulation in a typically developing adolescent, as well as changes occurring during depression, we need to ask: to what extent is the brain shaped by the

(a)   (b)

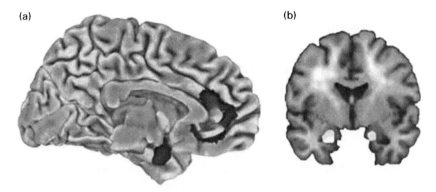

Figure 6.5. This figure is also reproduced in color between pages 144 and 145. Effect of genotype (5-HTTLPR) on the amount of gray matter in the anterior cingulate cortex (a) and amygdala (b) in healthy adult volunteers. Reprinted with permission from Pezawas *et al.* (2004).

genes or by the individual's environment and experiences? This final section provides background information relevant to interpretation of previous and future studies of affect and depression along the gene–environment continuum.

Let us begin with an example of two recent studies. In one study, genetic variation in the promotor region of the serotonin transporter gene (5-HTTLPR) was associated with variations in brain morphology, namely in the amount of gray matter in the anterior cingulate cortex and amygdala, in healthy adult volunteers (Pezawas *et al.*, 2004; Figure 6.5). The two structures also showed significant inter-regional correlations both in their morphology (i.e. gray-matter density) and in the degree of their "activation" during the perceptual processing of fearful and threatening facial expressions (Pezawas *et al.*, 2004). The latter (functional connectivity) relationship predicted 30% of variance in harm avoidance (Pujol *et al.*, 2002). This set of findings could be interpreted as suggesting that this particular genetic variation "causes" changes in brain structure and function, potentially increasing the probability of individuals with the "disadvantageous" genotype (short 5-HTTLPR allele in this case) to develop depressive illness. But could it be the other way around? The second study explored the effect of adverse environment, namely the number of stressful life events, on the number of episodes of major depression; the 5-HTTLPR genotype was also taken into account (Caspi *et al.*, 2003; Figure 6.6). The genotype (i.e. having a short allele of the 5-HTTLPR gene) played no role unless the individual experienced at least three stressful events in over the past 5 years, a clear example of gene–environment interaction.

Putting together the above two studies, two possibilities exist: (1) structural and functional differences between individuals with the two different 5-HTTLPR genotypes will be present irrespective of the number of stressful life events; or (2) such differences will only be present when comparing

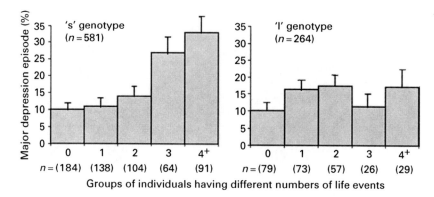

Figure 6.6. Effect of a genotype (5-HTTLPR) by environment (number of adverse life events) interaction on the incidence of major depression episodes. Reprinted with permission from Caspi *et al.* (2003).

individuals who experienced a high number of stressful events. At this point, we do not know the answer to this question. In the following paragraphs, we will put forward evidence from other domains supporting the notion of experience influencing brain structure.

Conceptually, we often think of structure as leading to function. We tend to assume that some biological process, be it a gene or a hormone, initiates structural changes that, in turn, lead to (improved) function. This last section reviews evidence in favor of the opposite view, namely that a repeated (functional) engagement of a particular neural circuit leads to changes in its structural properties, which can be detected *in vivo* with MRI. Of course, determining directionality of such structure-function relationships is impossible in the majority of current studies. By reviewing evidence consistent with the notion of cumulative experience leading to changes in brain structure, we wish to stimulate a view that considers the role of experience when interpreting structural findings present in the literature on typically developing adolescents and adolescents suffering from a depressive illness.

Magnetic resonance imaging studies of musicians' brains were the first to describe a quantitative relationship between brain structure and function in healthy individuals. Although the directionality of the relationship cannot be inferred from such studies, it is quite likely that extensive practice plays a significant role in shaping musicians' auditory cortex, specifically Heschl's gyrus (Gaser & Schlaug, 2003; Schneider *et al.*, 2002), planum temporale (Aydin *et al.*, 2005; Schlaug *et al.*, 1995), motor cortex (Amunts *et al.*, 1997; Gaser & Schlaug, 2003), cerebellum [Hutchinson *et al.*, 2003], Broca's area (Sluming *et al.*, 2002), and the corpus callosum (Ozturk *et al.*, 2002; Schlaug *et al.*, 1995). Several factors have been noted to influence such structure-function relationships, including the onset of musical training, its duration, and musician's gender.

Linguistic experience represents another example of long-term engagement of specific neural circuits. Higher GM density was found in the left inferior parietal cortex in bilingual, compared with monolingual, subjects; this effect correlated positively with proficiency and negatively with the age of acquisition (Mechelli *et al.*, 2004). In yet another example, duration (in years) of navigation experience (i.e. driving a taxi in London) correlates with the volume of the posterior hippocampus (Maguire *et al.*, 2000); no relationship is observed between the hippocampal volume and "innate" navigational expertise (Maguire *et al.*, 2003).

But, perhaps, musical training, bilingualism, and years of taxi driving represent extreme cases of a repeated engagement of neural circuits involved in the given behaviors, often starting in childhood. Is it possible to detect changes in brain structure induced by a much shorter exposure to a particular experience and taking place in adulthood? It appears that three months of juggling practice is sufficient to increase GM density in the putative V5 in young (22 yr) healthy volunteers (Draganski *et al.*, 2004). This strongly suggests that MR is sensitive enough to detect, *in vivo*, cumulative effects of short-lasting experience on brain structure. What underlies such changes? Here we need to turn to research in experimental animals.

In his book *The Organization of Behavior*, Donald Hebb (1949) proposed that when one cell excites another repeatedly, a change takes place in one or both cells; we now know that multiple manifestations of such activity-induced (homosynaptic) plasticity can be observed at both functional and structural levels. Hebb was also the first to suggest that "enriched environment" affects behavior of experimental animals; rats that he brought home as pets showed higher problem-solving abilities when tested later (Hebb, 1947). Over the last 40 years, a number of studies showed that rats housed in an enriched environment, which provides "a combination of complex inanimate and social stimulation" (Rosenzweig *et al.*, 1978), differ from their "standard housing" counterparts in brain weight, cortical thickness, extent of dendritic branching, spine density, angiogenesis, gliogenesis, and neurogenesis (Kolb *et al.*, 1998; Lewis, 2004; van Praag *et al.*, 2000). Not surprisingly, many of these structural changes co-occur in the same animal. Sirevaag & Greenough (1988) used multivariate statistics to explore the relationship among 36 measures of synaptic, cellular and vascular morphological features of the occipital cortex in three groups of rats reared, respectively, in complex, social, and individual housing environments (for 30 days). They found a coordinated change in the "synaptic" and "metabolic" domains of the (occipital) cortex; rats housed in the complex (vs. individual) environment had more synapses per neuron, a lower neuronal density, a larger capillary and mitochondrial volume fraction, and more glial cells (Figure 6.2, right).

It is thus clear that increases in *synaptic* efficacy are accompanied by a "build-up" of the *metabolic* machinery. Are such effects generalized or do specific experiences influence specific brain regions relevant for a given function? It seems that the latter is the case. For example, dendritic changes were found in the visual cortex contralateral to the un-occluded (vs. occluded) eye in rats trained in a visual maze (Chang & Greenough, 1982), and in the motor cortex contralateral to the forelimb trained to retrieve food from tubes (Greenough et al., 1985; Kolb et al., 1998). A possible relationship between dendritic arborization and experience has also been demonstrated in the human cerebral cortex. Here, the approach has been necessarily indirect and one can certainly challenge the interpretation of the findings, namely those of higher dendritic arborization in Wernicke's area in individuals with a higher amount of education (Jacobs et al., 1993), and that of more complex dendritic trees in the putative finger area of the somatosensory cortex in individuals who used fingers in their professions, such as typists (Scheibel et al., 1990).

Overall, repeated engagement of a given neural circuit by relevant stimulation/experience leads to changes in multiple cellular compartments of the rat brain. In human subjects, the size of the structural effect appears large enough to be detected with MRI. It is therefore possible that some of the maturational changes in brain structure observed during adolescence, sex differences emerging later in life, or structural correlates of psychopathological states such as depression, may represent consequences of differential experience. It is of course possible that such structural changes may in turn lead to an "entrenchment" of the relevant functional processes.

Summary

The adolescent brain is work in progress. Over the past 10 years, a number of MRI studies revealed subtle quantitative changes in brain structure taking place during this period of human development. The most robust effects of age appear to involve white matter, both globally and locally, as well as the cortical gray-matter in fronto-parietal and temporal regions. The exact timing and, in some cases, the extent of growth differ in boys and girls. The exact nature of such age- and sex-related changes in shaping the structure of the human brain during adolescence is unknown. It is likely, however, that the individual's experience/environment exerts a powerful influence on brain structure, not only during the early development but also later in life.

REFERENCES

Adleman, N.E., Menon, V., Blasey, C.M. et al. (2002). A developmental fMRI study of the Stroop color-word task. *Neuroimage*, **16**, 61–75.

Allison, T., Puce, A., & McCarthy, G. (2000). Social perception from visual cues: role of the STS region. *Trends in Cognitive Sciences*, **4**(7), 267–278.

Amunts, K., Schlaug, G., Jancke, L. *et al.* (1997). Motor cortex and hand motor skills: structural compliance in the human brain. *Human Brain Mapping*, **5**, 206–215.

Amunts, K., Jancke, L., Mohlberg, H., Steinmetz, H., & Zilles, K. (2000). Interhemispheric asymmetry of the human motor cortex related to handedness and gender. *Neuropsychologia*, **38**(3), 304–312.

Angold, A., Costello, E.J., & Worthman, C.M. (1998). Puberty and depression: the roles of age, pubertal status and pubertal timing. *Psychological Medicine*, **28**(1), 51–61.

Angold, A., Costello, E.J., Erkanli, A., & Worthman, C.M. (1999). Pubertal changes in hormone levels and depression in girls. *Psychological Medicine*, **29**(5), 1043–1053.

Ankney, C.D. (1992). Differences in brain size. *Nature*, **358**(6387), 532.

Ashburner, J., & Friston, K.J. (2000). Voxel-based morphometry – the methods. *NeuroImage*, **11**(6 Pt 1), 805–821.

Aydin, K., Ciftci, K., Terzibasioglu, E. *et al.* (2005). Quantitative proton MR spectroscopic findings of cortical reorganization in the auditory cortex of musicians. *American Journal of Neuroradiology*, **26**(1), 128–136.

Baird, A.A., Gruber, S.A., Fein, D.A. *et al.* (1999). Functional magnetic resonance imaging of facial affect recognition in children and adolescents. *Journal of the American Academy of Child and Adolescent Psychiatry*, **38**, 195–199.

Beauchamp, M.S., Lee, K.E., Haxby, J.V., & Martin, A. (2002). Parallel visual motion processing streams for manipulable objects and human movements. *Neuron*, **34**, 149–159.

Beaulieu, C., Plewes, C., Paulson, L.A. *et al.* (2005). Imaging brain connectivity in children with diverse reading ability. *Neuroimage*, **25**(4), 1266–1271.

Bermudez, P., & Zatorre, R.J. (2001). Sexual dimorphism in the corpus callosum: methodological considerations in MRI morphometry. *Neuroimage*, **13**(6 Pt 1), 1121–1130.

Blanton, R.E., Levitt, J.G., Peterson, J.R. *et al.* (2004). Gender differences in the left inferior frontal gyrus in normal children. *Neuroimage*, **22**, 626–636.

Bonda, E., Petrides, M., Ostry, D., & Evans, A. (1996). Specific involvement of human parietal systems and the amygdala in the perception of biological motion. *Journal of Neuroscience*, **16**, 3737–3744.

Braitenberg, V. (2001). Brain size and number of neurons: an exercise in synthetic neuroanatomy. *Journal of Computational Neuroscience*, **10**, 71–77.

Brown, T.T., Lugar, H.M., Coalson, R.S. *et al.* (2004). Developmental changes in human cerebral functional organization for word generation. *Cerebral Cortex*, **15**(3), 275–290.

Bunge, S.A. (2002). Immature frontal lobe contributions to cognitive control in children: evidence from fMRI. *Neuron*, **33**, 301–311.

Carey, S., De Schonen, S., & Ellis, H.D. (1992). Becoming a face expert. *Philosophical Transactions: Biological Sciences*, **335**, 95–103.

Carne, R.P., Vogrin, S., Litewka, L., & Cook, M.J. (2006). Cerebral cortex: an MRI-based study of volume and variance with age and sex. *Journal of Clinical Neuroscience*, **13**(1), 60–72.

Caspi, A., Sugden, K., Moffitt, T.E. *et al.* (2003). Influence of life stress on depression: moderation by a polymorphism in the 5-HTT gene. *Science*, **301**(5631), 386–389.

Chang, F.L., & Greenough, W.T. (1982). Lateralized effects of monocular training on dendritic branching in adult split-brain rats. *Brain Research*, **232**(2), 283–292.

Cocosco, C.A., Zijdenbos, A.P., & Evans, A.C. (2003). A fully automatic and robust MRI tissue classification method. *Medical Image Analysis*, **7**, 513–527.

Collins, D.L., Neelin, P., Peters, T.M., & Evans, A.C. (1994). Automatic 3D intersubject registration of MR volumetric data in standardized Talairach space. *Journal of Computer Assisted Tomography*, **18**, 192–205.

Collins, D.L., Holmes, C.J., Peters, T.M., & Evans, A.C. (1995). Automatic 3D model-based neuroanatomical segmentation. *Human Brain Mapping*, **3**, 190–208.

Cowell, P.E., Allen, L.S., Zalatimo, N.S., & Denenberg, V.H. (1992). A developmental study of sex and age interactions in the human corpus callosum. *Brain Research. Developmental Brain Research*, **66**(2), 187–192.

Davidson, M.C., Thomas, K.M., & Casey, B.J. (2003). Imaging the developing brain with fMRI. *Mental Retardation and Developmental Disabilities Research Reviews*, **9**, 161–167.

De Bellis, M.D., Keshavan, M.S., Beers, S.R. *et al.* (2001). Sex differences in brain maturation during childhood and adolescence. *Cerebral Cortex*, **11**(6), 552–557.

Decety, J., Grezes, J., Costes, N. *et al.* (1997). Brain activity during observation of actions: influence of action content and subject's strategy. *Brain*, **120**, 1763–1777.

Dekaban, A.S. (1978). Changes in brain weights during the span of human life: relation of brain weights to body heights and body weights. *Annals of Neurology*, **4**(4), 345–356.

Deutsch, G.K., Dougherty, R.F., Bammer, R. *et al.* (2005). Children's reading performance is correlated with white matter structure measured by diffusion tensor imaging. *Cortex*, **41**(3), 354–363.

Draganski, B., Gaser, C., Busch, V., Schuierer, G., Bogdahn, U., & May, A. (2004). Neuroplasticity: changes in grey matter induced by training. *Nature*, **427**, 311–312.

Evans, A.C., Collins, D.L., Mills, S.R. *et al.* (1993). 3D statistical neuroanatomical models from 305 MRI volumes. *Proceedings of the IEEE-Nuclear Science Symposium and Medical Imaging Conference*, 1813–1817.

Fischl, B., & Dale, A.M. (2000). Measuring the thickness of the human cerebral cortex from magnetic resonance images. *Proceedings of the National Academy of Sciences USA*, **97**(20), 11050–11055.

Gaser, C., & Schlaug, G. (2003). Brain structures differ between musicians and non-musicians. *Journal of Neuroscience*, **23**(27), 9240–9245.

Giedd, J.N., Rumsey, J.M., Castellanos, F.X. *et al.* (1996a). A quantitative MRI study of the corpus callosum in children and adolescents. *Developmental Brain Research*, **91**, 274–280.

Giedd, J.N., Snell, J.W., Lange, N. *et al.* (1996b). Quantitative magnetic resonance imaging of human brain development: ages 4–18. *Cerebral Cortex*, **6**, 551–560.

Giedd, J.N., Vaituzis, A.C., Hamburger, S.D. *et al.* (1996c). Quantitative MRI of the temporal lobe, amygdala and hippocampus in normal human development: ages 4–18 years. *Journal of Comparative Neurology*, **366**, 223–230.

Giedd, J.N., Blumenthal, J., Jeffries, N.O. *et al.* (1999a). Brain development during childhood and adolescence: a longitudinal MRI study. *Nature Neuroscience*, **2**, 861–863.

Giedd, J.N., Blumenthal, J., Jeffries, N.O. *et al.* (1999b). Development of the human corpus callosum during childhood and adolescence: a longitudinal MRI study. *Progress in Neuro-Psychopharmacology and Biological Psychiatry*, **23**(4), 571–588.

Gogtay, N., Giedd, J.N., Lusk, L. *et al.* (2004). Dynamic mapping of human cortical development during childhood through early adulthood. *Proceedings of the National Academy of Sciences USA*, **101**, 8174–8179.

Good, C.D., Johnsrude, I., Ashburner, J. *et al.* (2001). Cerebral asymmetry and the effects of sex and handedness on brain structure: a voxel-based morphometric analysis of 465 normal adult human brains. *Neuroimage*, **14**(3), 685–700.

Goren, C.C., Sarty, M., & Wu, P.Y.K. (1975). Visual following and pattern discrimination of face-like stimuli by newborn infants. *Pediatrics*, **56**, 544–549.

Greenough, W.T., Larson, J.R., & Withers, G.S. (1985). Effects of unilateral and bilateral training in a reaching task on dendritic branching of neurons in the rat motor-sensory forelimb cortex. *Behavioral and Neural Biology*, **44**(2), 301–314.

Grezes, J., Costes, N., & Decety, J. (1999). The effects of learning and intention on the neural network involved in the perception of meaningless actions. *Brain*, **122**, 1875–1887.

Grosbras, M.H., & Paus, T. (2006). Brain networks involved in viewing angry hands or faces. *Cerebral Cortex*, **16**, 1087–1096.

Gur, R.C., Gunning-Dixon, F., Bilker, W.B., & Gur, R.E. (2002). Sex differences in temporo-limbic and frontal brain volumes of healthy adults. *Cerebral Cortex*, **12**(9), 998–1003.

Hagmann, P., Cammoun, L., Martuzzi, R. *et al.* (2006). Hand preference and sex shape the architecture of language networks. *Human Brain Mapping*, **27**, 828–835.

Han, X., Jovicich, J., Salat, D. *et al.* (2006). Reliability of MRI-derived measurements of human cerebral cortical thickness: the effects of field strength, scanner upgrade and manufacturer. *Neuroimage*, **32**(1), 180–194.

Hebb, D.O. (1947). The effects of early experience on problem solving at maturity. *American Psychologist*, **2**, 737–745.

Hebb, D.O. (1949). *The Organization of Behavior: A Neuropsychological Theory.* New York: John Wiley.

Heeger, D.J., Huk, A.C., Geisler, W.S., & Albrecht, D.G. (2000). Spikes versus BOLD: what does neuroimaging tell us about neuronal activity? *Nature Neuroscience*, **3**, 631–633.

Herba, C., & Phillips, M. (2004). Annotation: Development of facial expression recognition from childhood to adolescence: behavioral and neurological perspectives. *Journal of Child Psychology and Psychiatry*, **45**(7), 1185–1198.

Hutchinson, S., Lee, L.H., Gaab, N., & Schlaug, G. (2003). Cerebellar volume of musicians. *Cerebral Cortex*, **13**(9), 943–949.

Hwang, S.J., Ji, E.K., Lee, E.K. *et al.* (2004). Gender differences in the corpus callosum of neonates. *Neuroreport*, **15**(6), 1029–1032.

Jacobs, B., Schall, M., & Scheibel, A.B. (1993). A quantitative dendritic analysis of Wernicke's area in humans: II. Gender, hemispheric, and environmental factors. *Journal of Comparative Neurology*, **327**(1), 97–111.

Jancke, L., Schlaug, G., Huang, Y., & Steinmetz, H. (1994). Asymmetry of the planum parietale. *Neuroreport*, **5**(9), 1161–1163.

Jerison, H.J. (1987). Brain size. In G. Adelman (Ed.), *Encyclopedia of Neuroscience, Volume 1* (pp. 168–170). Boston, MA: Birkhauser.

Joffe, T.H., Tarantal, A.F., Rice, K. *et al.* (2005). Fetal and infant head circumference sexual dimorphism in primates. *American Journal of Physical Anthropology*, **126**(1), 97–110.

Kilts, C.D., Egan, G., Gideon, D.A., Ely, T.D., & Hoffman, J.M. (2003). Dissociable neural pathways are involved in the recognition of emotion in static and dynamic facial expressions. *Neuroimage*, **18**, 156–168.

Kimura, D. (1999). *Sex and Cognition*. Cambridge, MA: MIT Press.

Klingberg, T., Vaidya, C.J., Gabrieli, J.D.E., Moseley, M.E., & Hedehus, M. (1999). Myelination and organization of the frontal white matter in children: a diffusion tensor MRI study. *NeuroReport*, **10**, 2817–2821.

Kolb, B., Forgie, M., Gibb, R., Gorny, G., & Rowntree, S. (1998). Age, experience and the changing brain. *Neuroscience and Biobehavioural Reviews*, **22**, 143–159.

Kovalev, V.A., Kruggel, F., & von Cramon, D.Y. (2003). Gender and age effects in structural brain asymmetry as measured by MRI texture analysis. *Neuroimage*, **19**(3), 895–905.

Kulynych, J.J., Vladar, K., Jones, D.W., & Weinberger, D.R. (1994). Gender differences in the normal lateralization of the supratemporal cortex: MRI surface-rendering morphometry of Heschl's gyrus and the planum temporale. *Cerebral Cortex*, **4**(2), 107–118.

Kwon, H., Reiss, A.L., & Menon, V. (2002). Neural basis of protracted developmental changes in visuo-spatial working memory. *Proceedings of the National Academy of Sciences USA*, **99**, 13336–13341.

Lerch, J., & Evans, A.C. (2005). Cortical thickness analysis examined through power analysis and a population simulation. *Neuroimage*, **24**(1), 163–173.

Lewis, M.H. (2004). Environmental complexity and central nervous system development and function. *Mental Retardation and Developmental Disabilities Research Reviews*, **10**(2), 91–95.

Logothetis, N.K., Pauls, J., Augath, M., Trinath, T., & Oeltermann, A. (2001). Neurophysiological investigation of the basis of the fMRI signal. *Nature*, **412**, 150–157.

Luders, E., Steinmetz, H., & Jancke, L. (2002). Brain size and grey matter volume in the healthy human brain. *Neuroreport*, **13**(17), 2371–2374.

Luna, B., Thulborn, K.R., Munoz, D.P. *et al.* (2001). Maturation of widely distributed brain function subserves cognitive development. *Neuroimage*, **13**, 786–793.

Maguire, E.A., Gadian, D.G., Johnsrude, I.S. *et al.* (2000). Navigation-related structural change in the hippocampi of taxi drivers. *Proceedings of the National Academy of Sciences USA*, **97**(8), 4398–4403.

Maguire, E.A., Spiers, H.J., Good, C.D., Hartley, T., Frackowiak, R.S., & Burgess, N. (2003). Navigation expertise and the human hippocampus: a structural brain imaging analysis. *Hippocampus*, **13**(2), 250–259.

Mangin, J.F., Riviere, D., Cachia, A. *et al.* (2004). A framework to study the cortical folding patterns. *Neuroimage*, **23**(Suppl. 1), S129–S138.

Mathiessen, C., Caesar, K., Akgoren, N., & Lauritzen, M. (1998). Modification of activity-dependent increases of cerebral blood flow by excitatory synaptic activity and spikes in rat cerebellar cortex. *Journal of Physiology*, **512**, 555–566.

Matsuzawa, J., Matsui, M., Konishi, T. *et al.* (2001). Age-related volumetric changes of brain gray and white matter in healthy infants and children. *Cerebral Cortex*, **11**(4), 335–342.

McGivern, R.F., Andersen, J., Byrd, D., Mutter, K.L., & Reilly, J. (2002). Cognitive efficiency on a match to sample task decreases at the onset of puberty in children. *Brain and Cognition*, **50**, 73–89.

Mechelli, A., Crinion, J.T., Noppeney, U. *et al.* (2004). Neurolinguistics: structural plasticity in the bilingual brain. *Nature*, **431**(7010), 757.

Ozturk, A.H., Tascioglu, B., Aktekin, M., Kurtoglu, Z., & Erden, I. (2002). Morphometric comparison of the human corpus callosum in professional musicians and non-musicians by using in vivo magnetic resonance imaging. *Journal of Neuroradiology*, **29**(1), 29–34.

Paus, T. (2005). Mapping brain maturation and cognitive development during adolescence. *Trends in Cognitive Sciences*, **9**(2), 60–68.

Paus, T., Otaky, N., Caramanos, Z. *et al.* (1996a). In vivo morphometry of the intrasulcal gray matter in the human cingulate, paracingulate, and superior-rostral sulci: hemispheric asymmetries, gender differences and probability maps. *Journal of Comparative Neurology*, **376**(4), 664–673.

Paus, T., Tomaiuolo, F., Otaky, N. *et al.* (1996b). Human cingulate and paracingulate sulci: pattern, variability, asymmetry, and probabilistic map. *Cerebral Cortex*, **6**, 207–214.

Paus, T., Zijdenbos, A., Worsley, K. *et al.* (1999). Structural maturation of neural pathways in children and adolescents: in vivo study. *Science*, **283**, 1908–1911.

Perrin, J., Collins, L., Evans, A.C. *et al.* (2006, June). *Gender Differences in Brain Structure During Adolescence: The Saguenay Youth Study.* Paper presented at the 12th annual meeting of the Organization for Human Brain Mapping, Florence, Italy.

Peters, M., Jancke, L., Staiger, J.F. *et al.* (1998). Unsolved problems in comparing brain sizes in *Homo sapiens*. *Brain and Cognition*, **37**(2), 254–285.

Pezawas, L., Verchinski, B.A., Mattay, V.S. *et al.* (2004). The brain-derived neurotrophic factor val66met polymorphism and variation in human cortical morphology. *Journal of Neuroscience*, **24**(45), 10099–10102.

Pfefferbaum, A., Mathalon, D.H., Sullivan, E.V. *et al.* (1994). A quantitative magnetic resonance imaging study of changes in brain morphology from infancy to late adulthood. *Archives of Neurology*, **51**, 874–887.

Poythress, N., Lexcen, F.J., Grisso, T., & Steinberg, L. (2006). The competence-related abilities of adolescent defendants in criminal court. *Law and Human Behavior*, **30**(1), 75–92.

Preis, S., Jancke, L., Schmitz-Hillebrecht, J., & Steinmetz, H. (1999). Child age and planum temporale asymmetry. *Brain and Cognition*, **40**(3), 441–452.

Puce, A., Allison, T., Bentin, S., Gore, J.C., & McCarthy, G. (1998). Temporal cortex activation in humans viewing eye and mouth movements. *Journal of Neuroscience*, **18**, 2188–2199.

Pujol, J., Vendrell, P., Junque, C., Marti-Vilalta, J.L., & Capdevila, A. (1993). When does human brain development end? Evidence of corpus callosum growth up to adulthood. *Annals of Neurology*, **34**, 71–75.

Pujol, J., Lopez, A., Deus, J. *et al.* (2002). Anatomical variability of the anterior cingulate gyrus and basic dimensions of human personality. *Neuroimage*, **15**(4), 847–855.

Rauch, R.A., & Jinkins, J.R. (1994). Analysis of cross-sectional area measurements of the corpus callosum adjusted for brain size in male and female subjects from childhood to adulthood. *Behavioural Brain Research*, **64**, 65–78.

Rees, G., Friston, K., & Koch, C. (2000). A direct quantitative relationship between the functional properties of human and macaque V5. *Nature Neuroscience*, **3**, 716–723.

Reiss, A.L., Abrams, M.T., Singer, H.S., Ross, J.L., & Denckla, M.B. (1996). Brain development, gender and IQ in children. A volumetric imaging study. *Brain*, **119**, 1763–1774.

Rosenberg, D.R., Sweeney, J.A., Gillen, J.S. *et al.* (1997). Magnetic resonance imaging of children without sedation: preparation with simulation. *Journal of the American Academy of Child and Adolescent Psychiatry*, **36**(6), 853–859.

Rosenzweig, M.R., Bennett, E.L., Hebert, M., & Morimoto, H. (1978). Social grouping cannot account for cerebral effects of enriched environments. *Brain Research*, **153**(3), 563–576.

Rubia, K., Overmeyer, S., Taylor, E. *et al.* (2000). Functional frontalisation with age: mapping neurodevelopmental trajectories with fMRI. *Neuroscience and Biobehavioral Reviews*, **24**, 13–19.

Scheibel, A., Conrad, T., Perdue, S., Tomiyasu, U., & Wechsler, A. (1990). A quantitative study of dendrite complexity in selected areas of the human cerebral cortex. *Brain and Cognition*, **12**(1), 85–101.

Schlaggar, B.L., Brown, T.T., Lugar, H.M. *et al.* (2002). Functional neuroanatomical differences between adults and school-age children in the processing of single words. *Science*, **296**, 1476–1479.

Schlaug, G., Jancke, L., Huang, Y., Staiger, J.F., & Steinmetz, H. (1995). Increased corpus callosum size in musicians. *Neuropsychologia*, **33**, 1047–1055.

Schlaug, G., Jancke, L., Huang, Y., & Steinmetz, H. (1995). In vivo evidence of structural brain asymmetry in musicians. *Science*, **267**(5198), 699–701.

Schmithorst, V.J., Wilke, M., Dardzinski, B.J., & Holland, S.K. (2002). Correlation of white matter diffusivity and anisotropy with age during childhood and adolescence: a cross-sectional diffusion-tensor MR imaging study. *Radiology*, **222**(1), 212–218.

Schmithorst, V.J., Wilke, M., Dardzinski, B.J., & Holland, S.K. (2005). Cognitive functions correlate with white matter architecture in a normal pediatric population: a diffusion tensor MRI study. *Human Brain Mapping*, **26**(2), 139–147.

Schneider, P., Scherg, M., Dosch, H.G. *et al.* (2002). Morphology of Heschl's gyrus reflects enhanced activation in the auditory cortex of musicians. *Nature Neuroscience*, **5**(7), 688–694.

Sequeira Sdos, S., Woerner, W., Walter, C. *et al.* (2006). Handedness, dichotic-listening ear advantage, and gender effects on planum temporale asymmetry – a volumetric investigation using structural magnetic resonance imaging. *Neuropsychologia*, **44**(4), 622–636.

Shaw, P., Greenstein, D., Lerch, J. *et al.* (2006). Intellectual ability and cortical development in children and adolescents. *Nature*, **440**(7084), 676–679.

Sirevaag, A.M., & Greenough, W.T. (1988). A multivariate statistical summary of synaptic plasticity measures in rats exposed to complex, social and individual environments. *Brain Research*, **441**, 386–392.

Sisk, C.L., & Foster, D.L. (2004). The neural basis of puberty and adolescence. *Nature Neuroscience*, **7**(10), 1040–1047.

Skullerud, K. (1985). Variations in the size of the human brain. Influence of age, sex, body length, body mass index, alcoholism, Alzheimer changes, and cerebral atherosclerosis. *Acta Neurologica Scandinavica*, **102**(Suppl), 1–94.

Sluming, V., Barrick, T., Howard, M., Cezayirli, E., Mayes, A., & Roberts, N. (2002). Voxel-based morphometry reveals increased gray matter density in Broca's area in male symphony orchestra musicians. *Neuroimage*, **17**(3), 1613–1622.

Smith, S.M., Jenkinson, M., Johansen-Berg, H. *et al.* (2006). Tract-based spatial statistics: voxelwise analysis of multi-subject diffusion data. *Neuroimage*, **31**(4), 1487–1505.

Snook, L., Paulson, L.A., Roy, D., Phillips, L., & Beaulieu, C. (2005). Diffusion tensor imaging of neurodevelopment in children and young adults. *Neuroimage*, **26**(4), 1164–1173.

Sowell, E.R., Thompson, P.M., Tessner, K.D., & Toga, A.W. (2001). Mapping continued brain growth and gray matter density reduction in dorsal frontal cortex: inverse relationships during post-adolescent brain maturation. *Journal of Neuroscience*, **21**, 8819–8829.

Steinmetz, H., Jancke, L., Kleinschmidt, A. *et al.* (1992). Sex but no hand difference in the isthmus of the corpus callosum. *Neurology*, **42**(4), 749–752.

Suzuki, M., Hagino, H., Nohara, S. *et al.* (2005). Male-specific volume expansion of the human hippocampus during adolescence. *Cerebral Cortex*, **15**(2), 187–193.

Talairach, J., & Tournoux, P. (1988) *Co-planar Stereotaxic Atlas of the Human Brain.* New York: Thieme Medical Publishers.

Tamm, L., Menon, V., & Reiss, A.L. (2002). Maturation of brain function associated with response inhibition. *Journal of the American Academy of Child and Adolescent Psychiatry*, **41**, 1231–1238.

Taylor, M.J., McCarthy, G., Saliba, E., & Degiovanni, E. (1999). ERP evidence of developmental changes in processing of faces. *Clinical Neurophysiology*, **110**, 910–915.

Thomas, K.M., Drevets, W.C., Whalen, P.J. *et al.* (2001). Amygdala response to facial expressions in children and adults. *Biological Psychiatry*, **49**, 309–316.

van Praag, H., Kempermann, G., & Gage, F.H. (2000). Neural consequences of environmental enrichment. *Nature Reviews Neuroscience*, **1**(3), 191–198.

Wada, J.A., Clarke, R., & Hamm, A. (1975). Cerebral hemispheric asymmetry in humans. Cortical speech zones in 100 adults and 100 infant brains. *Archives of Neurology*, **32**(4), 239–246.

Witelson, S.F., & Pallie, W. (1973). Left hemisphere specialization for language in the newborn. Neuroanatomical evidence of asymmetry. *Brain*, **96**(3), 641–646.

Yang, T.T., Menon, V., Reid, A.J., Gotlib, I.H., & Reiss, A.L. (2003). Amygdalar activation associated with happy facial expressions in adolescents: A 3-T functional MRI study. *Journal of the American Academy of Child and Adolescent Psychiatry*, **42**, 979–985.

Yucel, M., Stuart, G.W., Maruff, P. *et al.* (2001). Hemispheric and gender-related differences in the gross morphology of the anterior cingulate/paracingulate cortex in normal volunteers: an MRI morphometric study. *Cerebral Cortex*, **11**(1), 17–25.

Zijdenbos, A.P., Forghani, R., & Evans, A.C. (2002). Automatic 'pipeline' analysis of 3D MRI data for clinical trials: Application to multiple sclerosis. *IEEE Transactions on Medical Imaging*, **21**, 1280–1291.

7

Neurobiological processes in depressive disorders: links with adolescent brain development

Erika E. Forbes, Jennifer S. Silk, and Ronald E. Dahl

Adolescence is a period of dynamic changes in a wide range of domains, including mood, motivation, behavior, and social context (Dahl & Spear, 2004). This is also a maturational period of increased vulnerability to various forms of psychopathology. One domain of change that has received a great deal of interest is the increased role of peers (Bukowski *et al.*, 1993), and tendencies for greater concerns about status in relation to peers. Another important dimension of change is the adolescent increase in sensation-seeking and reward-seeking that contributes to risk-taking, reckless behavior, and greater rates of accidents – the largest single source of mortality in adolescence (Dahl & Spear, 2004). Most relevant to the focus of this chapter, adolescence is also associated with a dramatic rise in rates of depression (Costello *et al.*, 2002). In tandem with these behavioral and clinical changes, the adolescent brain is continuing to develop. The volume of neuron-containing tissue decreases, the speed and efficiency of neuronal transmission of information rises, and the connections among neurons are undergoing refinement (Spear, 2000). In terms of function, the brain continues to improve its capacity for planning, executing, and modulating behavior during adolescence.

The central topic to be addressed in this chapter is the relation between brain development and depression during adolescent development. Relatively little is currently known about the intricacies of normal and abnormal structure and function in the adolescent brain, and virtually no research has attempted to understand the specific relationship between depression and brain development during this period. As a result, this chapter will consider several issues in attempting to connect the dots among three areas of research: neural systems involved in affect regulation, development of those neural systems during adolescence, and structural and functional brain characteristics

Adolescent Emotional Development and the Emergence of Depressive Disorders, ed. Nicholas B. Allen and Lisa B. Sheeber. Published by Cambridge University Press. © Cambridge University Press 2009.

observed in adult depression. The goal is not to imply definitive understanding of these areas, but rather to describe key conceptual links and point to promising candidates for current and future lines of investigation.

Adolescent depression and affect regulation

Adolescents with depression struggle with mood difficulties that are persistent, unpleasant, and resistant to change. They experience more negative affect, such as sadness and irritability, and they experience less positive affect, such as joy. These affective experiences create functional impairments – particularly in peer and family relationships, academic performance, and participation in rewarding activities (see Tompson, McKowen, and Asarnow, Chapter 15; LaGreca, Davila, and Siegel, Chapter 17).

Consistent with several conceptual accounts of depression, we propose that adolescent depression is primarily a disorder of affect regulation. More specifically, the disorder appears to involve problems with initiating, maintaining, or modifying the quality, intensity, or timing of affective responses (Cole et al., 2004; Forbes & Dahl, 2005). Key aspects of this disorder – especially the persistent low mood and anhedonia typical of depressive episodes – can be conceptualized as changes in affect regulation. Both the intensity and duration of affective states appear to be abnormal in depression, which also suggests alterations in affect regulation processes. Several behavioral studies have indicated that depressed adolescents evidence poor affect regulation and report using ineffective regulation strategies (Garber et al., 1995; Sheeber et al., 2000). Some frameworks of depression have also emphasized poor affective flexibility (Rottenberg et al., 2003). In other words, people with depression could have difficulty modulating their affect in an appropriate or timely way as circumstances change. For example, they might be slow to shift from a neutral to a pleasant affective state when a potentially rewarding event occurs, or they may appear "stuck" in a negative mood state after a challenge resolves.

Therefore, to understand crucial aspects of the neurobehavioral underpinnings of adolescent depression, we believe it is essential to consider the neural processes critical to regulating affect. This chapter seeks to place adolescent depression in the context of its neural substrates and the development of those substrates. Two approaches guide our efforts: affective neuroscience, which attempts to describe the neural substrates of affective states and disorders, and developmental psychopathology, which attempts to describe disorders within the context of normal and abnormal development.

Positive affect and adolescent depression

Within the realm of affect regulation, we propose that alterations in the regulation of *positive affect* are a critical feature of adolescent depression

(Forbes & Dahl, 2005). Though negative affect is almost certainly disrupted in depression, we view positive affect as also disrupted and as separate, to some extent, from negative affect. Whilst changes in the two affective systems can be difficult to disentangle based on clinical characteristics or behavioral observation, affective neuroscience provides a framework for understanding the unique contributions that each system might make to adolescent depression. An affective neuroscience perspective on positive affect emphasizes reward-motivated behavior and defines positive affect as an emotional state elicited by reward (Rolls, 1999; Schultz, 2000). Thus, understanding deficits in the regulation of positive affect in depression involves examining components of reward responding such as motivation to obtain reward, sensitivity to reward magnitude, and enjoyment of reward.

Our emphasis on positive affect has a history in several conceptual models of depression. Emotion-based (Clark & Watson, 1991), motivation-based (Depue & Iacono, 1989), behavioral (Lewinsohn et al., 1985), and evolutionary models (Allen & Badcock, 2003) of affective psychopathology all emphasize disturbance in positive affect as a central feature of depression. In general, these models posit that decreased pursuit of reward is a key characteristic and possibly a maintaining factor in depression. Similarly, behavioral treatments of depression, including those in adolescents, emphasize the activation of behavior that will likely result in reward (Lewinsohn & Clarke, 1999). Furthermore, models of affective behavior during adolescence have emphasized the influence of positive affect systems over aversive or negative affect systems in this period of life, as well as the relative immaturity of regulatory systems (Ernst et al., 2006).

Investigating the affective neuroscience of adolescent depression can also shed light on puberty-related changes in reward systems. Paradoxically, adolescence is remarkable both for the increase in incidence of depression and for the sharp increase in reward-related and risk-taking behavior that occurs. Increased reward-related behavior is evident in domains including substance use, sexual behavior, and accidents (Dahl & Spear, 2004; Steinberg, 2004). Affective intensity and reward responsiveness, in some conceptualizations of adolescence, also appear to be enhanced during this period (Steinberg, 2004). These developmental changes may indicate that neural systems underlying reward are undergoing important changes with pubertal development. In some, brain systems involved in positive affect may undergo atypical development, leading to the onset of depression. Developmental changes in these brain systems may take the opposite path in some adolescents, leading to reduced rather than enhanced reward motivation, suggesting that the *regulation* of positive affect, rather than its level per se, is undergoing significant developmental change during adolescence. This proposition remains to be examined in studies of brain development.

Neurobiology of affect regulation

In this section, we review several features of neural systems implicated in affect regulation. These systems have been identified in developmental research as well as research on typical adult brain function. We begin with a definition of affect regulation that will guide our review. Next, we describe systems implicated in affective reactivity, or the production of affective states. We then describe those systems implicated in affect regulation. Reactivity and regulation are closely related (Cole *et al.*, 2004), and neural systems of reactivity and regulation function together to influence behavior. Positive affect systems, negative affect systems, and regulatory systems have been proposed as the components of a triadic model of affective behavior during adolescence (Ernst *et al.*, 2006).

A working definition of affect regulation

Based on our approach to affect regulation in children and adolescents, we offer the following working definition: "affect regulation is a set of internal and external processes involved in the initiation, maintenance, or modification of the quality, intensity, or chronometry of affective responses" (Forbes & Dahl, 2005, p. 5). This definition is broad, and it intentionally includes several elements. Others as well as the self are seen as playing a role in affect regulation, automatic as well as effortful processes are involved, affect can increase or decrease and positive or negative affect can be the target of regulation. Finally, regulation can occur at several stages of the affective process, not simply after the onset of an affective state. Affect regulation involves behavioral, physiological, and subjective elements, and the first two of these are addressed by affective neuroscience.

Affect reactivity and regulation

Positive affect
The neural circuits involved in positive affect include the striatum, orbitofrontal cortex, and amygdala (see Figure 7.1). Because positive affect is linked to reward processing (Rolls, 1999), reward-related brain systems are relevant to the regulation of positive affect. Reward-related brain systems have functions such as detecting reward, predicting future reward, representing reward value, and representing goals (Schultz, 2000). The regions traditionally implicated in reward processing include the striatum and orbitofrontal cortex (Dalgleish, 2004; Rolls, 2000; Schultz, 2000). Activation in the ventral striatum, particularly in the area including the nucleus accumbens, occurs during the anticipation of reward (Knutson *et al.*, 2001, 2003). The ventral striatum, dorsal

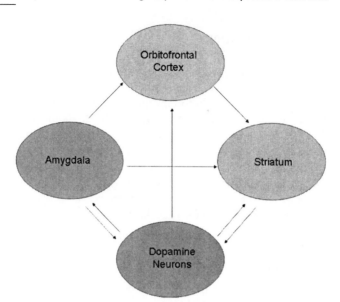

Figure 7.1. The neural circuits involved in positive affect include the striatum, orbitofrontal cortex, and amygdala.

striatum (especially caudate), amygdala, and ventromedial prefrontal cortex (PFC) exhibit enhanced activation during receipt of reward (Delgado *et al.*, 2000; Elliott *et al.*, 2002; Knutson *et al.*, 2001, 2003). The amygdala and orbitofrontal cortex exhibit sensitivity to predicted reward value (Gottfried *et al.*, 2003), and the orbitofrontal cortex is implicated in processing extremes of reward magnitude (Elliott *et al.*, 2003).

Recent studies of monetary reward also suggest that the amygdala, which is thought to respond to social signals of emotion (Dalgleish, 2004), appears to play a role in reward responding (Elliott *et al.*, 2003, 2004). Because the amygdala is also thought to play a role in representing stimulus-value associations involving reward (Baxter & Murray, 2002), amygdala activation may also accompany reward processing.

The dopamine system also is thought to play a central role in positive affect and has been implicated in depression (Drevets, 2001). Mesolimbic dopamine projections from the ventral tegmental area to reward-related regions such as the ventral striatum, amygdala, and orbitofrontal cortex appear to support a system critical to pleasant mood, motivation to obtain reward, and reward-related behavior (Spanagel & Weiss, 1999). In humans, feelings of euphoria are correlated with amphetamine-induced dopamine release in the ventral striatum (Drevets *et al.*, 2001). Thus, disturbances in this system may underlie reduced positive affect in depression.

Neuroscience research indicates that the components of reward processing must be examined separately. For example, motivation or "wanting" has a different neural substrate than enjoyment or "liking" (Berridge & Robinson, 2003). To determine the neural bases of reward processing in depression, it is necessary to examine brain activation during a variety of reward experiences. In our own work, we have approached the development of reward processing through investigations of reward-related decisions, reward anticipation, and reward outcome in young people with depression or at risk for depression (Forbes *et al.*, 2006a, 2006b, 2007).

Negative affect

The brain area most often associated with negative affect is the amygdala (Davidson & Irwin, 1999). The amygdala responds to facial expressions of fear and anger (e.g. Hariri *et al.*, 2002) and to self-generated sad mood (Schneider *et al.*, 1995). Lesions to the amygdala appear to produce abnormal generation of negative affect (Davidson & Irwin, 1999). Across studies of affective processing, the amygdala seems to be particularly related to fear (Murphy *et al.*, 2003). Other types of negative affect are more consistently associated with other brain areas: the insula and globus pallidus with disgust, and the orbitofrontal cortex with anger (Murphy *et al.*, 2003). The ventromedial PFC has been linked to sadness in studies of mood induction (Mayberg *et al.*, 1999). Finally, the anterior cingulate may play a role in negative affect, especially in situations involving pain or attention to one's own affective state (Davis *et al.*, 1997; Devinsky *et al.*, 1995; Lane *et al.*, 1998).

Among neurotransmitter systems, the serotonin system has been particularly implicated in negative affect and depression. Serotonin has important functions in modulating affective behavior (Lucki, 1998), and it has been linked to depression through the efficacy of pharmacologic agents such as fluoxetine that target the availability of serotonin in synapses (Blier & de Montigny, 1999; March *et al.*, 2004; Vasa *et al.*, 2006).

Studies of genetic influences on depression and anxiety in humans have emphasized the role of genes related to 5-HT and hypothalamic-pituitary-adrenal (HPA) axis function (Leonardo & Hen, 2006). For example, studies suggest that individuals homozygous for the 5-HTTLPR short allele are at increased risk for depressive disorders, but only in the context of environmental risk (Caspi *et al.*, 2003; Kendler *et al.*, 2005). This finding has been replicated in an adolescent sample, but only for girls (Eley *et al.*, 2004). Another recent developmental study suggests that severity of depression in maltreated children can be predicted by a more complicated gene–gene–environment interaction (Kaufman *et al.*, 2006). In this study, the 5-HTTLPR short allele and the met allele of the brain-derived neurotrophic factor (BDNF) val66met polymorphism interacted with the environment such that having both genes was associated with higher depression scores, but only among children who were maltreated.

Affect regulation

The regulation of emotion and motivation appears to involve interactions across several affective and cognitive systems. In particular, areas of the prefrontal cortex (PFC) – a region whose general role is to support executive functions such as planning, shifting attention, inhibiting behavior, and executing complex behavioral sequences – appear to be critical to regulate affect in ways that are adaptive and help to serve goal-directed behavior. A variety of areas and systems within the PFC are likely to contribute to affect regulation, and these are likely to interact in complex ways. Two areas that appear particularly important to affect regulation are the medial prefrontal cortex, including the anterior cingulate cortex, and the ventral PFC, including areas of orbitofrontal cortex. One function of anterior cingulate cortex is the monitoring of errors and conflict (Carter *et al.*, 1998; Kerns *et al.*, 2004). Other areas of the medial prefrontal cortex play a role in self-awareness and social cognition (Amodio & Frith, 2006). The ventral PFC inhibits prepotent behavioral responses and contributes to flexible responses in the face of changing stimulus conditions (Rolls, 1999). Finally, the coordination between dorsal and ventral areas of the PFC has been proposed as a means of regulating affect in the service of larger or long-term goals (Nelson *et al.*, 2005). Because affect regulation involves pursuing goals, monitoring behavior, and modulating the intensity and quality of affective responses according to circumstances and goals, these areas are likely to be important to affective functioning.

Development of affect reactivity and affect regulation brain systems

Below, we review the findings on brain development in the regions and circuits that appear to play a role in affect regulation. These findings have been generated by studies of healthy young people, and they illustrate the typical course of development in the neural substrates of affect.

Structural changes in relevant brain areas during adolescence

The changes in brain structure that occur during adolescence include changes in gray matter volume, increases in white matter, and synapse elimination. Gray matter is the gray-colored cortex of the brain and contains neuron bodies and supporting glial cells. White matter contains the myelinated axon fibers of neurons. Myelin is a fatty coating of neurons' axons by oligodentrocytes that increases the speed of transmission between neurons. Synapse elimination occurs as connections among neurons through dendrites are eliminated by pruning. During adolescence, brain systems continue to change as a result of modifying the strength and speed of neural connections that lead to improved efficiency of neuronal transmission.

Development does not occur uniformly throughout the brain. Areas involved in more sophisticated functions develop later than areas involved in basic functions (Gogtay *et al.*, 2004). In fact, areas involved in reward processing and affect regulation are among the last to mature, with development continuing through adolescence. For instance, the dorsolateral PFC, which plays a critical role in executive function, does not reach its adult volume until the late 20s (Giedd, 2004). The orbitofrontal cortex is among the last cortical areas to mature (Gogtay *et al.*, 2004). The caudate, a subcortical structure that is part of the striatum and participates in reward processing (Delgado *et al.*, 2000), decreases in volume during the teen years (Giedd, 2004). White matter in the brain increases linearly with development as a result of axon myelination, and its increases continue into early adulthood and do not appear to vary with brain region (Durston *et al.*, 2001; Giedd, 2004). Synapse elimination occurs through adolescence, and like gray matter decreases, continues longer in the PFC than in other areas of the brain (Huttenlocher, 1990; Huttenlocher & Dabholkar, 1997).

Areas of the cerebellum also evidence late maturational structural change (Keller *et al.*, 2003), with development continuing through adolescence and into early adulthood (Giedd, 2004). The cerebellum appears to contribute to a broad range of cognitive and affective functions. Work by Strick and colleagues has emphasized the role of cerebellar circuitry in fine-tuning the scaling of actions that require adaptive modulations (Hoshi *et al.*, 2005; Middleton & Strick, 2000). As there are many aspects of affect regulation that may require the scaling of emotional and/or motivational signals in adaptive ways, the late maturation of these regions may have significance for adolescents' ability to regulate affect adaptively.

Functional changes in relevant brain areas during adolescence

Studies of functional change with development have indicated that several brain areas important to affect regulation lag behind areas involved in affective reactivity in reaching adult-like patterns of function. Areas of the PFC that are critical to response inhibition, for example, are functionally immature in adolescents (Casey *et al.*, 2000; Luna & Sweeney, 2004). In a recent fMRI study of reward processing, adolescents' nucleus accumbens activation appeared similar to that of adults, while their orbitofrontal cortex activation appeared more similar to that of children (Galvan *et al.*, 2006). In other words, systems involved in responding to reward seemed to mature before systems that exert control over affective response. The later maturation of brain circuits critical to affect regulation could be especially challenging for adolescents given that some brain areas related to reward responding, such as the nucleus accumbens, are more active in response to reward in adolescents than in adults (Ernst *et al.*, 2005).

Neurobiology of affect dysregulation in adolescent depression

Because our framework emphasizes the development of brain areas relevant to affect regulation as underlying the onset of depression during adolescence, we will next discuss what appear to be structural and functional correlates of depression in those areas. Much of the work we address has been conducted with adults, and we therefore attempt to extrapolate findings to adolescents. In addition, because our conceptualization of alterations to affect regulation in depression emphasizes alterations to the neural substrates of positive affect, we will consider what is known about adolescents' brain function during reward processing and decision-making.

Brain regions implicated in adult depression

Studies of structural and functional alterations of brain regions have revealed that a number of affect-related regions are unusual in people with depressive disorder. These studies have focused on adult depression, however, and their findings must be extended to adolescent depression cautiously. In some cases, changes in brain structure and function may be a consequence rather than a cause of depression.

In addition, developmental differences between adult brains and adolescent brains suggest that findings for adult depression cannot simply be generalized to adolescent depression. For instance, a meta-analysis of research on amygdala volume in depression concluded that studies with children and adults have reported opposite findings: larger-than-typical amygdala volume in children but smaller-than-typical amygdala volume in adults with depression (Haggerty, unpublished manuscript). This discrepancy could be related to variability in definition of anatomical boundaries, as a study including a broad range of ages found consistently smaller amygdala volumes in people with depression (Haggerty, unpublished manuscript).

Neuroimaging studies of depression have indicated disruption in the structure and function of several areas related to affect regulation (Drevets, 2001). Ventromedial brain areas appear to be smaller in adults with familial depression (Drevets *et al.*, 1998). Functionally, studies of depression in adults have indicated a pattern of increased activation in ventral brain regions considered important for affect perception and affective response (Phillips *et al.*, 2003). For example, depressed adults exhibit increased resting blood flow in the amygdala (Drevets *et al.*, 1992) and the ventromedial PFC (Mayberg *et al.*, 1999). Right frontal electroencephalogram asymmetry, a pattern of brain electrical activity evident in adults with depression and children of depressed mothers, has been hypothesized to be a risk factor for depression (Davidson, 1994; Tomarken & Keener, 1998).

During affective contexts, depression is associated with unusual brain function. Depressed adults exhibit increased activation in the amygdala in response to faces displaying fear expressions (Sheline *et al.*, 2001) and more sustained amygdala activation in response to negatively valenced words (Siegle *et al.*, 2002). During an induced sad mood, adults with depression display decreased activation in ventromedial PFC (Keedwell *et al.*, 2005a) whereas healthy adults display increased activation in this region (Keedwell *et al.*, 2005a; Mayberg *et al.*, 1999).

Relevant to our focus on positive affect, adults with depression exhibit unusual neural response to pleasant stimuli. When viewing facial expressions of happiness, adults with unipolar depression fail to display the increased ventral striatal activation that is typical of healthy adults (Lawrence *et al.*, 2004; Surguladze *et al.*, 2005). While viewing happy faces and experiencing a happy autobiographical memory, adults with depression exhibited increased ventromedial PFC activation, while healthy adults exhibited decreased activation in this region (Keedwell *et al.*, 2005a). In a study using stimuli with increasing intensity of happy facial expressions, adults with depression failed to show enhanced activation in the putamen (part of the striatum) as intensity of stimuli increased (Surguladze *et al.*, 2005). These same adults showed enhanced activation in this region to facial expressions of increasing sadness, however. In addition, depression symptoms reflecting altered positive affect are associated with activation in reward-related areas. Specifically, adults' anhedonia was inversely correlated with amygdala and ventral striatum activation during pleasant contexts (Keedwell *et al.*, 2005b).

In one recent study conducted with adolescents depressive symptom scores were positively correlated with activation in the ventromedial PFC and anterior cingulate cortex during viewing of fearful faces (Killgore & Yurgelun-Todd, 2006). These findings suggest that adolescent depression is similar to adult depression in its pattern of brain function during affective picture-viewing. Whether this is the case in other affective contexts or in response to positive affect must be addressed by future studies.

A recent study in our group addressed reward-related decision-making in children and adolescents with major depressive disorder (Forbes *et al.*, 2006b). During both the anticipation phase and the outcome phase of a task with varying probability and magnitude of receiving reward, young people with depression exhibited less neural activation in areas such as the amygdala, orbitofrontal cortex, and caudate (dorsal striatum). Thus, it appears that reward processing is altered in child and adolescent depression.

Impact of brain development on vulnerability to depression

In short, brain regions that are critical to affect regulation, reward processing, and decision-making mature relatively late. Taken with the evidence that these regions are functionally disrupted in depression and the increased incidence of depression during adolescence, it is likely that the timing of brain maturation contributes to depression in those who are vulnerable. Specifically, the abnormal maturation of these areas could be linked to depression. Longitudinal studies are needed to investigate whether changes in function in brain regions such as the ventral PFC, the striatum, and the amygdala develop differently in young people with depression. Whether the course of development goes awry with the experience of depressive episodes or precedes the onset of depression is an issue for these studies to address.

Potential impact of depression on brain development

Although we have assumed until now that brain development plays a role in the development and course of adolescent depression, the opposite direction of influence is also worthy of consideration. That is, does depression influence the course of brain development? Few studies have adopted this perspective, but the literatures on brain plasticity and normal brain development during adolescence suggest that an atypical experience such as depression could exert an influence on the structure and function of brain systems.

If one accepts the working model that adolescence is a crucial time in normal development for the refinement of neural circuitry underpinning the regulation of emotion and motivation, some compelling questions arise about the consequences of going through this maturational interval under the influence of a depressive disorder. Might the diminishment of rewarding activities result in more enduring effects on neural systems of reward? Could the experience of depression during a period in which social behavior changes dramatically have consequences for social and affective development? Conversely, could this period of plasticity in neural systems of affect regulation also create a window of opportunity for interventions, before a chronic course of disorder emerges?

Influence of depression on brain structure and function

An extensive literature on temporal lobe structure in depression indicates that the hippocampus, an area important to memory and learning, is smaller in adults who have experienced depression (Videbech & Ravnkilde, 2004). This seems to be particularly the case for those with a recurrent course of depression. In addition, there is some evidence that early-onset depression is associated with reduced hippocampal volume (Campbell *et al.*, 2004). The findings on changes in amygdala volume with depression have been inconsistent across studies, but there is evidence that other brain areas involved in affect regulation are smaller in people with depression. The subgenual prefrontal cortex appears to be smaller in adults with depression (Drevets *et al.*, 1997), and some studies have reported smaller volume in orbitofrontal cortex with depression (Cotter *et al.*, 2005; Lacerda *et al.*, 2004).

Decreased hippocampal volume is thought to be influenced by increased stress reactivity among people with depression (Plotsky *et al.*, 1998). Those who are high in stress reactivity mount excessively vigorous or persistent responses to stressors in the corticotropin-releasing hormone system and the locus coeruleus norepinephrine system (McEwen, 1998). Chronic elevated glucocorticoid secretion is associated with adverse effects on neural structure and function, particularly in the hippocampus, including decreased dendritic branching, neuronal loss, changes in synaptic terminal structure, and inhibition of the neuron regeneration (Bremner & Vermetten, 2001; Sapolsky, 1996). Extension of findings of dysregulation of the hypothalamic-pituitary-adrenal axis in major depressive disorder to child and adolescent populations has resulted in mixed findings, with some evidence of elevated cortisol secretion in child and adolescent depression around sleep onset (Dahl *et al.*, 1991; Forbes *et al.*, 2006c; Kaufman *et al.*, 1997). Longitudinal research is needed to examine the link between stress reactivity and long-term changes in brain structure and function in children and adolescents.

In addition, another model of brain structure in depression – the neurotrophic hypothesis – posits that decreased expression of growth factors in the brain plays an important role in depression. Specifically, brain-derived neurotrophic factor (BDNF) could also contribute to the decreases in volume in the hippocampus and areas of the PFC (Duman & Monteggia, 2006). Reduced BDNF expression is considered a response to stress, and increased BDNF expression could mediate the effects of antidepressant medications. Brain-derived neurotrophic factor gene polymorphisms have now been linked to early-onset depression (Strauss *et al.*, 2004, 2005), suggesting that BDNF could contribute to the onset of depression during adolescence as well.

Adolescence as a period for ameliorating effects of depression on brain development

Adolescence may also be a period of opportunities for intervention. Because brain development continues to occur during these years, there may be a chance of influencing the development of affect regulation skills, the neural bases of affect regulation, and the course of depression. Animal models of early life stress have indicated that enrichment in the social environment during adolescence appears to compensate for some (but not all) of the effects of early experience, especially maternal separation, on brain function (Francis *et al.*, 2002). Specifically, the abnormal HPA axis regulation and stress-related behaviors that occur with maternal separation (Meaney, 2001) appear to be reversed by environmental enrichment. These results are consistent with the model that one window of plasticity in these regulatory systems occurs very early in development, while puberty/adolescence provides another window of plasticity to continue to modify the impact of early experience.

It is also possible that treatment of adolescent depression can protect against the potentially damaging effects of depression. Studies of bipolar disorder in particular have demonstrated that pharmacologic agents such as lithium have neurotrophic effects (Brambilla *et al.*, 2005). For example, adults with bipolar disorder who have not been treated with lithium show decreased volume in the anterior cingulate, whereas those who have received treatment show volumes in this region that are similar to those of healthy controls (Sassi *et al.*, 2004). These questions have not been addressed in young people with depression, but it is possible that they would experience similar benefits from treatment. Furthermore, because treatment studies indicate that the combination of fluoxetine and cognitive-behavioral therapy appears more efficacious than fluoxetine alone in treating adolescent depression (March *et al.*, 2004), one might speculate that there could be neuroprotective effects for psychosocial treatments in combination with pharmacotherapy.

Conclusion

Brain development during adolescence appears to be closely related to the onset and consequences of adolescent depression. Not only is adolescence a period in which depression becomes more likely and in which behavioral and affective changes occur rapidly, it is a period in which brain systems involved in affect expression and affect regulation continue to develop. Furthermore, there is striking overlap among the neural systems developing during adolescence, those involved in affect regulation, and those associated with depression. This paper has attempted to describe links among these three topics of developmental affective neuroscience. By doing so, this paper aims to extend our thinking not only about the neural substrates of adolescent depression but about the implications of adolescent depression for future adjustment and brain development.

It will be especially important for future work to include longitudinal studies of brain structure and function in adolescents with depression. Because alterations to positive affect systems appear to play a key role in adolescent development and adolescent depression, studies that examine positive affect components such as reward processing are particularly valuable. In addition, studies of the development of typical brain structure and function are needed to provide a context for findings of abnormalities associated with depression. With such studies, we can begin to understand the interplay of brain development, affect regulation, and depression. This approach can lead not only to better description of the pathophysiology of depression but to treatments targeted to the long-term functioning and development of those with depression.

REFERENCES

Allen, N.B., & Badcock, P.B.T. (2003). The social risk hypothesis of depressed mood: evolutionary, psychosocial, and neurobiological perspectives. *Psychological Bulletin,* **129**(6), 1–28.

Amodio, D.M., & Frith, C.D. (2006). Meeting of minds: the medial frontal cortex and social cognition. *Nature Reviews Neuroscience,* **7**(4), 268–277.

Baxter, M.G., & Murray, E.A. (2002). The amygdala and reward. *Nature Reviews: Neuroscience,* **3**(7), 563–573.

Berridge, K.C., & Robinson, T.E. (2003). Parsing reward. *Trends in Neurosciences,* **26**(9), 507–513.

Blier, P., & de Montigny, C. (1999). Serotonin and drug-induced therapeutic responses in major depression, obsessive-compulsive and panic disorders. *Neuropsychopharmacology,* **21**(2 Suppl), 91S–98S.

Brambilla, P., Glahn, D.C., Balestrieri, M., & Soares, J.C. (2005). Magnetic resonance findings in bipolar disorder. *Psychiatric Clinics of North America,* **28**(2), 443–467.

Bremner, J., & Vermetten, E. (2001). Stress and development: behavioral and biological consequences. *Development and Psychopathology,* **13**(3), 473–489.

Bukowski, W.M., Hoza, B., & Boivin, M. (1993). Popularity, friendship, and emotional adjustment during early adolescence. In B. Laursen (Ed.), *Close Friendships in Adolescence* (pp. 23–37). San Francisco, CA: Jossey-Bass.

Campbell, S., Marriott, M., Nahmias, C., & MacQueen, G.M. (2004). Lower hippocampal volume in patients suffering from depression: a meta-analysis. *American Journal of Psychiatry,* **161**(4), 598–607.

Carter, C.S., Braver, T.S., Barch, D.M. *et al.* (1998). Anterior cingulate cortex, error detection, and the online monitoring of performance. *Science,* **280**(5364), 747–749.

Casey, B.J., Giedd, J.N., & Thomas, K.M. (2000). Structural and functional brain development and its relation to cognitive development. *Biological Psychology,* **54**, 241–257.

Caspi, A., Sugden, K., Moffitt, T.E. *et al.* (2003). Influence of life stress on depression: moderation by a polymorphism in the 5-htt gene. *Science,* **301**(5631), 386–389.

Clark, L.A., & Watson, D. (1991). Tripartite model of anxiety and depression: psychometric evidence and taxonomic implications. *Journal of Abnormal Psychology,* **100**, 316–336.

Cole, P.M., Martin, S.E., & Dennis, T.A. (2004). Emotion regulation as a scientific construct: methodological challenges and directions for child development research. *Child Development*, **75**(2), 317–333.

Costello, E.J., Pine, D.S., Hammen, C. *et al.* (2002). Development and natural history of mood disorders. *Biological Psychiatry*, **52**(6), 529–542.

Cotter, D., Hudson, L., & Landau, S. (2005). Evidence for orbitofrontal pathology in bipolar disorder and major depression, but not in schizophrenia. *Bipolar Disorder*, **7**(4), 358–369.

Dahl, R.E., & Spear, L.P. (2004). Adolescent brain development. *Annals of the New York Academy of Sciences*, **1021**, 1–22.

Dahl, R.E., Ryan, N.D., Puig-Antich, J. *et al.* (1991). 24-hour cortisol measures in adolescents with major depression: a controlled study. *Biological Psychiatry*, **30**(1), 25–36.

Dalgleish, T. (2004). The emotional brain. *Nature Reviews: Neuroscience*, **5**(7), 583–589.

Davidson, R.J. (1994). Asymmetric brain function, affective style, and psychopathology: the role of early experience and plasticity. *Development and Psychopathology*, **6**, 741–758.

Davidson, R.J., & Irwin, W. (1999). The functional neuroanatomy of emotion and affective style. *Trends in Cognitive Sciences*, **3**(1), 11–21.

Davis, K.D., Taylor, S.J., Crawley, A.P., Wood, M.L., & Mikulis, D.J. (1997). Functional MRI of pain- and attention-related activations in the human cingulate cortex. *Journal of Neurophysiology*, **77**(6), 3370–3380.

Delgado, M.R., Nystrom, L.E., Fissell, C., Noll, D.C., & Fiez, J.A. (2000). Tracking the hemodynamic responses to reward and punishment in the striatum. *Journal of Neurophysiology*, **84**(6), 3072–3077.

Depue, R.A., & Iacono, W.G. (1989). Neurobehavioral aspects of affective disorders. *Annual Review of Psychology*, **40**, 457–492.

Devinsky, O., Morrell, M.J., & Vogt, B.A. (1995). Contributions of anterior cingulate cortex to behaviour. *Brain*, **118**(Pt 1), 279–306.

Drevets, W.C. (2001). Neuroimaging and neuropathological studies of depression: implications for the cognitive-emotional features of mood disorders. *Current Opinion in Neurobiology*, **11**, 240–249.

Drevets, W.C., Videen, T.O., Price, J.L. *et al.* (1992). A functional anatomical study of unipolar depression. *Journal of Neuroscience*, **12**(9), 3628–3641.

Drevets, W.C., Price, J.L., Simpson, J.R., Jr. *et al.* (1997). Subgenual prefrontal cortex abnormalities in mood disorders. *Nature*, **386**(6627), 824–827.

Drevets, W.C., Ongur, D., & Price, J.L. (1998). Neuroimaging abnormalities in the subgenual prefrontal cortex: Implications for the pathophysiology of familial mood disorders. *Molecular Psychiatry*, **3**(3), 220–226, 190–221.

Drevets, W.C., Gautier, C., Price, J.C. *et al.* (2001). Amphetamine-induced dopamine release in human ventral striatum correlates with euphoria. *Biological Psychiatry*, **49**(2), 81–96.

Duman, R.S., & Monteggia, L.M. (2006). A neurotrophic model for stress-related mood disorders. *Biological Psychiatry*, **59**(12), 1116–1127.

Durston, S., Hulshoff Pol, H.E., Casey, B.J. *et al.* (2001). Anatomical MRI of the developing human brain: what have we learned? *Journal of the American Academy of Child and Adolescent Psychiatry*, **40**(9), 1012–1020.

Eley, T., Sugden, K., Corsico, A. *et al.* (2004). Gene-environment interaction analysis of serotonin system markers with adolescent depression. *Molecular Psychiatry*, 9(10), 908–915.

Elliott, R., Rubinsztein, J.S., Sahakian, B.J., & Dolan, R.J. (2002). The neural basis of mood-congruent processing biases in depression. *Archives of General Psychiatry*, 59, 597–604.

Elliott, R., Newman, J.L., Longe, O.A., & Deakin, J.F. (2003). Differential response patterns in the striatum and orbitofrontal cortex to financial reward in humans: a parametric functional magnetic resonance imaging study. *Journal of Neuroscience*, 23(1), 303–307.

Elliott, R., Newman, J.L., Longe, O.A., & William Deakin, J.F. (2004). Instrumental responding for rewards is associated with enhanced neuronal response in subcortical reward systems. *Neuroimage*, 21(3), 984–990.

Ernst, M., Nelson, E.E., Jazbec, S. *et al.* (2005). Amygdala and nucleus accumbens in responses to receipt and omission of gains in adults and adolescents. *Neuroimage*, 25(4), 1279–1291.

Ernst, M., Pine, D.S., & Hardin, M. (2006). Triadic model of the neurobiology of motivated behavior in adolescence. *Psychological Medicine*, 36(3), 299–312.

Forbes, E.E., & Dahl, R.E. (2005). Neural systems of positive affect: relevance to understanding child and adolescent depression. *Development and Psychopathology*, 17(3), 827–850.

Forbes, E.E., Fox, N.A., Cohn, J.F., Galles, S.J., & Kovacs, M. (2006a). Children's affect regulation during a disappointment: psychophysiological responses and relation to parent history of depression. *Biological Psychology*, 71, 264–277.

Forbes, E.E., May, J.C., Ladouceur, C.D. *et al.* (2006b). Reward-related decision-making in pediatric major depressive disorder: an fMRI study. *Journal of Child Psychology and Psychiatry and Allied Disciplines*, 47(10), 1031–1040.

Forbes, E.E., Williamson, D.E., Ryan, N.D. *et al.* (2006c). Peri-sleep-onset cortisol levels in children and adolescents with affective disorders. *Biological Psychiatry*, 59(1), 24–30.

Forbes, E.E., Shaw, D.S., & Dahl, R.E. (2007). Alterations in reward-related decision making in boys with current and future depressive disorders. *Biological Psychiatry*, 61, 633–639.

Francis, D.D., Diorio, J., Plotsky, P.M., & Meaney, M.J. (2002). Environmental enrichment reverses the effects of maternal separation on stress reactivity. *Journal of Neuroscience*, 22, 7840–7843.

Galvan, A., Hare, T.A., Parra, C.E. *et al.* (2006). Earlier development of the accumbens relative to orbitofrontal cortex might underlie risk-taking behavior in adolescents. *Journal of Neuroscience*, 26(25), 6885–6892.

Garber, J., Braafladt, N., & Weiss, B. (1995). Affect regulation in depressed and nondepressed children and young adolescents. *Development and Psychopathology*, 7(1), 93–115.

Giedd, J.N. (2004). Structural magnetic resonance imaging of the adolescent brain. *Annals of the New York Academy of Sciences*, 1021, 77–85.

Gogtay, N., Giedd, J.N., Lusk, L. *et al.* (2004). Dynamic mapping of human cortical development during childhood through early adulthood. *Proceedings of the National Academy of Sciences USA*, 101(21), 8174–8179.

Gottfried, J.A., O'Doherty, J., & Dolan, R.J. (2003). Encoding predictive reward value in human amygdala and orbitofrontal cortex. *Science*, **301**, 1104–1107.

Hariri, A.R., Tessitore, A., Mattay, V.S., Fera, F., & Weinberger, D.R. (2002). The amygdala response to emotional stimuli: a comparison of faces and scenes. *Neuroimage*, **17**(1), 317–323.

Hoshi, E., Tremblay, L., Feger, J., Carras, P.L., & Strick, P.L. (2005). The cerebellum communicates with the basal ganglia. *Nature Neuroscience*, **8**(11), 1491–1493.

Huttenlocher, P.R. (1990). Morphometric study of human cerebral cortex development. *Neuropsychologia*, **28**(6), 517–527.

Huttenlocher, P.R., & Dabholkar, A.S. (1997). Regional differences in synaptogenesis in human cerebral cortex. *Journal of Comparative Neurology*, **387**(2), 167–178.

Kaufman, J., Birmaher, B., Perel, J. *et al.* (1997). The corticotropin-releasing hormone challenge in depressed abused, depressed nonabused, and normal control children. *Biological Psychiatry*, **42**(8), 669–679.

Kaufman, J., Yang, B.-Z., Douglas-Palumberi, H. *et al.* (2006). Brain-derived neurotrophic factor-5-HTTLPR gene interactions and environmental modifiers of depression in children. *Biological Psychiatry*, **59**, 673–680.

Keedwell, P.A., Andrew, C., Williams, S.C., Brammer, M.J., & Phillips, M.L. (2005a). A double dissociation of ventromedial prefrontal cortical responses to sad and happy stimuli in depressed and healthy individuals. *Biological Psychiatry*, **58**(6), 495–503.

Keedwell, P.A., Andrew, C., Williams, S.C., Brammer, M.J., & Phillips, M.L. (2005b). The neural correlates of anhedonia in major depressive disorder. *Biological Psychiatry*, **58**(11), 843–853.

Keller, A., Castellanos, F.X., Vaituzis, A.C., Jeffries, N.O., Giedd, J.N., & Rapoport, J.L. (2003). Progressive loss of cerebellar volume in childhood-onset schizophrenia. *American Journal of Psychiatry*, **160**(1), 128–133.

Kendler, K.S., Kuhn, J.W., Vittum, J., Prescott, C.A., & Riley, B. (2005). The interaction of stressful life events and a serotonin transporter polymorphism in the prediction of episodes of major depression. *Archives of General Psychiatry*, **62**(5), 529–535.

Kerns, J.G., Cohen, J.D., MacDonald, A.W., III *et al.* (2004). Anterior cingulate conflict monitoring and adjustments in control. *Science*, **303**(5660), 1023–1026.

Killgore, W.D., & Yurgelun-Todd, D.A. (2006). Ventromedial prefrontal activity correlates with depressed mood in adolescent children. *Neuroreport*, **17**(2), 167–171.

Knutson, B., Fong, G.W., Adams, C.M., Varner, J.L., & Hommer, D. (2001). Dissociation of reward anticipation and outcome with event-related fMRI. *Neuroreport*, **12**(17), 3683–3687.

Knutson, B., Fong, G.W., Bennett, S.M., Adams, C.M., & Hommer, D. (2003). A region of mesial prefrontal cortex tracks monetarily rewarding outcomes: characterization with rapid event-related fMRI. *Neuroimage*, **18**(2), 263–272.

Lacerda, A.L., Keshavan, M.S., Hardan, A.Y. *et al.* (2004). Anatomic evaluation of the orbitofrontal cortex in major depressive disorder. *Biological Psychiatry*, **55**(4), 353–358.

Lane, R.D., Reiman, E.M., Axelrod, B. *et al.* (1998). Neural correlates of levels of emotional awareness. Evidence of an interaction between emotion and attention in the anterior cingulate cortex. *Journal of Cognitive Neuroscience*, **10**(4), 525–535.

Lawrence, N.S., Williams, A.M., Surguladze, S. *et al.* (2004). Subcortical and ventral prefrontal cortical neural responses to facial expressions distinguish patients with bipolar disorder and major depression. *Biological Psychiatry,* **55**(6), 578–587.

Leonardo, E.D., & Hen, R. (2006). Genetics of affective and anxiety disorders. *Annual Review of Psychology,* **57**, 117–137.

Lewinsohn, P.M., & Clarke, G.N. (1999). Psychosocial treatments for adolescent depression. *Clinical Psychology Review,* **19**(3), 329–342.

Lewinsohn, P.M., Hoberman, H.M., Teri, L., & Hautzinger, M. (1985). An integrative theory of unipolar depression. In S. Reiss & R.R. Bootzin (Eds.), *Theoretical Issues in Behavior Therapy* (pp. 331–359). Orlando, FL: Academic Press.

Lucki, I. (1998). The spectrum of behaviors influenced by serotonin. *Biological Psychiatry,* **44**(3), 151–162.

Luna, B., & Sweeney, J.A. (2004). *Adolescent Brain Development: Vulnerabilities and Opportunities* (Vol. XII). New York, NY: New York Academy of Sciences.

March, J., Silva, S., Petrycki, S. *et al.* (2004). Fluoxetine, cognitive-behavioral therapy, and their combination for adolescents with depression: treatment for adolescents with depression study (TADS) randomized controlled trial. *Journal of the American Medical Association,* **292**(7), 807–820.

Mayberg, H.S., Liotti, M., Brannan, S.K. *et al.* (1999). Reciprocal limbic-cortical function and negative mood: converging PET findings in depression and normal sadness. *American Journal of Psychiatry,* **156**(5), 675–682.

McEwen, B.S. (1998). Protective and damaging effects of stress mediators. *New England Journal of Medicine,* **338**(3), 171–179.

Meaney, M.J. (2001). The development of individual differences in behavioral and endocrine responses to stress. *Annual Review of Neuroscience,* **24**, 1161–1192.

Middleton, F.A., & Strick, P.L. (2000). Basal ganglia and cerebellar loops: motor and cognitive circuits. *Brain Research. Brain Research Reviews,* **31**(2–3), 236–250.

Murphy, F.C., Nimmo-Smith, I., & Lawrence, A.D. (2003). Functional neuroanatomy of emotions: a meta-analysis. *Cognitive, Affective, and Behavioral Neuroscience,* **3**(3), 207–233.

Nelson, E.E., Leibenluft, E., McClure, E.B., & Pine, D.S. (2005). The social re-orientation of adolescence: a neuroscience perspective on the process and its relation to psychopathology. *Psychological Medicine,* **35**(2), 163–174.

Phillips, M.L., Drevets, W.C., Rauch, S.L., & Lane, R. (2003). Neurobiology of emotion perception II: implications for major psychiatric disorders. *Biological Psychiatry,* **54**(5), 515–528.

Plotsky, P.M., Owens, M.J., & Nemeroff, C.B. (1998). Psychoneuroendocrinology of depression: hypothalamic-pituitary-adrenal axis. *Psychiatric Clinics of North America,* **21**(2), 293–307.

Renouf, A.G., Kovacs, M., & Mukerji, P. (1997). Relationship of depressive, conduct, and comorbid disorders and social functioning in childhood. *Journal of the American Academy of Child and Adolescent Psychiatry,* **36**(7), 998–1004.

Rohde, P., Lewinsohn, P.M., & Seeley, J.R. (1991). Comorbidity of unipolar depression: II. Comorbidity with other mental disorders in adolescents and adults. *Journal of Abnormal Psychology,* **100**(2), 214–222.

Rolls, E.T. (1999). *The Brain and Emotion.* New York, NY: Oxford.

Rolls, E.T. (2000). The orbitofrontal cortex and reward. *Cerebral Cortex*, **10**, 284–294.

Rottenberg, J., Wilhelm, F.H., Gross, J.J., & Gotlib, I.H. (2003). Vagal rebound during resolution of tearful crying among depressed and nondepressed individuals. *Psychophysiology*, **40**, 1–6.

Sapolsky, R.M. (1996). Why stress is bad for your brain. *Science*, **273**(5276), 749–750.

Sassi, R.B., Brambilla, P., Hatch, J.P. *et al.* (2004). Reduced left anterior cingulate volumes in untreated bipolar patients. *Biological Psychiatry*, **56**(7), 467–475.

Schneider, F., Gur, R.E., Mozley, L.H. *et al.* (1995). Mood effects on limbic blood flow correlate with emotional self-rating: a PET study with oxygen-15 labeled water. *Psychiatry Research*, **61**(4), 265–283.

Schultz, W. (2000). Multiple reward signals in the brain. *Nature Reviews: Neuroscience*, **1**(3), 199–207.

Sheeber, L., Allen, N., Davis, B., & Sorensen, E. (2000). Regulation of negative affect during mother-child problem-solving interactions: adolescent depressive status and family processes. *Journal of Abnormal Child Psychology*, **28**(5), 467–479.

Sheline, Y.I., Barch, D.M., Donnelly, J.M. *et al.* (2001). Increased amygdala response to masked emotional faces in depressed subjects resolves with antidepressant treatment: an fMRI study. *Biological Psychiatry*, **50**(9), 651–658.

Siegle, G.J., Steinhauer, S.R., Thase, M.E., Stenger, V.A., & Carter, C.S. (2002). Can't shake that feeling: event-related fMRI assessment of sustained amygdala activity in response to emotional information in depressed individuals. *Biological Psychiatry*, **51**(9), 693–707.

Spanagel, R., & Weiss, F. (1999). The dopamine hypothesis of reward: past and current status. *Trends in Neurosciences*, **22**(11), 521–527.

Spear, L.P. (2000). The adolescent brain and age-related behavioral manifestations. *Neuroscience and Biobehavioral Reviews*, **24**, 417–463.

Steinberg, L. (2004). Risk-taking in adolescence: what changes, and why? *Annals of the New York Academy of Sciences*, **1021**, 51–58.

Strauss, J., Barr, C.L., George, C.J. *et al.* (2004). Association study of brain-derived neurotrophic factor in adults with a history of childhood onset mood disorder. *American Journal of Medical Genetics. Part B Neuropsychiatric Genetics*, **131**(1), 16–19.

Strauss, J., Barr, C.L., George, C.J. *et al.* (2005). Brain-derived neurotrophic factor variants are associated with childhood-onset mood disorder: confirmation in a Hungarian sample. *Molecular Psychiatry*, **10**(9), 861–867.

Surguladze, S., Brammer, M.J., Keedwell, P. *et al.* (2005). A differential pattern of neural response toward sad versus happy facial expressions in major depressive disorder. *Biological Psychiatry*, **57**, 201–209.

Tomarken, A.J., & Keener, A.D. (1998). Frontal brain asymmetry and depression: a self-regulatory perspective. *Cognition and Emotion*, **12**(3), 387–420.

Vasa, R.A., Carlino, A.R., & Pine, D.S. (2006). Pharmacotherapy of depressed children and adolescents: current issues and potential directions. *Biological Psychiatry*, **59**(11), 1021–1028.

Videbech, P., & Ravnkilde, B. (2004). Hippocampal volume and depression: a meta-analysis of MRI studies. *American Journal of Psychiatry*, **161**(11), 1957–1966.

The development of executive cognitive function and emotion regulation in adolescence

Amanda Kesek, Philip David Zelazo, and Marc D. Lewis

Adolescence is a time of great physical and psychological change, often accompanied by challenging emotional experiences. Many adolescents find themselves in conflict with parents and other adults as they struggle with powerful new feelings. However, adolescents also isolate themselves, sometimes for days at a time, and struggle with sadness, loneliness, shame, self-doubt, and other feelings associated with depression. The dramatic emotional states that adolescents experience challenge their developing abilities to regulate these emotions. Indeed, emotion regulation (i.e. the deliberate self-regulation of feelings, impulses, and appraisals) is one of the most important developmental processes of adolescence.

The capacity for emotion regulation increases throughout adolescence, as does the intensity of emotions themselves. However, these changes do not always occur in parallel. When the advent of novel emotional states precedes the development of the capacity to regulate them, adolescents may resemble unskilled drivers trying to maneuver a car that has just been turbo-charged by puberty (Dahl, 2004). In fact, many theorists consider it typical for regulatory capacities to lag behind increases in the intensity and range of emotions. This lag may explain the normative increase in negative emotion and family conflict reported by many researchers (e.g. Paikoff & Brooks-Gunn, 1991). For these reasons, understanding the neurocognitive bases of emotion regulation in adolescence is an important objective for developmental psychologists.

The ability to regulate emotions and behavior depends, in large part, on cognitive capacities that do not reach maturity until early adulthood. As adolescents develop, they show improvements in a variety of cognitive domains, including learning, reasoning, information processing and memory (for reviews see Byrnes, 2003; Kuhn, 2006). Many higher order cognitive

Adolescent Emotional Development and the Emergence of Depressive Disorders, ed. Nicholas B. Allen and Lisa B. Sheeber. Published by Cambridge University Press. © Cambridge University Press 2009.

functions are encompassed by the construct of executive function (EF) – the psychological processes involved in the deliberate self-regulation of thought, action, and emotion. These functions include, among others, cognitive flexibility, goal-setting, and online performance monitoring (Zelazo & Müller, 2002). The goal of this chapter is to review the neural underpinnings of self-regulatory capacity – studied under the rubric of EF – as it develops through late childhood and adolescence.

Overview

Historically, it was believed that the adolescent brain resembled the brain of an adult, with no significant changes occurring after childhood. However, recent research using neuroimaging techniques has revealed that although the brain has reached about 95% of its total volume by middle childhood (Caviness *et al.*, 1996; Reiss *et al.*, 1996), it continues to undergo considerable development until young adulthood – particularly in regions such as prefrontal cortex (PFC), the part of cerebral cortex anterior to premotor cortex and the supplementary motor area. The development of PFC that takes place during this period may underlie improvement in various fundamental cognitive capacities, including EF. The successes and failures that adolescents experience in regulating their emotions may depend largely on developmental and individual differences in PFC-mediated EF abilities.

Executive function emerges early in development and continues to develop through adolescence, in parallel with changes in PFC. The close connection between EF and the PFC is now well established (Luria, 1966; Stuss & Benson, 1986). Early studies on patients with prefrontal damage revealed a peculiar pattern of impairments despite preservation of basic cognitive functions, including many aspects of language, memory, and intelligence (Luria, 1973). The impairments, which have a family resemblance, include (but are not limited to) failures to make "wise" judgments, poor planning of future actions, and difficulty inhibiting inappropriate responses (Stuss & Benson, 1986). The construct of EF is intended to capture the psychological abilities whose impairment is presumed to underlie these manifest deficits: the ability to make wise judgments, the ability to plan, the ability to inhibit inappropriate responses, and the ability to monitor and modify cognitive appraisals. The development of these abilities during adolescence will be reviewed below, along with some speculations as to their role in emotion regulation. First, however, we begin with a brief discussion of the development of the prefrontal cortex during this period.

Development of prefrontal cortex in adolescence

Until recently, examination of brain structure and function depended on autopsy and lesion work, and it was, therefore, difficult to study the adolescent brain (Casey *et al.*, 2000). Recent technological advances, however, have allowed unprecedented opportunities to track developmental changes in the brain. One of the most exciting developments is functional magnetic resonance imaging (fMRI), which measures changes in the ratio of oxygenated and deoxygenated blood that occur as a result of activity in specific brain regions. Although fMRI has relatively poor temporal resolution (when compared with electrophysiological techniques), it can provide excellent anatomical resolution, as well as a fairly accurate estimate of the location of the neural activity associated with a specific task. Through cross-sectional and longitudinal studies, fMRI has provided us with a much clearer picture of the structural and functional changes that occur over the course of childhood and adolescence.

There is a great deal of variability within brain structures, even among healthy, typically developing populations (Giedd *et al.*, 1996). However, there are some relatively consistent patterns of structural change that are seen over the course of adolescence. One well-documented change in neural structure during late childhood and adolescence is the shift in the ratio of white to gray matter in brain. Cell bodies, dendrites, and synapses comprise most of the gray matter, whereas white matter is made up of axons covered by myelin, which insulates axons and facilitates the conduction of electrical impulses. Among the white matter tracts is the corpus callosum, which connects the two cerebral hemispheres. Typically, white matter volume increases linearly over the course of childhood, as a function of myelination. In contrast, gray matter volume increases in most regions until early or middle childhood and then declines (Huttenlocher, 1990), with lateral PFC being among the last regions to reach adult levels of gray matter volume (Gogtay *et al.*, 2004; O'Donnell *et al.*, 2005). More recent research suggests that there is another transitory increase in gray matter volume around puberty (Giedd *et al.*, 1999; Gogtay *et al.*, 2004). Reductions in gray matter volume are typically attributed to synaptic pruning, which may occur as a function of learning and experience (Casey *et al.*, 2000; Durston *et al.*, 2001). The over-production and subsequent pruning around puberty may reflect the experience-dependent reorganization of cognitive functions believed to take place at this time (Spear, 2000).

The PFC itself is a heterogenous region, and it comprises several distinct subregions, including orbitofrontal cortex (OFC), anterior cingulate cortex (ACC), and ventrolateral (VL-PFC), dorsolateral (DL-PFC), and rostrolateral prefrontal cortices (RL-PFC; Figure 8.1). Evidence for the functional specificity of various regions of PFC has been established by a number of different neuropsychological approaches. These regions differ on a cellular level and vary in the way in which they are connected to other brain regions. Studies involving both human patients and primates have demonstrated that unique patterns of cognitive impairment accompany lesions in various regions of

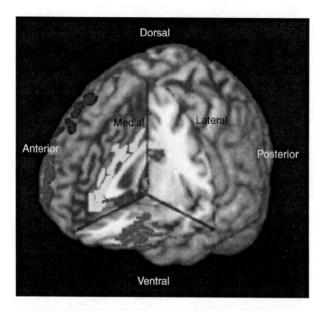

Figure 8.1. This figure is also reproduced in color between pages 144 and 145. The human brain, showing various regions of prefrontal cortex. Green: orbitofrontal cortex; Yellow: anterior cingulate cortex; Blue: dorsolateral prefrontal cortex (DL-PFC); Red: rostrolateral prefrontal cortices. Ventrolateral prefrontal cortex, which is more ventral than DL-PFC, is not shown. (Reprinted with permission from Bunge, S., & Zelazo, P.D. (2006). A brain-based account of the development of rule use in childhood. *Current Directions in Psychological Science*, **15**, 118–121).

the PFC. As well, researchers have used fMRI to investigate more directly the brain regions recruited by children and adults as they perform diverse tasks designed to assess various aspects of cognitive functioning. Within PFC, there is evidence that more ventral regions develop more rapidly than more anterior and more dorsal regions (Gogtay *et al.*, 2004).

The neural maturation that occurs over the course of adolescence is associated with general changes in patterns of neural recruitment. Specifically, several researchers have noted a shift from more diffuse to more focal activation of PFC (Bunge *et al.*, 2002; Casey *et al.*, 1997). This increasing focalization suggests more specialized and efficient processing with development, which can lead to improvements in EF. Older children and children who perform better on measures of EF show more focal patterns of neural activation (i.e. more activation in areas related to EF in adults, less activation in unrelated areas). For example, Durston *et al.* (2006), in a combined longitudinal and cross-sectional design, had children perform a target detection task. Older children tended to recruit a more focused range of brain regions, and this shift was accompanied by an improvement in performance.

Another general trend in neural maturation is increasing reliance on more anterior regions of cortex (i.e. frontalisation). Rubia *et al.* (2000) had adolescents and young adults perform a stop signal task and a motor synchronization task, and found a general pattern of increased frontal activation with age. For example, in the motor synchronization task, the better performance demonstrated by adults was accompanied by increased activity in a fronto-striato-parietal network. This trend is also seen using electroencephalography (EEG), which measures the electrical activity generated at the scalp. Event-related potentials (ERPs) are EEG components time-locked to particular stimuli and/or responses. Lamm *et al.* (2006) measured ERPs as children and adolescents performed a Go/No-Go task, and collected a number of behavioral measures of EF. The N2 component of the ERP, an index of cognitive control, was source localized to the cingulate cortex and to VL-PFC. However, the source of the N2 in those children who performed well on the EF tasks was more anterior than that of children who performed poorly. This suggests that children rely more heavily on more anterior regions of PFC as performance on measures of EF increases.

Age-related changes in executive function

Traditionally, conceptualizations of EF have focused on its relatively "cool" aspects, often associated with lateral PFC, which primarily involve cognitive, abstract, and decontextualized reasoning (Happaney *et al.*, 2004; Zelazo & Müller, 2002). Recently, however, there has been growing interest in the interaction of cognition and emotion, including the development of relatively "hot" aspects of EF, which predominate in situations that are emotionally and motivationally significant, often involving rewards, or the re-appraisal of previously rewarding stimuli. Emotion regulation may be a function of both hot and cool EF. Currently felt or more intense emotions may require regulation by EF processes we describe as hot. Inhibiting emotional impulses would epitomize this sort of self-control. In contrast, the ability to compare events, update the context of events, and avoid or adjust situations that might lead to negative emotions involves a kind of self-regulation that requires cool EF processes. These more sophisticated aspects of emotion regulation appear to be precisely what adolescents often lack.

Orbitofrontal cortex is part of a fronto-striatal circuit that has strong connections to the amygdala and other parts of the limbic system. It also receives input from taste, olfactory, and somatosensory areas, which process information about primary reinforcers, and so it is uniquely positioned to be highly involved in learning and evaluating reward contingencies and regulating emotional behavior (Rolls, 2004). Although PFC develops later than other areas of the brain, there is some evidence that OFC develops earlier than areas associated with more relatively cool aspects of EF, such as DL-PFC (Gogtay *et al.*, 2004). Thus, adolescents may be able to exert OFC-mediated regulatory processes, through hot EF, but remain unable to adopt cool EF for modifying emotional decisions using higher-order strategies.

Although different contexts may evoke relatively hot or cool aspects of EF, there is a constant dynamic interaction between cognition and emotion. The PFC is an integrated system, and both affective and cognitive aspects of EF may be elicited in a single situation. Zelazo & Cunningham (2007) have proposed a model integrating hot and cool EF, suggesting that these two constructs represent a continuum rather than a dichotomy. This model follows the course of information processing from the thalamus and amygdala, which generate quick emotional response tendencies that are then fed into the OFC. The orbitofrontal cortex then generates simple approach-avoidance (stimulus-reward) rules and is also involved in learning to reverse these rules. If these relatively unreflective processes fail to provide an adequate response to the situation, anterior cingulate cortex (ACC), thought to act as a performance monitor, signals the need for further, higher-level processing in lateral PFC. Different regions of lateral PFC are involved in representing rules at different levels of complexity – from sets of conditional rules (VL-PFC and DL-PFC), to explicit consideration of task sets (RL-PFC), as proposed by Bunge & Zelazo (2006).

Work on the development of rule use in children suggests that children first acquire the ability to use a single rule, then a pair of rules, and then a hierarchical system of rules that allows them to select among incompatible pairs of rules (Zelazo *et al.*, 2003). According to the Levels of Consciousness Model (Zelazo, 2004) and the Cognitive Complexity and Control-Revised theory (Zelazo *et al.*, 2003), these increases in the complexity of children's rule systems are made possible by age-related increases in the highest degree of conscious reflection that children can muster in response to situational demands, where conscious reflection is modeled as re-entrant signaling of information via thalamo-cortical circuits involving the PFC. Reflection on rules formulated at one level of complexity is required in order to formulate higher-order rules that control the application of these lower-order rules.

Figure 8.2 illustrates the way in which regions of PFC may correspond to rule use at different levels of complexity. As should be clear, the function of PFC is proposed to be hierarchical in a way that corresponds to the hierarchical complexity of the rule use underlying EF. As individuals engage in reflective processing, ascend through levels of consciousness, and formulate more complex rule systems, they recruit an increasingly complex hierarchical

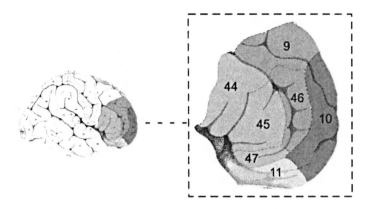

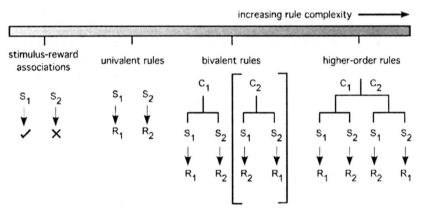

Figure 8.2. A hierarchical model of rule representation in prefrontal cortex (PFC). A lateral view of the human brain is depicted at the top of the figure, with regions of PFC identified by the Brodmann areas (BA) that comprise them: Orbitofrontal cortex (BA 11), ventrolateral PFC (BA 44, 45, 47), dorsolateral PFC (BA 9, 46), and rostrolateral PFC (BA 10). The PFC regions are shown in various shades of gray, indicating which types of rules they represent. Rule structures are depicted below, with darker shades of gray indicating increasing levels of rule complexity. The formulation and maintenance in working memory of more complex rules depends on the reprocessing of information through a series of levels of consciousness, which in turn depends on the recruitment of additional regions of PFC into an increasingly complex hierarchy of PFC activation. Note: S = stimulus; check (✓) = reward; cross (×) = non-reward; R = response; C = context, or task set. Brackets indicate a bivalent rule that is currently being ignored. (Reprinted with permission from Bunge, S., & Zelazo, P. D. (2006). A brain-based account of the development of rule use in childhood. *Current Directions in Psychological Science*, **15**, 118–121).

network of PFC regions. This can be viewed as a shift from hotter to cooler aspects of EF.

Developmental research suggests that the order of acquisition of rule types corresponds to the order in which each of these regions matures. In particular, gray matter volume reaches adult levels earliest in OFC, followed by VL-PFC, and then by DL-PFC (Giedd *et al.*, 1999). Measures of cortical thickness suggest that DL-PFC and RL-PFC exhibit similar, slow rates of structural change (Nagy *et al.*, 2004). On the basis of this evidence, Bunge & Zelazo (2006) hypothesized that the pattern of developmental changes in rule use reflects the different rates of development of specific regions within PFC. The use of relatively complex rules is acquired late in development because it involves the hierarchical coordination of regions of PFC – a hierarchical coordination that parallels the hierarchical structure of children's rule systems and develops in a bottom-up fashion, with higher levels in the hierarchy operating on the products of lower levels.

In the following sections, we will elaborate on these processes and their development in adolescence, consider their role in emotion regulation, and then consider briefly how atypical development of EF may be associated with emotional problems that have clinical relevance.

Orbitofrontal cortex: approach-avoidance decisions

Delay of gratification

Orbitofrontal cortex function has been assessed using a variety of related paradigms (Monterosso *et al.*, 2001), and several of these paradigms have been used with young children. For example, delay of gratification tasks measure a child's ability to refuse an immediate reward in favor of a larger reward later. In one classic version, developed by Mischel *et al.* (1972), children are told they can wait for two treats, or they can choose to end their wait and have only one treat. In a modified version of this task, where children were asked to decide if they would like a small reward now or a larger reward later, age-related changes in the tendency to delay gratification were observed between 3 and 5 years (Prencipe & Zelazo, 2005; Thompson *et al.*, 1997). Although young children have a tendency to approach the treat they are presented, they must avoid this treat if they wish to reach their goal of having two treats. The ability to inhibit behavioral responses based on immediate desires is a capacity that develops with age, and likely depends on the development of the OFC. This ability is clearly necessary for processes of emotion regulation that pave the way for normal social development.

This delay of gratification paradigm is a powerful predictor of many later outcomes. In longitudinal studies of children who performed this task in preschool, the amount of time children were able to wait was predictive of later outcomes, including academic achievement and parent-rated competence in a number of domains, such as attentiveness, verbal ability, ability to plan, and coping skills (Mischel et al., 1988, 1989). The ability to delay gratification in preschool is also a predictor of EF as assessed by a Go/No-Go paradigm administered 14 years later. Eigsti and colleagues (2006) divided children who had performed the standard delay of gratification task in preschool into two groups: children who were highly focused on the reward or on the bell that would enable them to end their wait, and children who did not focus on these items. Children in the low-temptation group were able to execute responses more quickly on the go trials, with no reduction in accuracy, than children in the high-temptation group. This suggests that both the tendency to direct one's attention from a tempting treat at the age of 4 years and performance on Go/No-Go at age 18 years reflect the development of relatively general aspects of attentional control.

Although the standard delay of gratification tasks used in research with young children do not immediately lend themselves to work with adolescents, the tendency to delay rewards in adolescence can be assessed using the delay-discounting paradigm. Typically, people prefer immediate rewards; the value of a future reward tends to be systematically discounted and children tend to discount the value of future rewards more quickly than adults (Green et al., 1999). Just as individual differences in the ability to delay gratification in children are predictors of later outcomes, delay discounting is a predictor of behavior and academic success in adolescents (Duckworth & Seligman, 2006). The predictive power of the relatively simple decision to delay gratification in anticipation of a later, greater reward suggests that this process is a foundational one. The ability to apply simple approach-avoidance rule systems in childhood may serve as the basis for the hierarchical development of more complex rule systems in adolescence. Individual differences in the ability to manipulate these rule systems may correspond with differences in the capacity to think one's way out of threatening or dangerous situations characterized by conflicting emotions.

Decision making and reward learning

Delay of gratification paradigms require relatively simple decision making: a larger reward is guaranteed, if one is willing to wait. However, more complex decision-making often requires individuals to use probabilistic and ambiguous information. One of the most commonly used measures to assess complex decision-making is the Iowa Gambling Task, which requires participants to make approach-avoidance decisions in the face of uncertainty (Bechara et al., 1994). In this task, participants are presented with two decks of cards, one advantageous and one disadvantageous in the long run.

Typically, adults begin by selecting from the decks at random. Over the course of the task, adults are able to use the information they gain to modify their pattern of responding, and they begin to favor the more advantageous decks.

Kerr & Zelazo (2004) developed a version of this task for children and presented reward and loss information in the form of happy and sad faces. Three-year-olds performed poorly on this task, failing to develop a preference for the advantageous decks. Four- and 5-year-olds, on the other hand, were able to make advantageous decisions. The ability to make advantageous decisions in an affective context increases dramatically in the preschool years, but it continues to improve throughout childhood. Crone *et al.* (2005) examined the performance of children aged 7–12 on a gambling task, and found that children between the ages of 7 and 12 were able to make advantageous decisions on a gambling task when punishment, in the form of losses, was presented frequently. However, when punishment was infrequent, and children had to regulate their behavior more independently, they tended to make decisions resembling those made by patients with OFC damage; the tendency to make advantageous choices with infrequent punishment improved with age.

A number of studies have examined adolescents' performance on various gambling tasks; throughout adolescence the tendency to make advantageous decisions increases (Hooper *et al.*, 2004; Overman *et al.*, 2004). For example, Crone & van der Molen (2004), in a task similar to the Iowa Gambling Task, observed increasingly advantageous patterns of responding observable throughout childhood and adolescence. Overman *et al.* (2004) found that older adolescents not only made more advantageous decisions, they also modified their responding after fewer trials than younger children. Whether these improvements are mediated by continued development of OFC circuits, or by connections between OFC and other prefrontal regions, remains to be determined.

Medial PFC: performance monitoring

A crucial element of EF is the ability to recognize when actions do not have the intended effect, necessitating further processing. Although the OFC is able to generate approach-avoidance response rules, and plays a key role in learning to reverse these rules, these relatively simple rule systems may not be able to deal successfully with more complex or ambiguous situations and stimuli. Within the context of Zelazo & Cunningham's model (2007), a performance monitoring system, mediated by medial PFC (Ridderinkhof *et al.*, 2004), may signal the need for more elaborate processing dependent on lateral PFC. The anterior cingulate cortex (ACC) is considered a key component of

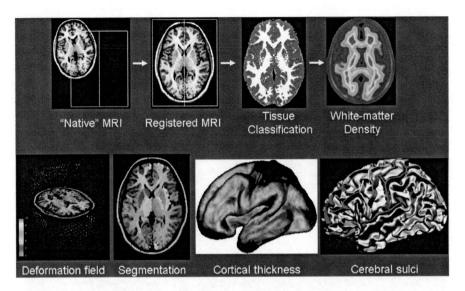

Figure 6.1

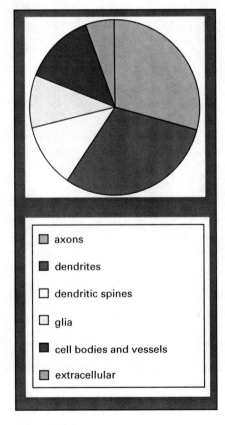

Figure 6.2 (a)

These figures are available for download in colour from www.cambridge.org/9781107406599

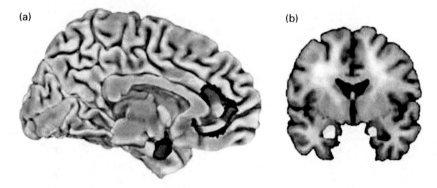

Figure 6.5

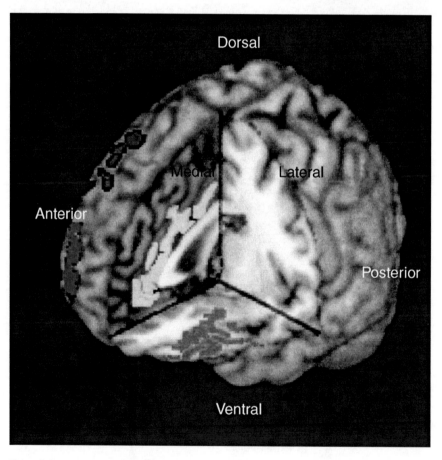

Figure 8.1

this system. Medial PFC, including ACC, may begin to develop earlier than dorsal and lateral PFC, but still follow a protracted developmental course.

Typically, younger children make more errors on tasks requiring EF than adults, and may be less aware of them. One way to assess performance monitoring is using ERPs. The ERN (error-related negativity) is a negative-going ERP component, probably originating in the ACC, which is associated with the realization that an error has been committed (Segalowitz & Davies, 2004). There is also a smaller negativity associated with correct responses (Ford, 1999), and both negativities are often considered part of a class of medial frontal negativities (MFNs) that reflect performance monitoring (e.g. Ridderinkhof et al., 2004). The N2, discussed earlier, is considered a member of this class of ERPs as well (Tucker et al., 2003). Often, very young children display no post-error ERN, or one that is much smaller in amplitude than is typically observed in adults.

Segalowitz et al. (2004) measured the ERN in participants from age 10 to age 25 as they completed the Eriksen flanker task. This task requires participants to identify the letter in the center of a string of either congruent (e.g. SSSSS) or incongruent flankers (e.g. SSHSS). The results suggest that the development of ACC follows a protracted course, which may be related to puberty. In general, ERN amplitude increased with age. In addition, however, Davies et al. (2004) examined ERPs during a flanker task and found a U-shaped drop in the amplitude of the ERN that was maximal for boys at age 13 years and maximal for girls at age 10 years, which is consistent with what one would expect if this dip were related to puberty.

A number of other studies have also found similar increases in ERN amplitude in older adolescents (Hogan et al., 2005; Ladouceur et al., 2004). The observed changes in the ERN correspond to improved task performance, including fewer errors and quicker response times, suggesting that the ability to perform online error monitoring is an important element in the development of EF. The role of the medial PFC, including ACC, in managing conflict, as well as its relatively late maturation, suggest that this brain region may be an important mediator of developmental changes in the ability to resolve conflict by recognizing the need for more elaborate processing.

Not only is performance monitoring a key element of EF, but it is one that can readily be seen to apply to emotion regulation. In real life, situations that involve conflict and require resolution through the formulation of rule hierarchies almost always involve emotions, and these generally include negative emotions. Thus, the development of ACC-mediated performance monitoring to adjust one's thought or behavior must be a critical step along the developmental path of emotion regulation abilities. If these abilities are still developing during the adolescent years, as suggested by research on ERN amplitudes, then younger teenagers may often be unable to adjust their thought and behavior when emotional demands are highly salient.

Lateral PFC: rule use at various levels of complexity

The activation of medial PFC, signaling that the simple approach-avoidance tendencies generated by the OFC have not resolved the present situation, may lead to more elaborate processing in lateral areas of PFC, including the formulation of increasingly complex rules for controlling behavior. In contrast to OFC, which represents simple approach-avoidance tendencies, both VL-PFC and DL-PFC have been consistently implicated in the retrieval, maintenance, and use of more complex sets of conditional rules in both lesion studies and fMRI studies (Bunge, 2004). For example, using fMRI, Crone *et al.* (2006) found that both VL-PFC and DL-PFC are active during the maintenance of sets of conditional rules, and that they are sensitive to rule complexity, showing more activation for bivalent rules than for univalent rules. Bunge *et al.* (2003) observed that these two regions are also more active for more abstract conditional rules ("match" or "non-match" rules, whereby different actions are required depending on whether two objects match or not) than for specific stimulus-response associations.

The ability to use rules flexibly to guide behavior often requires the use of one set of bivalent rules while ignoring competing alternatives. fMRI data suggest that DL-PFC may be especially important when participants must resist interference from a previously relevant rule. For example, MacDonald *et al.* (2000) found that as participants completed a Stroop task, the left DL-PFC was more active when participants had to name the color of the word, overriding the tendency to read the word. Further, the level of activation in DL-PFC in individual participants was predictive of the size of their Stroop-interference effect (the difference in response time between word reading and color-naming trials).

Bivalent rule use in young children has often been assessed using the Dimensional Change Card Sort (DCCS; Zelazo *et al.*, 1996, 2003). In this task, children are presented with cards that vary on two dimensions, shape and color. In what is termed the pre-switch phase of the task, the child is instructed to sort the cards by one of these dimensions. After a number of pre-switch trials, the child is told that he or she is now going to play a new game, and is instructed to sort by the previously irrelevant dimension. Even though children appear to understand the rules, and can successfully answer questions about which dimension they should use for sorting, the majority of 3-year-olds continue to sort by the pre-switch dimension.

By the age of 4, most children no longer perseverate on the DCCS and are able to successfully switch from sorting by color to sorting by shape. However, difficulties associated with switching between rule sets continue to persist across the lifespan. The well-documented increase in reaction time associated with switching between tasks is referred to as switch cost (e.g. Rogers & Monsell, 1995). Using a task similar to the DCCS, but modified for older participants, Zelazo *et al.* (2004) found that performance improved substantially between about 9 years of age and early adulthood. Moreover, these improvements were related to estimates of conscious control of memory generated by Jacoby's (1991) process dissociation procedure.

Lifespan studies of the ability to switch rapidly between rules and/or responses suggest that the development of switching follows a U-shaped curve, with reductions in switch cost throughout childhood and adolescence, and subsequent increases in older adults (Cepeda *et al.*, 2001; Zelazo *et al.*, 2004). Crone *et al.* (2004) administered a task similar to the Wisconsin Card Sorting Test that required children and adolescents to adjust their responses on the basis of negative feedback. There was a large decrease in the tendency to make perseverative errors (i.e. continuing to sort by the same rule after receiving negative feedback) between the ages of 8 and 12. However, errors due to distraction were not reduced to adult levels until 13 to 15 years. This study demonstrates that a number of factors may be responsible for the observed differences in EF across the age span of late childhood and adolescence.

The hypothesis that DL-PFC plays a key role in following bivalent rules – using one pair of rules while ignoring a competing alternative – is consistent with its well-documented role in working memory, the ability to maintain and manipulate information to control responding. That is, working memory involves working on some information (e.g. trial-unique information) while ignoring other information (e.g. information from previous trials). Working memory has been linked to DL-PFC function using a number of different neuropsychological methods, including fMRI and lesion studies (Braver *et al.*, 1997; Diamond & Goldman-Rakic, 1989). To examine whether DL-PFC also underlies working memory in children, Casey and colleagues (1995) had children complete a working memory task in an fMRI scanner. Participants between 9 and 11 years completed a task that required them to respond to a target letter only if an identical letter had been presented two trials previously. Neural activation was observed in DL-PFC and ACC, which mirrors the pattern of activation observed in adults who performed an identical task of working memory (Cohen *et al.*, 1997).

Studies involving children in early and middle childhood have found marked improvement in working memory capacity over this age range, but there is limited behavioral research with young people over the age of 12 years. The developmental trajectory of working memory is often inferred from research involving young children and older adults, with relatively little work on adolescence. The research that has been done suggests that increases in working memory capacity continue through adolescence. Luciana *et al.* (2005) administered several different tasks with varying level of difficulty, designed to assess various aspects of working memory, to participants age 9 to 20 years. More difficult applications of working memory were associated with different developmental trajectories. Memory for faces matured early, with little observable improvement after the age of 9 years, whereas the ability to develop a strategy for visual search continued to improve until the age of 16.

Whereas VL-PFC is thought to be important for the representation and maintenance of rules, and DL-PFC is thought to play an important role in implementing rules in the face of interference, RL-PFC is hypothesized to be involved in reflection on task sets, as when switching between two abstract rules (Bunge *et al.*, 2005; Crone *et al.*, 2006), integrating information in the context of analogical reasoning (Christoff *et al.*, 2001), or coordinating hierarchically embedded goals (Koechlin *et al.*, 1999). Indeed, there is evidence that RL-PFC may interact with different parts of prefrontal cortex (i.e. VL-PFC or DL-PFC) depending on the type of task involved (Sakai & Passingham, 2003, 2006), and hence, we would argue, depending on the complexity of the rule systems involved. Little is known about the development of RL-PFC, but it seems likely that, like DL-PFC, RL-PFC does not complete its development until late adolescence or early adulthood (O'Donnell *et al.*, 2005).

The slow development of lateral PFC is likely to have profound implications for emotion regulation. Adolescents who have difficulty switching between higher-order rules, or set-shifting in general, will also have difficulty regulating their interpretations of emotion-eliciting situations when more than one interpretation is available. For example, the decision to take drugs can be looked at as a function of one's growing independence or as a risk that is not worth taking. Emotions of excitement, shame, and anxiety have to be regulated by switching between these interpretations effectively. Similarly, sophisticated working memory abilities are necessary for regulating emotions related to one's self-concept, which may be particularly unstable for youths with depressive tendencies. It is important to hold in mind an image of one's positive qualities, admirable deeds, and so forth, perhaps in comparison with those of one's peers, in order to regulate feelings of shame, sadness, and self-blame. As before, major developmental changes in these emotion-regulatory capacities point to important normative advances and milestones, with critical implications for parenting practices and other forms of social support. However, they also point to the likelihood of wide-ranging individual differences during the adolescent years, and these differences have ramifications for developing behavior problems and serious clinical disorders.

Adjustment outcomes

Difficulties with EF are typical in childhood and adolescence, but they are especially pronounced in children who are diagnosed with particular disorders such as conduct disorder, anxiety, attention deficit hyperactivity disorder (ADHD), and depression. Children with these disorders may have particular difficulty with rule use – they may know rules and be able to articulate them, but nonetheless have considerable difficulty putting them into practice. Because EF develops so slowly, and is associated with the PFC, which continues to develop into adulthood, it is perhaps not surprising that impairments in EF (albeit slightly different patterns of impairment) are associated with so many different disorders with childhood onset. The model presented here provides a framework for considering these impairments. For example, children may have difficulty detecting conflict (and hence, detecting the need for elaborative rule processing), or they may detect conflict but have difficulty formulating more complex rule systems to control their responding.

With the development of PFC and EF, children and adolescents are typically better able to monitor their own actions, focus on alternative appraisals or strategies, disengage from distressing cues, and inhibit impulses. The initial emotional responses generated by more subcortical and ventral areas of PFC can be processed further, reducing the influence of relatively "hot" situations. As children mature, they are typically able to regulate negative emotions more efficiently. Lewis *et al.* (2006) examined developmental differences in two inhibitory ERPs, the N2 and frontal P3, before and after negative emotion induction. Typically developing children between the ages 5 and 16 performed a Go/No-Go task with the goal of maintaining a high level of points to win a desirable prize. However, after some initial success, a change in the algorithm caused the children to lose all their points. It was hypothesized that these two ERP amplitudes would diminish with age, consistent with fMRI and ERP studies suggesting that cortical efficiency improves with development, but that amplitudes would increase with the emotion induction, indicating greater efforts at inhibitory control. Indeed, both the frontal N2 and frontal P3 components decreased in amplitude as well as latency across five age points in a fairly linear profile. Amplitudes were also greater following the emotion induction phase of the task, suggesting increased EF in the service of emotion regulation.

Given that EF is required in the service of affect regulation, deficits in EF may underlie mood disorders. Depressed adolescents may tend to ruminate on particular higher-order rules, impairing their ability to switch flexibly between task sets. Depressed adults and adolescents show deficits in a number of set-shifting paradigms, including the WCST, which requires the ability to shift flexibly between abstract rules (Merriam *et al.*, 1999; Purcell *et al.*, 1997). The deficits in cognitive flexibility demonstrated by depressed patients are often accompanied by distinct attention biases and increased activation of the amygdala in response to negative stimuli (Siegle *et al.*, 2002). The symptoms associated with depression may be due, in part, to deficits in the ability to employ top-down control in choosing among tasks sets, accompanied by the tendency to attend selectively to negative stimuli.

Summary

The development of EF in childhood and adolescence follows a protracted course that mirrors the slow development of PFC. Future research should continue to elucidate the exact nature of the neural and cognitive processes involved in EF. On the account presented here, stimuli in the environment are processed through a hierarchical circuit, starting with a relatively automatic subcortical amygdala response; this amygdala response feeds into OFC and, if further processing is necessary, this is signaled by ACC activation which recruits more lateral areas of PFC. Although some situations and problems may be addressed with the relatively simple response tendencies generated by OFC, more complex or ambiguous situations require more reflective, top-down control. These processes develop throughout childhood and adolescence, mirroring the developmental course of the PFC.

With the development of PFC, adolescents are able to use increasingly complex rule hierarchies to guide their actions. Age-related improvements in working memory allow several relevant rule sets to be kept in mind, and leading to the ability to select among competing task sets, and improvements in the ability to ignore irrelevant information. Adolescents are increasingly able to implement top-down control, reducing the influence of bottom-up, automatic processing that often dominates in children. However, EF appears to be a fragile, complex developmental achievement that is vulnerable to disruption from a variety of sources, ranging from genetic abnormalities to environmental stressors.

Deficits in EF may have implications for the ability to successfully regulate emotions, leading to disorders such as anxiety and depression. Neurocognitive work on different developmental disorders may reveal distinct patterns of impairment in EF. Children and adolescents with anxiety or depression may experience intense emotional reactions to negative stimuli, and have difficulty mediating these reactions with higher-order processing. Depressed adolescents, for example, may tend to ruminate on particular higher-order rules, impairing their ability to switch flexibly between task sets.

Further research remains to be done, of course. Our hope is that with knowledge of the course of typical development of EF, and what happens when this development goes awry, we will be better positioned to develop interventions that help children to acquire the EF skills they need to regulate their emotions effectively.

REFERENCES

Bechara, A., Damasio, A. R., Damasio, H., & Anderson S. W. (1994). Insensitivity to future consequences following damage to human prefrontal cortex. *Cognition*, **50**, 7–15.

Braver T.S., Cohen J.D., Nystron, L.E. *et al.* (1997). A parametric study of prefrontal cortex involvement in human working memory. *Neuroimage*, **5**, 49–62.

Bunge, S.A. (2004). How we use rules to select actions: a review of evidence from cognitive neuroscience. *Cognitive, Affective, and Behavioral Neuroscience*, **4**, 564–579.

Bunge, S., & Zelazo, P.D. (2006). A brain-based account of the development of rule use in childhood. *Current Directions in Psychological Science*, **15**, 118–121.

Bunge, S.A., Dudukovic, N.M., Thomason, M.E., Vaidya, C.J., & Gabrieli, J.D.E. (2002). Development of frontal lobe contributions to cognitive control in children: evidence from fMRI. *Neuron*, **33**, 301–311.

Bunge, S.A., Kahn, I., Wallis, J.D., Miller, E.K., & Wagner, A.D. (2003). Neural circuits subserving the retrieval and maintenance of abstract rules. *Journal of Neurophysiology*, **90**, 3419–3428.

Bunge, S.A., Wallis, J.D., Parkers, A. *et al.* (2005). Neural circuitry underlying rule use in humans and nonhuman primates. *Journal of Neuroscience*, **25**, 10347–10350.

Byrnes, J.P. (2003). Cognitive development during adolescence. In G.R. Adams & M.D. Berzonsky (Eds.), *Blackwell Handbook of Adolescence* (pp. 227–246). Malden, MA: Blackwell Publishing.

Casey, B.J., Cohen, J.D., Jezzard, P. *et al.* (1995). Activation of prefrontal cortex in children during a nonspatial working memory task with functional MRI. *Neuroimage*, **2**, 221–229.

Casey, B.J., Trainor, R.J., Orendi, J.L. *et al.* (1997). A developmental functional MRI study of prefrontal activation during performance of a Go/No-Go task. *Journal of Cognitive Neuroscience*, **9**, 835–847.

Casey, B.J., Giedd, J.N., & Thomas, K.M. (2000). Structural and functional brain development and its relation to cognitive development. *Biological Psychology*, **54**, 241–257.

Caviness, V.S., Kennedy, D.N., Richelme, C., Rademacher, J., & Filipek, P.A. (1996). The human brain age 7–11 years: a volumetric analysis based on magnetic resonance images. *Cerebral Cortex*, **6**, 726–736.

Cepeda, N.J., Kramer, A.F., & Gonzalez de Sather, J.C.M. (2001). Changes in executive control across the life span: examination of task-switching performance. *Developmental Psychology*, **37**, 715–730.

Christoff, K., Prabhankaran, V., Dorfman, J. *et al.* (2001). Rostrolateral prefrontal cortex involvement in relational integration during reasoning. *Neuroimage*, **14**, 1136–1149.

Cohen, J.D., Perlstein, W.M., Braver, T.S. *et al.* (1997). Temporal dynamics of brain activation during a working memory task. *Nature*, **386**, 604–608.

Crone, E.A., & van der Molen, M.W. (2004). Developmental changes in real life decision making: performance on the gambling task previously shown to depend on the ventromedial prefrontal cortex. *Developmental Neuropsychology*, **25**, 251–279.

Crone, E.A., Ridderinkhof, K.R., Worm, M., Somsen, R.J.M., & van der Molen, M.W. (2004). Switching between stimulus-response mappings: a developmental study of cognitive flexibility. *Developmental Science*, **7**, 443–455.

Crone, E.A., Bunge, S.A., Latenstein, H., & van der Molen, M.W. (2005). Characterization of children's decision making: sensitivity to punishment frequency, not task complexity. *Child Neuropsychology*, **11**, 245–263.

Crone, E.A., Wendelken, C., Donohue, S., van Leijenhorst, L., & Bunge, S.A. (2006). Neurocognitive development of the ability to manipulate information in working memory. *Proceedings of the National Academy of Sciences*, **103**, 9315–9320.

Dahl, R.E. (2004). Adolescent brain development: a period of vulnerabilities and opportunities. Keynote address. *Annals of the New York Academy of Sciences*, **1021**, 1–22.

Davies, P.L., Segalowitz, S.J., & Gavin, W.J. (2004). Development of response-monitoring ERPs in 7- to 25-year-olds. *Developmental Neuropsychology*, **25**, 355–376.

Diamond, A., & Goldman-Rakic, P.S. (1989). Comparison of human infants and rhesus monkeys on Piaget's AB task: evidence for dependence on dorsolateral prefrontal cortex. *Experimental Brain Research*, **74**, 24–40.

Duckworth, A.L., & Seligman, M.E.P. (2006). Self-discipline gives girls the edge: gender in self-discipline, grades and achievement test scores. *Journal of Educational Psychology*, **98**, 198–208.

Durston, S., Hulshoff Pol, H.E., Casey, B.J. *et al.* (2001). Anatomical MRI of the developing human brain: what have we learned? *Journal of the American Academy of Child and Adolescent Psychiatry*, **40**, 1012–1020.

Durston, S., Davidson, M.C., Tottenham, N. *et al.* (2006). A shift from diffuse to focal cortical activity with development. *Developmental Science*, **9**, 1–20.

Eigsti, I.M., Zayas, V., Mischel, W. *et al.* (2006). Predicting cognitive control from preschool to late adolescence and young adulthood. *Psychological Science*, **17**, 478–484.

Ford, J.M. (1999). Schizophrenia: the broken P300 and beyond. *Psychophysiology*, **36**, 667–682.

Giedd, J.N., Snell, J.W., Lange, N. *et al.* (1996). Quantitative magnetic resonance imaging of human brain development: ages 4–18. *Cerebral Cortex*, **6**, 551–560.

Giedd, J.N., Blumenthal, J., Jeffries, N.O. *et al.* (1999). Brain development during childhood and adolescence: a longitudinal MRI study. *Nature Neuroscience*, **2**, 861–863.

Gogtay, N., Giedd, J.N., Lusk, L. *et al.* (2004). Dynamic mapping of human cortical development during childhood through early adulthood. *Proceedings of the National Academy of Sciences*, **101**, 8174–8179.

Green, L., Myerson, J., & Ostaszewski, P. (1999). Discounting of delayed rewards across the lifespan: age differences in individual discounting functions. *Behavioral Processes*, **46**, 89–96.

Happaney, K., Zelazo, P.D., & Stuss, D.T. (2004). Development of orbitofrontal function: current themes and future directions. *Brain and Cognition*, **55**, 1–10.

Hogan, A.M., Vargha-Khadem, F., Kirkham, F.J., & Baldeweg, T. (2005). Maturation of action monitoring from adolescence to adulthood: an ERP study. *Developmental Science*, **8**, 525–534.

Hooper, C.J., Luciana, M., Conklin, H.M., & Yarger, R.S. (2004). Adolescents' performance on the Iowa gambling task: implications for the development of decision making and ventromedial prefrontal cortex. *Developmental Psychology*, **40**, 1148–1158.

Huttenlocher, P.R. (1990). Morphometric study of human cerebral cortex development. *Neuropsychologia*, **28**, 517–527.

Jacoby, L.L. (1991). A process dissociation framework: separating automatic from intentional uses of memory. *Journal of Memory and Language*, **30**, 513–541.

Kerr, A., & Zelazo, P.D. (2004). Development of "hot" executive function: The Children's Gambling Task. *Brain and Cognition*, **55**, 148–157.

Koechlin, E., Basso, G., Pietrini, P., Panzer, S., & Grafman, J. (1999). The role of the anterior prefrontal cortex in human cognition. *Nature*, **399**, 148–151.

Kuhn, D. (2006). Do cognitive changes accompany developments in the adolescent brain? *Perspectives on Psychological Science*, **1**, 59–67.

Ladouceur, C.D., Dahl, R.E., & Carter, C.S. (2004). ERP correlates of action monitoring in adolescence. *Annals of the New York Academy of Science*, **1021**, 329–336.

Lamm, C., Zelazo, P.D., & Lewis, M.D. (2006). Neural correlates of cognitive control in childhood and adolescence: disentangling the contributions of age and executive function. *Neuropsychologia*, **44**, 2139–2148.

Lewis, M.D., Lamm, C., Segalowitz, S.J., Stieben, J., & Zelazo, P.D. (2006). Neurophysiological correlates of emotion regulation in children and adolescents. *Journal of Cognitive Neuroscience*, **18**, 430–443.

Luciana, M., Conklin, H., Hooper, C.J., & Yarger, R.S. (2005). The development of nonverbal working memory and executive control processes in adolescents. *Child Development*, **76**, 697–712.

Luria, A.R. (1966). *Higher Cortical Functions in Man* (2nd edn). New York: Basic Books. (Original work published in 1962).

Luria, A.R. (1973). *The Working Brain: An Introduction to Neuropsychology* (B. Haigh, Trans.). New York: Basic Books.

MacDonald A.W., Cohen J.D., Stenger V.A., & Carter C.S. (2000). Dissociating the role of dorsolateral prefrontal cortex and anterior cingulate cortex in cognitive control. *Science*, **288**, 1835–1837.

Merriam, E.P., Thase, M.E., Haas, G.L., Keshavan, M.S., & Sweeney, J.A. (1999). Prefrontal cortical dysfunction in depression determined by Wisconsin Card Sorting Test performance. *American Journal of Psychiatry*, **156**, 780–782.

Mischel, W., Ebbesen, E.B., & Zeiss, A.R. (1972). Cognitive and attentional mechanisms in delay of gratification. *Journal of Personality and Social Psychology*, **21**, 204–218.

Mischel, W., Shoda, Y., & Peake, P.K. (1988). The nature of adolescent competencies by preschool delay of gratification. *Journal of Personality and Social Psychology*, **54**, 687–696.

Mischel, W., Shoda, Y., & Rodriguez, M.L. (1989). Delay of gratification in children. *Science*, **244**, 933–938.

Monterosso, J., Ehrman, R., Napier, K.L., O'Brien, C.P., & Childress, A.R. (2001). Three decision-making tasks in cocaine-dependent patients: do they measure the same construct? *Addiction*, **96**, 1825–1837.

Nagy, Z., Westerberg, H., & Klingberg, T. (2004). Maturation of white matter is associated with the development of cognitive functions during childhood. *Journal of Cognitive Neuroscience*, **16**, 1227–1233.

O'Donnell, S., Noseworthy, M., Levine, B., Brandt, M., & Dennis, M. (2005). Cortical thickness of the frontopolar area in typically developing children and adolescents. *Neuroimage*, **24**, 948–954.

Overman, W.H., Frassrand, K., Ansel, S. *et al.* (2004). Performance on the Iowa card task by adolescents and adults. *Neuropsychologia*, **42**, 1838–1851.

Paikoff, R.L., & Brooks-Gunn, J. (1991). Do parent-child relationships change during puberty? *Psychological Bulletin*, **110**, 47–66.

Prencipe, A., & Zelazo, P.D. (2005). Development of affective decision-making for self and other: evidence for the integration of first- and third-person perspectives. *Psychological Science*, **16**, 501–505.

Purcell, R., Maruff, P., Kyrios, M., & Pantelis, C. (1997). Neuropsychological function in young patients with unipolar major depression. *Psychological Medicine*, **27**, 1277–1285.

Reiss, A.L., Abrams, M.T., Singer, H.S., Ross, J.L., & Denckla, M.B. (1996). Brain development, gender and IQ in children: a volumetric imaging study. *Brain*, **119**, 1763–1774.

Ridderinkhof, K.R., Ullsperger, M., Crone, E.A., & Nieuwenhuis, S. (2004). The role of the medial frontal cortex in cognitive control. *Science*, **306**, 443–447.

Rogers, R.D., & Monsell, S. (1995). Costs of a predictable switch between simple cognitive tasks. *Journal of Experimental Psychology: General*, **124**, 207–231.

Rolls, E.T. (2004). The functions of the orbitofrontal cortex. *Brain and Cognition*, **55**, 11–29.

Rubia, K., Overmeyer, S., Taylor, E. *et al.* (2000). Functional frontalisation with age: mapping neurodevelopmental trajectories with fMRI. *Neuroscience and Biobehavioral Reviews*, **24**, 13–19.

Sakai, K., & Passingham, R.E. (2003). Prefrontal interactions reflect future task operations. *Nature Neuroscience*, **6**, 75–81.

Sakai, K., & Passingham, R.E. (2006). Prefrontal set activity predicts rule-specific neural processing during subsequent cognitive performance. *Journal of Neuroscience*, **26**, 1211–1218.

Segalowitz, S.J., & Davies, P.L. (2004). Charting the maturation of the frontal lobe: An electrophysiological strategy. *Brain and Cognition*, **55**, 116–133.

Segalowitz, S.J., Davies, P.L., Santesso, D., Gavin, W.J., & Schmidt, L.A. (2004). The development of the error negativity in children and adolescents. In M. Ullsperger & M. Falkstein (Eds.), *Errors, Conflicts, and the Brain: Current Opinions on Performance Monitoring* (pp. 177–184). Leipzig, Germany: Max Planck Institute for Cognition and Neurosciences.

Siegle, G.J., Steinhauer, S.R., Thase, M.E., Stenger, V.A., & Carter, C.S. (2002). Can't shake that feeling: event-related fMRI assessment of sustained amygdala activity in response to emotional information in depressed individuals. *Biological Psychiatry*, **51**, 693–707.

Spear, L.P. (2000). Neurobehavioral changes in adolescence. *Current Directions in Psychological Science*, **9**, 111–114.

Stuss, D.T., & Benson, D.F. (1986). *The Frontal Lobes*. New York: Raven Press.

Thompson, C., Barresi, J., & Moore, C. (1997). The development of future-oriented prudence and altruism in preschoolers. *Cognitive Development*, **12**, 199–212.

Tucker, D.M., Luu, P., Desmond, R.E. *et al.* (2003). Corticolimbic mechanisms in emotional decisions. *Emotion*, **3**, 127–49.

Zelazo, P.D. (2004). The development of conscious control in childhood. *Trends in Cognitive Sciences*, **8**(1), 12–17.

Zelazo, P.D., & Cunningham, W. (2007). Executive function: Mechanisms underlying Emotion Regulation. In J. Gross (Ed.), *Handbook of Emotion Regulation*. New York: Guilford.

Zelazo, P.D., & Müller, U. (2002). Executive functions in typical and atypical development. In U. Goswami (Ed.), *Handbook of Childhood Cognitive Development* (pp. 445–469). Oxford: Blackwell.

Zelazo, P.D., Frye, D., & Rapus, T. (1996). An age-related dissociation between knowing rules and using them. *Cognitive Development*, **11**, 37–63.

Zelazo, P.D., Müller, U., Frye, D., & Marcovitch, S. (2003). The development of executive function in early childhood. *Monographs of the Society for Research on Child Development*, **68**(3), VII–137.

Zelazo, P.D., Craik, F.I.M., & Booth, L. (2004). Executive function across the lifespan. *Acta Psychologica*, **115**, 167–183.

9

Cognitive factors in depressive disorders: a developmental perspective

Christopher S. Monk and Daniel S. Pine

A multitude of studies has firmly established that depressed adults and children have disturbances in cognitive functioning (Beck, 1967, 1976). However, despite many studies on this topic, it is still not clear how best to use cognitive measures to characterize depression and understand its etiology. Moreover, major questions have emerged concerning the boundaries of depression and other disorders. The current chapter focuses on issues pertinent to the diagnosis of major depressive disorder (MDD). However, we also briefly describe studies of risk factors for major depression, including anxiety disorders, and we summarize the available literature on pediatric bipolar disorder.

This chapter proceeds in a series of stages. We first discuss approaches that have been used to uncover aspects of depressive symptomatology. Two approaches that we will focus on are the endophenotype approach, and an alternative strategy that we call "symptom-based." The endophenotype approach is presently widely used within psychiatry. However, we argue that the symptom-based approach may complement endophenotype strategy and be superior when studying the development of depression in youth. We then review behavioral and neuroimaging studies that reveal depression-related perturbations in cognitive processing in adults and children. Finally, we propose a strategy for using cognition to better understand the development of depression. Specifically, following the symptom-based approach, we propose the use of cognitive tasks in conjunction with neuroimaging to better understand the development of psychopathology and, in particular, the development of depression. For each of these three stages, we focus on data pertinent to MDD but also discuss data for other conditions, including bipolar disorder.

Adolescent Emotional Development and the Emergence of Depressive Disorders, ed. Nicholas B. Allen and Lisa B. Sheeber. Published by Cambridge University Press. © Cambridge University Press 2009.

Approaches to understanding depression

Although originally described over 30 years ago (Gottesman & Shields, 1973), there has been increasing enthusiasm about the use of endophenotypes for understanding all forms of psychopathology, including depression (Gottesman & Gould, 2003; Hasler *et al.*, 2004). An endophenotype describes a phenotype that is not detectable by the unaided eye but is associated both with overt expression of a disorder as well as underlying risk for the disorder. An endophenotype may be cognitive, neurophysiological, or neuroanatomical (Hasler *et al.*, 2004). Examples of endophenotypes include a selective impairment in cognitive function, a morphological difference in brain structure, or an abnormal pattern of neurotransmitter receptor density in the brain. The concept of an endophenotype has gained favor as the field struggles with methods for mapping genetic variation with specific psychiatric disorders. The rationale is that disorders, as defined by the *Diagnostic and Statistical Manual IV*, are heterogenous and do not reflect the result of single forms of pathophysiology and genetic variation (Hasler *et al.*, 2004). In contrast, endophenotypes are associated with narrower classes of syndromes, and their underlying neural substrates therefore may relate more clearly to genetic variation. Therefore, endophenotypes may be able to more effectively bridge the gap between genetic variation and disorders.

The principal tenets of the endophenotype approach are: (1) the endophenotype relates more strongly to the disorder of interest than to other disorders; (2) the endophenotype is stable across time including when the disorder remits spontaneously or following treatment; (3) the endophenotype occurs with greater frequency among the non-ill relatives of ill probands; and (4) the nature of the specific endophenotype relates to the core features of the specific disorder (Hasler *et al.*, 2004; Tsuang *et al.*, 1993).

The endophenotype concept is problematic within developmental psychopathology, particularly for depression. This is because a diagnosis of depression and other forms of psychopathology are often not stable during development. Moreover, similar overt phenotypes may arise from divergent causes ("equifinality") or different phenotypes may arise from the same cause ("multi-finality") (Rutter *et al.*, 2006). For example, distinct clinical classifications may be made for manifestations of the same underlying problem, as clinical aspects of the problem change across development. During the prepubertal stage, the child may be classified as having separation anxiety disorder; when the child enters late adolescence separation anxiety may wane but panic attacks may emerge; then in adulthood the individual experiences episodes of depression. Using the endophenotype perspective, one would search for stable markers (tenet 2) that relate meaningfully to the core features of the disorder (tenet 4). However, in the above scenario, it is difficult to determine what type of marker would relate to all three conditions while also adhering to the tenet of disorder specificity (tenet 1). Thus, using a developmental psychopathology approach, the endophenotype concept may not be particularly useful, at least when considering disorders, such as depression, that exhibit heterotypic pathways.

A complementary approach is to consider targeting symptoms through cognitive and brain-based probes. As stated above, we will call this the *symptom-based approach*. Like the endophenotype strategy, this approach considers the disorder from multiple levels (behavioral, neurophysiological, and molecular). However, the endophenotype approach does not consider symptoms, because symptoms are episodic and only stable markers are considered to be potential endophenotypes. The symptom-based approach considers symptoms to be a crucial level for understanding psychopathology. Symptoms are the behavioral manifestation of the underlying neural disturbance. Understanding how symptoms map onto cognitive and neural function may provide insight into the disorder from multiple levels.

Using the symptom-based approach, cognitive tasks are designed to tap symptoms by attempting to induce a low-level symptom response in a laboratory environment. If one were to use this approach to examine social phobia, for example, one could develop a cognitive task that captures the symptom of feeling negatively evaluated by peers. Such a task could involve the presentation of disgust or fearful facial expressions when the participant is performing a task. For depression, an executive function task in which subjects attempt to inhibit a negative thought process could be implemented to evaluate rumination. As is described in the third section of the chapter, the inclusion of a symptom-based approach may be an important component to the overall strategy for elucidating the mechanisms of developmental psychopathology.

The symptom-based approach allows for the scrutiny of relationships between specific cognitive profiles and symptom patterns. Thus, this approach requires a careful evaluation of symptomatic differences among disorders and their behavioral and biological correlates. Symptoms of MDD can be differentiated from related syndromes such as anxiety. Whereas MDD involves perturbations in mood, as reflected in sadness and irritability, anxiety involves perturbations in fear, as reflected in avoidance of fear objects and high levels of distress.

Despite relatively clear distinctions in phenomenology among MDD and anxiety disorders, other clinical aspects of these conditions appear related. Major depressive disorder shows a strong association with anxiety, both concurrently as well as prospectively. In fact, the longitudinal association between adolescent anxiety and adult MDD is equally as strong as that between adolescent MDD and adult MDD (Pine et al., 1998). Moreover, from a genetic perspective, MDD emerges from a shared diathesis both for mood disorders and for some anxiety disorders, particularly generalized anxiety disorder (Kendler, 1996). Given this strong overlap, major questions emerge concerning the degree to which an endophenotype for MDD can be differentiated from that for anxiety disorders.

As with the anxiety disorders, questions arise concerning the boundary between MDD and bipolar disorder, both of which involve predominant mood symptoms. The clearest difference in terms of phenomenology is that bipolar disorder requires the occurrence of mania at some point, which is characterized, in its classic form, by an elevation in mood, increases in energy, and associated symptoms. While classic mania can be distinguished from MDD relatively easily, the boundaries between MDD and bipolar disorder are less clear (Leibenluft *et al.*, 2003). Specifically, both MDD and bipolar disorder involve episodic perturbations in mood with associated changes in neurovegetative symptoms. While the precise nature of these changes differs in MDD and bipolar disorder in adults, the distinction may be more subtle in children and adolescents. For example, in youth, irritability is considered a sign either of MDD or of mania, whereas in adults irritability is considered a sign of mania but not MDD. From the symptom-based perspective, cognitive processes associated with bipolar disorder actually appear quite distinct from those associated with MDD, as reviewed below.

Behavioral and neural evidence that cognitive processes are disturbed in MDD in adults and juveniles

Aaron Beck (Beck, 1967, 1976) posited that depression arises from negative schemas that permeate one's thoughts about self and the surroundings. From this model, cognitive investigations have consistently found that individuals with depression show a bias for negative information (Gotlib *et al.*, 2004; Kyte *et al.*, 2005; Mogg *et al.*, 2000). In considering cognitive function in depression, it is useful to take an information processing approach. That is, to systematically examine depression-related perturbations in cognitive functioning across the stages of attention, executive function (rumination, decision making, and planning) and memory.

From this perspective, at least four major questions may be posed. First, what stages of information processing (attention, executive processes, or memory) are affected by negative biases? Second, are the biases specific to one type of emotion (e.g. sadness) or do they generalize to all negative emotions or even a broader class of valenced experiences (e.g. negative and positive emotions)? Third, do these cognitive biases cause depression, maintain the disorder, or represent merely downstream byproducts that are adaptations to having the illness? Fourth, how specific are these cognitive disturbances to depression or do they relate more generally to multiple forms of psychopathology? Answers to such questions are crucial for developing a full account of the relationship between cognition and depression. Furthermore, such answers may also have implications for cognitive–behavioral therapy-based treatment strategies that involve targeting symptom-based cognitions. Finally, the study of youth with depression may be particularly useful for answering these questions. Since depression often first appears before adulthood (Pine *et al.*, 1998), studying youth with depression allows one to look at the manifestation of the disorder when it is more proximal to the onset. Therefore, through the examination of depressed children's and adolescents' performance on cognitive tasks, it may be possible to gain a better understanding of the role of these cognitive processes on the development and maintenance of depression.

In addition to behavioral findings, we also discuss neuroimaging work. Results from neuroimaging provide another way to look at perturbations in information processing. Such an approach may be helpful in pinpointing which aspects of cognitive function are impaired.

Behavioral studies of attention

Behavioral studies of information processing that measure negative bias report equivocal results for early stages in depressed individuals (attention interference, attention orienting) and more consistent results for later stages (attention orienting when the stimulus is presented for a long duration, executive function and memory). An emotional version of the Stroop task is commonly used to examine attentional interference. In this task, subjects view emotional and non-emotional words in different colors and are asked to name the color as quickly as possible. Using these procedures, some have found that adult patients with depression show greater interference and are therefore slower to identify the color when words have a depressed content (Gotlib & Cane, 1987) and others have found that quantitative measures of depression are positively associated with interference to negative emotional words (Gotlib & McCann, 1984; Nulty *et al.*, 1987). However, several studies have found no such relationship between depression and attentional interference to any emotional stimulus (Hill & Knowles, 1991; Mogg *et al.*, 1993).

Studies of attention orienting to emotion-based stimuli report equally mixed findings. A widely used procedure for measuring attention orienting is the probe detection task (Bradley *et al.*, 1999; Monk *et al.*, 2006). In this procedure, two stimuli (e.g. a threatening word and neutral word) are presented briefly in two quadrants of a computer monitor (e.g. left or right side). Following the word presentation, a probe (e.g. an asterisk) is displayed in the location where one of the words previously appeared. Subjects are instructed to press one of two buttons to indicate the location of the probe as quickly as possible. This task captures the spatial location the subject is attending at the moment the two words disappear and the probe is displayed. If a threatening word orients attention to a greater degree than the neutral word, the subject will be a little faster at pressing the button to the probe when it follows the threatening word than when it follows the neutral word.

Using these procedures, depressed subjects did not show an attention bias for negative words presented for 750 ms (Hill & Dutton, 1989). However, when the exposure duration was increased to 1000 ms, dysphoric and depressed individuals showed an attention bias to negative words (Bradley et al., 1997). Emotional faces have also been widely used. When faces were presented for 500 ms, subjects with dysphoria showed reduced attention bias to happy faces (Bradley et al., 1998). In another study when faces were presented for 1000 ms, depressed subjects showed an attention bias toward sad faces and greater symptom severity positively correlated with attention bias away from happy faces (Gotlib et al., 2004). In summary, while the results are not entirely consistent, depressed adults show greater attention bias toward negatively valenced stimuli and possibly away from positively valenced stimuli. Moreover, while anxiety disorders are associated with disturbances in attention to briefly presented threatening stimuli (Mogg et al., 2004; Monk et al., 2006; Pine et al., 2005), depressed individuals show attention perturbations when the stimuli are presented for longer durations. These findings suggest that depression may not be associated with attentional disturbances in the initial orienting to negative stimuli, but rather disturbances appear at longer presentation durations when further processing is possible.

For children and adolescents, depression is related to difficulty in inhibiting irrelevant information as measured in the Stroop task (Cataldo et al., 2005). Impairments in inhibition have also been found in bipolar disorder (McClure et al., 2005; Pavuluri et al., 2005). However, it remains unclear the degree to which these findings appear for any form of irrelevant information across disorders or whether they reflect specific perturbations with emotional stimuli. Thus, with regard to whether specific types of emotional stimuli interfere with attention in depressed youth, the data are inconsistent. Dalgleish and colleagues found that children and adolescents with depression do not show an attention bias toward or away from depression-related or threatening words that were presented for 1500 ms (Dalgleish et al., 2003; Neshat-Doost et al., 2000). However, recently, in a variant of the Go/No-Go paradigm in which emotional faces were presented and participants were asked to press a button to specific emotions (Hare et al., 2005), juveniles with depression, relative to the controls, were faster to respond to sad faces that were presented for 500 ms (Ladouceur et al., 2006). As with adults, depressed youth may manifest specific attentional biases to specific types of stimuli at specific points in the information processing stream. Further work is necessary to more precisely identify the variables that most strongly relate to depression.

Neuroimaging studies of attention

Brain-imaging techniques complement the behavioral measures in specifying depression-related disturbances in information processing. In adults, Sheline and colleagues conducted an fMRI study in which they used a masking paradigm with emotional faces (fearful and happy) on adults with depression (Sheline *et al.*, 2001). The faces were presented briefly and then a masked stimulus was displayed, making it difficult if not impossible to perceive the faces. Subjects passively viewed the faces. The presentation of masked emotional faces was associated with increased amygdala activation relative to controls and this effect was particularly pronounced for fearful faces. Moreover, treatment with sertraline, a selective serotonin reuptake inhibitor, normalized the amygdala response to the faces. The amygdala, an almond-shaped structure within the limbic system, is particularly responsive to stimuli that may impact the well-being of an organism (Davis & Whalen, 2001). The findings from Sheline *et al.* suggest that depressed individuals evidence enhanced sensitivity to emotional stimuli at a very early stage of processing. When faces were presented for a longer period (2 seconds) and subjects were asked to respond to a non-emotional aspect of the face (gender identification), depressed adults showed greater amygdala activation to sad faces (Surguladze *et al.*, 2005). Furthermore, as in the treatment study when faces were briefly presented, 8 weeks of antidepressant medication was associated with decreased activation of the amygdala to faces presented for 3 seconds (Fu *et al.*, 2004). Thus, at very brief and longer durations, depression is associated with increased amygdala activation to negatively valenced stimuli. In addition, the abnormal activation of the amygdala is attenuated with antidepressant medication. These neurophysiological findings may relate to the behavioral data described above showing that depressed individuals have attentional biases toward negative stimuli. However, it may be that only the longer stimuli-presentation durations yield differences in behavioral performance. Further neuroimaging work is necessary to better understand the neural basis of depression-related attention biases.

There is little work examining brain function and attention in depressed youth. In one seminal study, a small sample of depressed children ($n=5$) viewed blocks of fearful and neutral faces (Thomas *et al.*, 2001). The faces were presented for 200 ms, but fearful and neutral faces were presented separately in blocks of 42 seconds. Thus, in this design, it was not possible to disentangle the early attention to the fearful face from the emotional response that could be induced from seeing a long train of emotional faces. Using these procedures, depressed children showed less amygdala activation to the fearful faces relative to controls, a finding that is inconsistent with the adult literature. Future studies in this area will help to clarify if these disparate findings are due to age-related changes or they are the result of methodological differences.

Interestingly, in studies beyond MDD, two recent studies do document associations among attention, psychopathology, and amygdala engagement in children and adolescents. First, McClure and colleagues found enhanced amygdala activation in a study of face-processing, with amygdala activation emerging specifically during fear-face viewing events, when subjects attended to their internal fear state (McClure *et al.*, 2007). Second, Rich and colleagues, using the same task, found similar signs of amygdala hyperactivation in bipolar disorder (Rich *et al.*, 2006). However, in bipolar disorder, this perturbation emerged for a different class of event, where neutral faces were viewed and internal fear state was the focus of attention. In a recent data analysis, we found that MDD adolescents studied with this task show that amygdala hyperactivation is not attention specific; rather, adolescent patients with MDD show increased amygdala activation to fearful faces across multiple attention tasks. Thus, attention dysfunction and associated brain circuitry engagement appears to differ among pediatric MDD, anxiety, and bipolar disorder. All three conditions are associated with perturbed amygdala activation, but the manifestation of the perturbation varies based on the cognitive task.

Behavioral studies of executive function

Executive function is a term that is poorly defined in the literature. For the present purposes it will be used to describe cognitive processes that are involved in the effortful control of thoughts and action (Kesek, Zelazo, and Lewis, see Chapter 8, this volume; Zelazo & Mueller, 2002). Executive function is part of and impacts many aspects of cognitive function, including inhibitory control, planning, and decision-making. Adults with depression are impaired on a range of executive function abilities, including behavioral inhibition (Murphy *et al.*, 1999), decision making (Murphy *et al.*, 2001; Rahman *et al.*, 2001), and planning (Beats *et al.*, 1996). Thus, depressed adults have difficulty with many aspects of executive function.

Furthermore, as in attention, disturbances in executive function often manifest as a bias toward greater processing of negative stimuli and reduced processing of positive stimuli. Using the affective Go/No-Go task in which participants alternate between selectively pressing the button to either happy or sad words, depressed subjects were faster at pressing to the sad words than happy words and made more omission errors to happy words (Erickson *et al.*, 2005). In contrast, healthy comparisons were slower to respond to sad words and faster to happy words. In addition, in another example of negative bias, the tendency to ruminate about negative events can be thought of as a failure of executive functioning. Specifically, depressed individuals may show executive function impairment in switching from or inhibiting a stream of ruminative thought. Depressed individuals have a greater tendency to ruminate and rumination may relate to the persistence of the disorder

(Nolen-Hoeksema *et al.*, 1992, 1993). Thus, as in attention, disturbances in executive function for depressed adults allows for greater cognitive resources to be dedicated to negative events and fewer resources are given to positive events.

Initial investigations suggest that executive function impairments among depressed children and adolescents may be more circumscribed than in adults. Adolescents with a recent history of depression showed impaired behavioral inhibition as measured with the Go/No-Go task involving emotional words (Kyte *et al.*, 2005). However, other areas of executive function were comparable to controls. In particular, no impairments were found in attentional flexibility and decision making. Furthermore, depressed youth were not more impulsive relative to controls as measured with several neuropsychological tasks (Cataldo *et al.*, 2005). Finally, Ladouceur and colleagues (Ladouceur *et al.*, 2006) reported some evidence of perturbed attention regulation in pediatric MDD on a task that taps aspects of executive function, but again the deficits were limited. Taken together, these studies suggest that impairments in executive function may be more limited early in youth relative to adults with MDD. Such developmental differences may be attributable to the accumulating effects of the disorder over time, long-term effects of treatment, or immature executive functioning in youth that temporarily masks the effects.

To the extent that data have been examined in the anxiety disorders, findings also appear relatively weak and inconsistent for these conditions. However, findings in pediatric bipolar disorder clearly implicate perturbed executive function in this condition. This association has been reported in at least three studies (Dickstein *et al.*, 2004; McClure *et al.*, 2005; Pavuluri *et al.*, 2005).

Neuroimaging studies of executive function

Following their neuropsychological work, Elliott and colleagues conducted a neuroimaging study of the emotional Go/No-Go study with adults diagnosed with depression (Elliott *et al.*, 2002). When sad words were the targets, patients showed greater activation relative to controls in the anterior cingulate, a structure involved in processing emotion. Furthermore, when sad words were the distractors, depressed adults showed greater activation relative to controls in the orbitofrontal cortex, another region that is principally involved in processing emotional stimuli. These findings indicate that between group differences in brain function varies as a result of whether the emotional words necessitate a motoric response (target) or inhibition (distractor). Among the depressed, both conditions revealed abnormal responses in regions involved in affective process. Furthermore, in both conditions, greater activation was dedicated to sad words among the depressed relative to controls. These findings are in line with neuropsychological work demonstrating that depressed individuals show a cognitive bias toward negatively valenced stimuli and events.

In another fMRI study with depressed adults, a gambling task that involved correct and incorrect responses was used to probe neural correlates of error processing (Steele *et al.*, 2004). The anterior cingulate showed greater activation to errors among the depressed adults. Activation in this structure has been implicated in detecting errors (Carter *et al.*, 1998) and processing monetary loss (Gehring & Willoughby, 2002). These findings suggest that the anterior cingulate is involved in the process of learning from suboptimal outcomes. Therefore, activation in this region appears to be involved in a form of executive function. Similar to the Go/No-Go results, the finding that depressed adults show greater activation in the anterior cingulate in response to errors is consistent with other work demonstrating that depressed people show a cognitive bias toward negative stimuli and events.

As described above, the ability to control rumination may also involve executive function. In a paradigm that has implications for the neural basis rumination, Siegle and colleagues found that depressed adults evidenced a sustained amygdala response (up to 30 seconds) following the presentation of negative words. This activation was maintained even when the depressed individuals performed a non-emotional cognitive task (Siegle *et al.*, 2002). In contrast, healthy participants showed amygdala activation to the stimuli, but the response subsided within 10 seconds. Furthermore, among the depressed adults, amygdala activation was associated with degree of rumination. Thus, these findings suggest that depressed individuals are impaired in the ability to cognitively control negative thought processes and this is in part manifested as hyperactivation in the amygdala.

We are aware of only one published study to examine brain correlates of executive function in depressed youth. This study used a decision-making task that involved winning and losing money (Forbes *et al.*, 2006). During the decision-making phase, depressed children and adolescents showed less activation in the anterior cingulate, orbitofrontal cortex, and the caudate relative to healthy youth. In the outcome phase, when subjects learn whether they won or lost money, depressed youth showed less activation in the anterior cingulate, orbitofrontal cortex, and caudate, but increased activation in the amygdala compared with healthy youth. This study implicates disturbed functioning in many of the same structures that were reported in the adult neuroimaging studies of depression. However, with the exception of the amygdala, the group differences in activation were in the opposite direction. There are at least three possible reasons for these cross-development inconsistencies. First, differences related to the tasks given to adults and youth could account for the inconsistent findings. Second, as most depressed adults experienced depression when they were young (Pine *et al.*, 1998), there may be a cumulative effect of the condition that leads to a switch in the neural response. Third, compared with depression in adults, depression in youth may be a distinct neurobiological phenomenon. In order to better understand these developmental differences, it is necessary to use the same task cross-sectionally in youth and adults as well as longitudinally with juveniles.

As with findings for behavioral investigations, neuroimaging studies implicate distinct processes and underlying neural architecture in MDD versus related conditions. For the anxiety disorders, Guyer and colleagues found that adolescents formerly characterized as behaviorally inhibited exhibited enhanced striatal activation during a reward task (Guyer *et al.*, 2006). As behavioral inhibition is a major risk factor for anxiety, this study does provide some evidence of differences between MDD and anxiety. Specifically, whereas Forbes *et al.* (in press) found reduced striatal activation in MDD, Guyer *et al.* (2006) found increased activation in behavioral inhibition. Similarly, Leibenluft *et al.* (2007) also found signs of reduced striatal activation in bipolar disorder during an executive function task. These data are consistent with other evidence of striatal perturbations in both pediatric and adult bipolar disorder (Blumberg *et al.*, 2000, 2003).

Behavioral studies of memory bias

Studies of adults consistently find that healthy controls show a memory bias for positive stimuli (e.g. words) whereas depressed adults exhibit a bias for negative stimuli (Bradley & Mathews, 1983, 1988). Depressed children, too, exhibit a memory bias for negative information (Bishop *et al.*, 2004; Neshat-Doost *et al.*, 1998; Zupan *et al.*, 1987). However, in contrast to these findings, children and adolescents with a history of depression showed a selective memory *deficit* for fearful faces, but not happy or angry faces (Pine *et al.*, 2004). These associations may be specific to MDD, as data in pediatric anxiety disorders often find no differences from healthy subjects (Gunther *et al.*, 2004; Ladouceur *et al.*, 2005). Studies in pediatric bipolar disorder also show evidence of memory perturbations (Pavuluri *et al.*, 2005). However, in bipolar disorder, evidence of perturbed memory emerges on standardized tasks. In pediatric MDD, perturbed memory only emerges in the context of emotional tasks. Given the potential specificity of these findings, further work is necessary to better understand how memory biases relate to aspects of depression.

Neuroimaging studies of memory bias

Surprisingly, there is very little imaging research exploring the relationship among memory, brain function, and depression. Since the most consistent cognitive correlate of depression appears to involve memory bias for negative stimuli, this is particularly unfortunate. Recently, our group used fMRI to examine brain correlates of memory for emotional and non-emotional faces in depressed adolescents (Roberson-Nay *et al.*, 2006). Behaviorally, depressed subjects were impaired in face memory performance, but the effects were not specific to any particular emotion. Thus, surprisingly, no memory bias for negative facial expressions was found. Neurophysiologically, the comparison of remembered to forgotten faces yielded greater activation of the amygdala among depressed adolescents relative to controls and those with anxiety disorders. While these findings require replication, they suggest that depressed adolescents relative to the other groups rely to a greater extent on the amygdala during successful memory encoding. Further work in this area is needed to understand the implications of these findings.

A strategy for better understanding developmental psychopathology

The field of developmental psychopathology has an opportunity to harness the recent advances in interdisciplinary approaches to better understand the mechanisms that underlie the emergence and course of all forms of psychopathology, including depression. As described in the first section, the endophenotype approach is valuable for understanding psychopathology from a multi-level (genes, molecules, brain function, and disorders) perspective. The endophenotype approach seeks to uncover disturbances that are independent of the status of the disorder (i.e. the disturbance is present when the patient is symptomatic or not). A virtue to this requirement is that the disturbance would probably not simply be a byproduct of the symptoms of the disorder. Instead, the endophenotype approach attempts to identify disturbances that *cause* the disorder.

However, as described above, identifying stable disturbances over time is a particular challenge for the study of depression. Transitioning from childhood to adolescence and on to adulthood, depression may be stable, it may follow another disorder (e.g. generalized anxiety disorder), it may precede another disorder, or it may develop independent of any other disorder. It would be difficult to locate a single disturbance that would be present across all four scenarios and development. Indeed, as proponents of the endophenotype approach stress, depression may be a heterogenous constellation of disorders that must be separated out if we are to effectively reveal endophenotypes for depression. Unfortunately, the field is far off from being able to identify endophenotypes that are stable across development and it is presently not possible to re-organize the definition of depression into meaningful subgroups. Therefore, to help bridge this gap, complementary approaches should also be considered. One complementary approach is to treat the symptoms not as downstream byproducts of the core disturbances, but rather as a valuable focus for analysis that can help to uncover mechanisms of the disorder. We call this the symptom-based approach.

Like the endophenotype strategy, the symptom-based approach examines mental disorders from multiple levels: (1) the disorder, (2) the symptoms that comprise the disorder, (3) cognitive-affective disturbances that bias one to develop symptoms, (4) brain function that subserves cognitive-affective processes, (5) the molecular architecture of the brain (e.g. receptors and neurotransmitters) that permits brain function, and (6) the genes that code for the molecular architecture. There are two advantages to considering symptoms. First, it allows for the examination of the relationship between cognitive disturbance and symptoms. As described above, there is an existing literature on cognitive studies of depression from which to draw. Thus, the cognitive findings can be used to bridge work between symptoms and brain function. Furthermore, clarification of the relationship between cognitive disturbance and symptoms has implications for treatment. Cognitive–behavioral therapy (CBT) is a form of treatment that attempts to alter disturbed cognitive functioning in patients (Beck, 1967, 1976). This is an effective form of treatment for depressed adults (Beck, 1976). For adolescents, the effectiveness of CBT is less clear, but in a multi-site, double-blind randomized clinical trial it appears to enhance the efficacy of fluoxetine (March et al., 2004). Further understanding of the relationship between cognition and symptoms may lead to improved forms of CBT.

Second, the symptom-based approach allows for a link to work on animal models. While existing animal models of depression are far from ideal (Berton & Nestler, 2006), animals have the capacity to exhibit many behaviors that are relevant to the symptoms of depression. Examples of these behaviors include learned helplessness (Seligman & Beagley, 1975; Seligman et al., 1968), reduced responsivity to reward (Nestler & Carlezon, 2006), and social defeat (Berton et al., 2006). Thus, by including symptomatology in attempting to better understand depression, it is possible to consider the mechanistic findings from animal models in the overall framework.

Therefore, in addition to using the endophenotype approach, it may be fruitful to use a symptom-based strategy to better understand the development of depression. In the latter strategy, tasks can be devised to mildly provoke symptoms and the impact on aspects of cognition can be examined. Furthermore, neuroimaging can be performed with the symptom-based task to gain a brain-based understanding of the processes that underlie the symptoms and cognitive function. As discussed in Section II, this approach has been used with adults and to some extent with children and adolescents. We propose to extend this strategy to more systematically probe for perturbations along the information processing stream (attention, executive function, and memory) during juvenile development. This will permit specific cognitive perturbations to be linked to specific symptoms. Finally, brain imaging can be utilized to understand how symptoms and cognitive perturbations relate to neurophysiology. Thus, it is possible to gain a multi-level (symptom, behavior, and brain function) understanding of the disorder. Furthermore, by also considering age, it is possible to explore how these multi-level factors relate to symptoms in ontogeny and how the prevalence of symptoms may change at different developmental stages.

Conclusions

The present chapter (1) discusses different approaches to understanding depression; (2) reviews the literature on cognitive processes that are disturbed in depression as measured with behavioral and neuroimaging methods; and (3) proposes a strategy for using cognition to better understand developmental psychopathology. We suggest that the approach of using cognitive function to bridge symptoms of psychopathology with brain function complements the widely accepted endophenotype approach. The use of this approach may be particularly valuable in the realm of developmental psychopathology where disorders and symptoms change over time, making it difficult to identify stable markers as required in the endophenotype approach. Pinpointing cognitive and brain-based disturbances that relate to symptoms may be a valuable step in understanding depression and other forms of psychopathology from a developmental perspective.

REFERENCES

Beats, B.C., Sahakian, B.J., & Levy, R. (1996). Cognitive performance in tests sensitive to frontal lobe dysfunction in the elderly depressed. *Psychological Medicine*, **26**, 591–603.

Beck, A.T. (1967). *Depression: Clinical, Experimental, and Theoretical Aspects.* New York: Harper & Row.

Beck, A.T. (1976). *Cognitive Therapy and the Emotional Disorders.* New York: International Universities Press.

Berton, O., & Nestler, E.J. (2006). New approaches to antidepressant drug discovery: beyond monoamines. *Nature Reviews Neuroscience*, **7**, 137–151.

Berton, O., McClung, C.A., Dileone, R.J. et al. (2006). Essential role of BDNF in the mesolimbic dopamine pathway in social defeat stress. *Science*, **311**, 864–868.

Bishop, S.J., Dalgleish, T., & Yule, W. (2004). Memory for emotional stories in high and low depressed children. *Memory*, **12**, 214–230.

Blumberg, H.P., Stern, E., Martinez, D. et al. (2000). Increased anterior cingulate and caudate activity in bipolar mania. *Biological Psychiatry*, **48**, 1045–1052.

Blumberg, H.P., Martin, A., Kaufman, J. et al. (2003). Frontostriatal abnormalities in adolescents with bipolar disorder: preliminary observations from functional MRI. *American Journal of Psychiatry*, **160**, 1345–1347.

Bradley, B., & Mathews, A. (1983). Negative self-schemata in clinical depression. *British Journal of Clinical Psychology*, **22**(Pt 3), 173–181.

Bradley, B., & Mathews, A. (1988). Memory bias in recovered clinical depressives. *Cognition and Emotion*, **2**, 235–245.

Bradley, B.P., Mogg, K., & Lee, S.C. (1997). Attentional biases for negative information in induced and naturally occurring dysphoria. *Behaviour Research and Therapy*, **35**, 911–927.

Bradley, B.P., Mogg, K., Falla, S.J., & Hamilton, L.R. (1998). Attentional bias for threatening facial expressions in anxiety. *Cognition and Emotion*, **12**, 737–753.

Bradley, B.P., Mogg, K., White, J., Groom, C., & de Bono, J. (1999). Attentional bias for emotional faces in generalized anxiety disorder. *British Journal of Clinical Psychology*, **38**, 267–278.

Carter, C.S., Braver, T.S., Barch, D.M. *et al.* (1998). Anterior cingulate cortex, error detection, and the online monitoring of performance. *Science*, **280**, 747–749.

Cataldo, M.G., Nobile, M., Lorusso, M.L., Battaglia, M., & Molteni, M. (2005). Impulsivity in depressed children and adolescents: a comparison between behavioral and neuropsychological data. *Psychiatry Research*, **136**, 123–133.

Dalgleish, T., Taghavi, R., Neshat-Doost, H. *et al.* (2003). Patterns of processing bias for emotional information across clinical disorders: a comparison of attention, memory, and prospective cognition in children and adolescents with depression, generalized anxiety, and posttraumatic stress disorder. *Journal of Clinical Child and Adolescent Psychology*, **32**, 10–21.

Davis, M., & Whalen, P.J. (2001). The amygdala: vigilance and emotion. *Molecular Psychiatry*, **6**, 13–34.

Dickstein, D.P., Treland, J.E., Snow, J. *et al.* (2004). Neuropsychological performance in pediatric bipolar disorder. *Biological Psychiatry*, **55**, 32–39.

Elliott, R., Rubinsztein, J.S., Sahakian, B.J., & Dolan, R.J. (2002). The neural basis of mood-congruent processing biases in depression. *Archives of General Psychiatry*, **59**, 597–604.

Erickson, K., Drevets, W.C., Clark, L. *et al.* (2005). Mood-congruent bias in affective Go/No-Go performance of unmedicated patients with major depressive disorder. *American Journal of Psychiatry*, **162**, 2171–2173.

Forbes, E.E., May, J.C., Siegle, G.J. *et al.* (2006). Reward-related decision-making in pediatric major depressive disorder: an fMRI study. *Journal of Child Psychology and Psychiatry*, **47**, 1031–1040.

Fu, C.H., Williams, S.C., Cleare, A.J. *et al.* (2004). Attenuation of the neural response to sad faces in major depression by antidepressant treatment: a prospective, event-related functional magnetic resonance imaging study. *Archives of General Psychiatry*, **61**, 877–889.

Gehring, W.J., & Willoughby, A.R. (2002). The medial frontal cortex and the rapid processing of monetary gains and losses. *Science*, **295**, 2279–2282.

Gotlib, I.H., & Cane, D.B. (1987). Construct accessibility and clinical depression: a longitudinal investigation. *Journal of Abnormal Psychology*, **96**, 199–204.

Gotlib, I.H., & McCann, C.D. (1984). Construct accessibility and depression: an examination of cognitive and affective factors. *Journal of Personality and Social Psychology*, **47**, 427–439.

Gotlib, I.H., Kasch, K.L., Traill, S. *et al.* (2004). Coherence and specificity of information-processing biases in depression and social phobia. *Journal of Abnormal Psychology*, **113**, 386–398.

Gottesman, II, & Gould, T.D. (2003). The endophenotype concept in psychiatry: etymology and strategic intentions. *American Journal of Psychiatry*, **160**, 636–645.

Gottesman, II, & Shields, J. (1973). Genetic theorizing and schizophrenia. *British Journal of Psychiatry*, **122**, 15–30.

Gunther, T., Holtkamp, K., Jolles, J., Herpertz-Dahlmann, B., & Konrad, K. (2004). Verbal memory and aspects of attentional control in children and adolescents with anxiety disorders or depressive disorders. *Journal of Affective Disorders*, **82**, 265–269.

Guyer, A.E., Nelson, E.E., Perez-Edgar, K. *et al.* (2006). Striatal functional alteration in adolescents characterized by early childhood behavioral inhibition. *Journal of Neuroscience*, **26**, 6399–6405.

Hare, T.A., Tottenham, N., Davidson, M.C., Glover, G.H., & Casey, B.J. (2005). Contributions of amygdala and striatal activity in emotion regulation. *Biological Psychiatry*, **57**, 624–632.

Hasler, G., Drevets, W.C., Manji, H.K., & Charney, D.S. (2004). Discovering endophenotypes for major depression. *Neuropsychopharmacology*, **29**, 1765–1781.

Hill, A.B., & Dutton, F. (1989). Depression and selective attention to self-esteem threatening words. *Personality and Individual Differences*, **10**, 915–917.

Hill, A.B., & Knowles, T.H. (1991). Depression and the "emotional" Stroop effect. *Personality and Individual Differences*, **12**, 481–485.

Kendler, K.S. (1996). Major depression and generalised anxiety disorder. Same genes, (partly) different environments – revisited. *British Journal of Psychiatry. Supplement*, 68–75.

Kyte, Z.A., Goodyer, I.M., & Sahakian, B.J. (2005). Selected executive skills in adolescents with recent first episode major depression. *Journal of Child Psychology and Psychiatry and Allied Disciplines*, **46**, 995–1005.

Ladouceur, C.D., Dahl, R.E., Williamson, D.E. *et al.* (2005). Altered emotional processing in pediatric anxiety, depression, and comorbid anxiety-depression. *Journal of Abnormal Child Psychology*, **33**, 165–177.

Ladouceur, C.D., Dahl, R.E., Williamson, D.E. *et al.* (2006). Processing emotional facial expressions influences performance on a Go/No-Go task in pediatric anxiety and depression. *Journal of Child Psychology and Psychiatry*, **47**(11), 1107–1115.

Leibenluft, E., Charney, D.S., & Pine, D.S. (2003). Researching the pathophysiology of pediatric bipolar disorder. *Biological Psychiatry*, **53**, 1009–1020.

Leibenluft, E., Rich, B., Vinton, D. *et al.* (2007). Neural circuitry engaged during unsuccessful motor inhibition in pediatric bipolar disorder vs. controls. *American Journal of Psychiatry*, **164**(1), 52–60.

March, J., Silva, S., Petrycki, S. *et al.* (2004). Fluoxetine, cognitive-behavioral therapy, and their combination for adolescents with depression: treatment for Adolescents With Depression Study (TADS) randomized controlled trial. *Journal of the American Medical Association*, **292**, 807–820.

McClure, E.B., Treland, J.E., Snow, J. *et al.* (2005). Deficits in social cognition and response flexibility in pediatric bipolar disorder. *American Journal of Psychiatry*, **162**, 1644–1651.

McClure, E.B., Monk, C.S., Nelson, E.E. *et al.* (2007). Abnormal attention modulation of fear circuit function in pediatric generalized anxiety disorder. *Archives of General Psychiatry*, **64**(1), 97–106.

Mogg, K., Bradley, B.P., Williams, R., & Mathews, A. (1993). Subliminal processing of emotional information in anxiety and depression. *Journal of Abnormal Psychology*, **102**, 304–311.

Mogg, K., Millar, N., & Bradley, B.P. (2000). Biases in eye movements to threatening facial expressions in generalized anxiety disorder and depressive disorder. *Journal of Abnormal Psychology*, **109**, 695–704.

Mogg, K., Philippot, P., & Bradley, B.P. (2004). Selective attention to angry faces in clinical social phobia. *Journal of Abnormal Psychology*, **113**, 160–165.

Monk, C.S., Nelson, E.E., McClure, E.B. *et al.* (2006). Ventrolateral prefrontal cortex activation and attentional bias in response to angry faces in adolescents with generalized anxiety disorder. *American Journal of Psychiatry*, **163**, 1091–1097.

Murphy, F.C., Sahakian, B.J., Rubinsztein, J.S. *et al.* (1999). Emotional bias and inhibitory control processes in mania and depression. *Psychological Medicine*, **29**, 1307–1321.

Murphy, F.C., Rubinsztein, J.S., Michael, A. *et al.* (2001). Decision-making cognition in mania and depression. *Psychological Medicine*, **31**, 679–693.

Neshat-Doost, H.T., Taghavi, M.R., Moradi, A.R., Yule, W., & Dalgleish, T. (1998). Memory for emotional trait adjectives in clinically depressed youth. *Journal of Abnormal Psychology*, **107**, 642–650.

Neshat-Doost, H.T., Moradi, A.R., Taghavi, M.R., Yule, W., & Dalgleish, T. (2000). Lack of attentional bias for emotional information in clinically depressed children and adolescents on the dot probe task. *Journal of Child Psychology and Psychiatry and Allied Disciplines*, **41**, 363–368.

Nestler, E.J., & Carlezon, W.A., Jr. (2006). The mesolimbic dopamine reward circuit in depression. *Biological Psychiatry*, **59**, 1151–1159.

Nolen-Hoeksema, S., Girgus, J.S., & Seligman, M.E. (1992). Predictors and consequences of childhood depressive symptoms: a 5-year longitudinal study. *Journal of Abnormal Psychology*, **101**, 405–422.

Nolen-Hoeksema, S., Morrow, J., & Fredrickson, B.L. (1993). Response styles and the duration of episodes of depressed mood. *Journal of Abnormal Psychology*, **102**, 20–28.

Nulty, D.D., Wilkins, A.J., & Williams, J.M. (1987). Mood, pattern sensitivity and headache: a longitudinal study. *Psychological Medicine*, **17**, 705–713.

Pavuluri, M.N., Birmaher, B., & Naylor, M.W. (2005). Pediatric bipolar disorder: a review of the past 10 years. *Journal of the American Academy of Child and Adolescent Psychiatry*, **44**, 846–871.

Pine, D.S., Cohen, P., Gurley, D., Brook, J., & Ma, Y. (1998). The risk for early-adulthood anxiety and depressive disorders in adolescents with anxiety and depressive disorders. *Archives of General Psychiatry*, **55**, 56–64.

Pine, D.S., Lissek, S., Klein, R.G. *et al.* (2004). Face-memory and emotion: associations with major depression in children and adolescents. *Journal of Child Psychology and Psychiatry and Allied Disciplines*, **45**, 1199–1208.

Pine, D.S., Mogg, K., Bradley, B.P. *et al.* (2005). Attention bias to threat in maltreated children: implications for vulnerability to stress-related psychopathology. *American Journal of Psychiatry*, **162**, 291–296.

Rahman, S., Sahakian, B.J., Cardinal, R.N., Rogers, R.D., & Robbins, T.W. (2001). Decision making and neuropsychiatry. *Trends in Cognitive Science*, **5**, 271–277.

Rich, B.A., Vinton, D.T., Roberson-Nay, R. *et al.* (2006). Limbic hyperactivation during processing of neutral facial expressions in children with bipolar disorder. *Proceedings of the National Academy of Sciences USA*, **103**, 8900–8905.

Roberson-Nay, R., McClure, E.B., Monk, C.S. *et al.* (2006). Increased amygdala activity during successful memory encoding in adolescent major depressive disorder: an fMRI study. *Biological Psychiatry*, **60**, 966–973.

Rutter, M., Kim-Cohen, J., & Maughan, B. (2006). Continuities and discontinuities in psychopathology between childhood and adult life. *Journal of Child Psychology and Psychiatry and Allied Disciplines*, **47**, 276–295.

Seligman, M.E., & Beagley, G. (1975). Learned helplessness in the rat. *Journal of Comparative Physiology and Psychology*, **88**, 534–541.

Seligman, M.E., Maier, S.F., & Geer, J.H. (1968). Alleviation of learned helplessness in the dog. *Journal of Abnormal Psychology*, **73**, 256–262.

Sheline, Y.I., Barch, D.M., Donnelly, J.M. *et al.* (2001). Increased amygdala response to masked emotional faces in depressed subjects resolves with antidepressant treatment: an fMRI study. *Biological Psychiatry*, **50**, 651–658.

Siegle, G.J., Steinhauer, S.R., Thase, M.E., Stenger, V.A., & Carter, C.S. (2002). Can't shake that feeling: event-related fMRI assessment of sustained amygdala activity in response to emotional information in depressed individuals. *Biological Psychiatry*, **51**, 693–707.

Steele, J.D., Meyer, M., & Ebmeier, K.P. (2004). Neural predictive error signal correlates with depressive illness severity in a game paradigm. *Neuroimage*, **23**, 269–280.

Surguladze, S., Brammer, M.J., Keedwell, P. *et al.* (2005). A differential pattern of neural response toward sad versus happy facial expressions in major depressive disorder. *Biological Psychiatry*, **57**, 201–209.

Thomas, K.M., Drevets, W.C., Dahl, R.E. *et al.* (2001). Amygdala response to fearful faces in anxious and depressed children. *Archives of General Psychiatry*, **58**, 1057–1063.

Tsuang, M.T., Faraone, S.V., & Lyons, M.J. (1993). Identification of the phenotype in psychiatric genetics. *European Archives of Psychiatry and Clinical Neuroscience*, **243**, 131–142.

Zelazo, P.D., & Mueller, U. (2002). Executive functions in typical and atypical development. In U. Goswami (Ed.), *Handbook of Childhood Cognitive Development* (pp. 445–469). Oxford: Blackwell.

Zupan, B.A., Hammen, C., & Jaenicke, C. (1987). The effects of current mood and prior depressive history on self-schematic processing in children. *Journal of Experimental Child Psychology*, **43**, 149–158.

10

Empathy and moral emotions

Nancy Eisenberg, Amanda Sheffield Morris, and Julie Vaughan

Moral emotions are presumed to play an important role in socioemotional development and social behavior (e.g. Hoffman, 2000; Eisenberg, 2000). Children and adolescents who experience others' emotions, concern for others, and emotions such as guilt and shame are expected to behave in ways that are responsive to others' feelings, social cues, norms, and cultural values regarding interactions with others. In this chapter, we review research on the normative development of empathy/sympathy, shame, and guilt and on their sociocognitive and socioemotional correlates in non-clinical samples. We generally do not discuss embarrassment and pride as they are likely less important in moral development, and because research on pride has most often concerned achievements (Eisenberg, 2000). Much of the research on moral emotions and normative socioemotional development has been conducted with children rather than adolescents, whereas research on the relations of moral emotions to psychological problems such as depression tends to be conducted with adolescent participants (see Gilbert and Irons, Chapter 11, this volume). In this chapter research on both childhood and adolescence is reviewed.

The relative dearth of empirical research on the development and correlates of moral emotions in typical adolescents (rather than those prone to depression) is not surprising given the tendency for social and behavioral scientists, as well as the press, to emphasize negative aspects of adolescence such as "raging" hormones, defiance of authority, and delinquency (Steinberg & Morris, 2001). Nonetheless, adolescence has been identified as a time in which individuals are relatively sophisticated in terms of self development (Harter, 2006) and in their abilities to understand a multitude of perspectives and their mutuality (Selman, 1980) – both of which would be expected to play a role in

Adolescent Emotional Development and the Emergence of Depressive Disorders, ed. Nicholas B. Allen and Lisa B. Sheeber. Published by Cambridge University Press. © Cambridge University Press 2009.

moral emotions. It has been argued that the surge of gonadal steroids at puberty induces changes within the limbic system that alter adolescents' emotional attributions about social stimuli while, at the same time, the maturation of the prefrontal cortex enables increasingly complex and controlled responses to social information (Nelson *et al.*, 2005). Thus, changes in social behavior and in emotional reactions during this period may have some neural basis, and such changes in brain development might affect emotional experience, the processing of emotional stimuli and ways in which youth regulate emotional reactions. Thus, the moral emotions may relate somewhat differently to social behavior in childhood than in adolescence, although this topic seldom has been addressed in empirical studies of socioemotional and moral development. Consequently, it is difficult to identify unique developmental changes relevant to moral emotions in adolescence and we must rely on the larger developmental literature to provide an understanding of the development and correlates of these emotions.

Empathy-related emotional reactions

Although definitions of empathy vary somewhat in subtle (and sometimes not so subtle) ways, we define *empathy* as an affective response that stems from the apprehension or comprehension of another's emotional state or condition, and that is similar to what the other person is feeling or would be expected to feel in the given situation. Thus, if a person views someone else who is sad and consequently also feels sad, that person is experiencing empathy. According to most theorists, true empathy must involve at least a modicum of self-other differentiation (e.g. Hoffman, 2000), such that the empathizer is aware at some level that the emotion or emotion-eliciting context is associated with another person, not the self. Thus, empathy involves both some cognition and an emotional response. Empathy can be evoked by direct exposure to another person or by information regarding that person's state or condition and can involve varying degrees of accessing stored information about the effects of being in the given situation and/or mentally putting oneself in the other's situation. Although empathy involves some degree of cognitive perspective taking (i.e. cognitively trying to understand another's internal states), empathy differs from the latter because it explicitly involves emotion.

Often, empathy is likely to lead to sympathy, personal distress, or perhaps both sequentially. *Sympathy* is an emotional response stemming from the apprehension of another's emotional state or condition that is not the same as the other's state or condition but consists of feelings of sorrow or concern for the other. Thus, if a child feels concern for a sad peer, he or she is experiencing sympathy. Sympathy is probably often based upon empathy although it is likely that it can also be evoked by cognitive perspective taking or accessing information from memory that is relevant to the other's experience.

Empathy also can lead to *personal distress*, a self-focused, aversive affective reaction to the apprehension of another's emotion (Batson, 1991). Personal distress often may stem from empathic overarousal – that is, high levels of vicariously induced aversive emotion (see Eisenberg *et al.*, 1996; Hoffman, 2000), although it is possible that personal distress sometimes stems from other emotion-related processes (e.g. shame), accessing relevant information from memory, or cognitively trying to take the perspective of others.

In brief, we view empathy as value-neutral, sympathy as a true moral emotion, and personal distress as an emotional reaction that may often lead to an egoistic orientation rather than an other-oriented, moral orientation. However, if empathy often engenders sympathy, it may be an indirect precursor of moral emotion and behavior in some contexts.

The development of empathy

Rudimentary forms of these abilities are present fairly early in life and are continually developed throughout childhood and into adolescence. Young infants typically cry in reaction to hearing another infant cry (see Eisenberg & Fabes, 1998; Hoffman, 2000). However, it is not until around their first birthday that infants show distress in the presence of another's distress, and may begin to show signs of attempting to help others in need. Children's empathic or sympathetic concern appears to increase during early childhood (Eisenberg & Fabes, 1998), likely in part due to advances in children's language, ability to label emotions, and perspective-taking skills (Denham, 1998; Jenkins & Ball, 2000).

As children mature, their abilities to decipher their own and other people's emotional states become more sophisticated, as does their cognitive understanding of the process of experiencing empathy. Bengtsson & Johnson (1987) examined age-related differences in children's thoughts about modulating the experience of empathy. When asked to increase or decrease their empathic arousal, second and fourth graders reported more mentalistic strategies (e.g. "I tried to imagine that I was she;" "I thought that it was really happening;" "Told myself not to be sad") than did kindergarteners. It seems that children between early and middle childhood develop a notion of the malleability of empathic arousal and awareness that they have some control over their own empathic reactions. Because sympathy is believed to be associated with optimal rather than empathic overarousal, such knowledge may increase the likelihood of children experiencing sympathy rather than personal distress.

The amount of empathic concern reported is generally higher for elementary school children compared with preschoolers (see Eisenberg, 2000). For example, in a study examining empathic concern in 5- to 9-year-olds,

Zahn-Waxler *et al.* (1990) found that older children exhibited more empathy than younger children. Age-related increases however, are often different depending on how empathy is measured, with larger effects emerging for observed behavioral reactions (not just facial) and self-reports than for physiological or facial indices (Eisenberg & Fabes, 1998).

Young children's empathic responses are usually confined to another's immediate, transitory, and situationally specific distress. However, as older children and adolescents acquire the ability to understand that people's situations can continue to exist over time, they are increasingly able to empathize and sympathize with others' general condition, such as having empathic concern for the impoverished or politically oppressed. Moreover, Hoffman (1982) proposed that cognitive maturation in late childhood provides children with the ability to experience empathy even when the person or group of persons in distress is not present.

Age-related increases in empathy-related responding appear to continue into adolescence. For example, in one study, sixth graders reported more empathic concern than second and fourth graders (Litvak-Miller & McDougall, 1997). Analogously, 13-year-olds evidenced higher levels of facial concern in response to empathy-inducing stimuli than did younger children (Strayer & Roberts, 1997). Increases in high school students' empathy across three time points have been reported (Davis & Franzoi, 1991), although age-related increases have not always been found in adolescence (see Eisenberg & Morris, 2002). For example, Hanson & Mullis (1985) found an increase in empathy for girls between early and middle adolescence but not between middle and late adolescence; for boys, there was no consistent increase in empathy. Eisenberg *et al.* (2005) found no age-related changes in sympathy from mid-adolescence into early adulthood. Empathy-related responding may be relatively stable by late adolescence.

In a cross-sectional study with 13- to 16-year-olds, manipulating the sex of the person in distress resulted in a differentiated pattern for girls' and boys' empathic concern (Olweus & Endresen, 1998). For girls, there was an increase, as a function of age, in empathic concern regardless of the sex of the person in distress; however, boys' empathic concern increased with age when the person in distress was a girl and decreased with age when the person in distress was a boy (Olweus & Endresen, 1998). Based on these findings, adolescents seem to be appraising the context of the situation when determining how they should feel in certain situations. The advancements in cognitive maturity in adolescents may contribute to the specificity and selectivity of their empathic concern.

Sex differences in empathy-related responding

For decades, researchers have investigated whether or not girls develop higher levels of empathic concern or sympathy than boys. In a meta-analytic review including findings with children of all ages, Eisenberg & Fabes (1998) found relatively large effects in self-reported empathy and sympathy, as well as in observed behavioral manifestations of sympathy (a combination of behavioral and facial reactions were scored), favoring girls. Sex differences with self-report measures were larger for older children. However, when the measure of empathy/sympathy was based on physiological responses or non-verbal facial expressions, no sex differences were found (also see Eisenberg & Lennon, 1983). Consequently, whether or not sex differences are found seems to depend on the method by which empathy/sympathy is measured (e.g. how easy it was to discern and control the sex-role consistent response) and, to a lesser degree, on the age of the child.

A related issue is whether there are sex differences versus gender differences in empathy-related responding. Karniol *et al.* (1998) examined whether sex or gender-orientation was a better predictor of sympathy in adolescence. Sympathy was unrelated to masculinity but was positively related to femininity and, when gender orientation was covaried, sympathy was unrelated to sex. In another study, Eisenberg *et al.* (2001) found that a feminine orientation predicted Brazilian adolescents' sympathy and perspective taking.

Relations of empathy-related responding to other socioemotional constructs

Empathy-related responding and perspective taking

For decades it has commonly been assumed that good perspective-taking skills increase the likelihood of individuals identifying, understanding, and sympathizing with others' distress or need (Batson, 1991; Eisenberg *et al.*, 1991c; Feshbach, 1978; Hoffman, 2000). Information about others' internal states is necessary for empathy and sympathy, and one way to obtain such information is by imagining oneself in another's position or accessing stored knowledge, mental associations, and social scripts or deduction (i.e. through perspective taking; Karniol, 1995).

There is some support for a positive relation between empathy-related responding and affective perspective taking across different age groups. For example, Strayer (1980) found a modest, positive correlation for observed empathy and affective perspective taking in preschoolers. Self-reported empathy and/or sympathy and affective perspective taking also have been positively related in studies of older children (Bengtsson & Johnson, 1992; see Eisenberg & Fabes, 1998; Eisenberg *et al.*, 2006).

Another type of perspective taking that has been investigated in relation to empathy is cognitive perspective taking. In various cultures, researchers have found a modest, positive relation between cognitive perspective taking and empathy or sympathy (usually the latter) in childhood and adolescence (Davis & Franzoi, 1991; Eisenberg *et al.*, 2001; Karniol *et al.*, 1998; McWhirter *et al.*, 2002). In addition, high-school students who are relatively high in sympathy are more likely than less sympathetic peers to use a variety of mental transformations to try to understand others' mental states (Karniol & Shomroni, 1999). Only a few researchers have found no relation between measures of cognitive perspective taking (including theory of mind) and empathy (Hughes *et al.*, 2000; Oswald, 2002).

Prosocial behavior, social competence, and emotion regulation

There is mounting evidence that sympathy and sometimes empathy are related to individual differences in the quality of children's and adolescents' social behavior. In numerous studies with children (Eisenberg *et al.*, 2006) and some with adolescents (Eisenberg, Miller, Shell, McNally, & Shea, 1991b; Estrada, 1995), investigators have found that youth prone to experience sympathy are more likely to assist other people, especially in situations that are less likely to evoke public approval (also see Carlo & Randall, 2002). Consistent with these findings, sympathy has been linked to higher-level moral reasoning about prosocial moral dilemmas in adolescence (Eisenberg *et al.*, 1991b). In addition, sympathy has been positively related to diverse measures of social competence, including popularity, socially appropriate behavior, and constructive social strategies during childhood (Eisenberg *et al.*, 1996; Zhou *et al.*, 2002) and adolescence (Laible *et al.*, 2000; Murphy *et al.*, 1999). Findings for the relation of empathy to social competence are less consistent, however, in adolescence than in childhood (Coleman & Byrd, 2003).

Eisenberg (2000) has argued that individual differences in the tendency to experience sympathy versus personal distress vary as a function of dispositional differences in individuals' abilities to regulate their emotional reactions. Well-regulated children (e.g. those who have control over their ability to focus and shift attention) are hypothesized to be relatively high in sympathy regardless of their emotional intensity because they can modulate their negative vicarious emotion to maintain an optimal level of emotional arousal – one that has emotional force and enhances attention, but is not so aversive and physiologically arousing that it engenders a self-focus. In contrast, children who are unable to regulate their emotions, especially if they are intense, are hypothesized to be low in dispositional sympathy and prone to personal distress. Individual differences in regulation have been linked to high sympathy and low personal distress in childhood and adolescence (Eisenberg *et al.*, 1996; Murphy *et al.*, 1999; Valiente *et al.*, 2004). In addition, during early adolescence sympathy has been correlated with the personality factor of conscientiousness (which partly taps regulation; Del Barrio *et al.*, 2004), as well as constructive modes of coping (McWhirter *et al.*, 2002), low aggression (see Eisenberg *et al.*, 2006), and self-reported efficacy in self-regulation (e.g. resisting peer pressure to engage in high-risk behaviors, use of alcohol and drugs, theft and other transgressive activities) and in managing negative emotions (Bandura *et al.*, 2003).

Moreover, Strayer (1993) found that children who experience more nega- tive emotion than the person who is eliciting their empathy (i.e. become overaroused) are relatively low in empathy/sympathy. In addition, there is limited evidence that unregulated children are low in sympathy regardless of their level of emotional intensity whereas, for moderately and highly regulated children, level of sympathy increases with level of emotional inten- sity (Eisenberg *et al.*, 1996; also see Eisenberg *et al.*, 1998). It appears that well-regulated children can modulate their vicarious arousal and therefore focus their attention on others' emotions and needs rather than on their own aversive vicarious emotion (Trommsdorff & Friedlmeier, 1999).

Indeed, Bengtsson (2003) found that Swedish elementary school children who were high in self-reported empathy and teacher-reported prosocial behavior tended to experience moderate rather than high levels of threat and modulate the emotional significance of empathy-eliciting stimuli through cognitive restructuring (which can be viewed as a mode of emotion regula- tion). If children and adolescents prone to sympathy are well regulated, it is not surprising that they are also more prosocial and socially skilled. This relation may be partly due to the effects of sympathy per se on social behavior, as well as to individual differences in self-regulation affecting both sympathy and youths' social behavior.

Socialization correlates of empathy-related responding

Researchers have found that supportive parenting that provides children with the understanding and tools for emotion regulation is associated with more sympathetic and prosocial behavior in children (Eisenberg *et al.*, 2006). Sympathetic children tend to have secure attachments (Kestenbaum *et al.*, 1989; Waters *et al.*, 1986). Moreover, their parents tend to be high in sympathy (Eisenberg *et al.*, 1991a), to express moderately high levels of positive emotion in the family (Eisenberg *et al.*, 1991a; Valiente *et al.*, 2004; Zhou *et al.*, 2002), and to buffer children from extremes of negative emotion (Fabes *et al.*, 1994). Parental warmth has been inconsistently related to children's sympathy; it seems likely that it is positively related when combined with other positive parenting practices (see Eisenberg & Fabes, 1998; Eisenberg *et al.*, 2004). In addition, sympathy and empathy appear to be linked to parental use of reasoning that points out the consequences of children's behavior for others (Eisenberg & Fabes, 1998; Hoffman, 2000; Krevans & Gibbs, 1996) and parental verbaliza- tions that help children understand others' perspectives (Eisenberg *et al.*, 1991a; Eisenberg & McNally, 1993).

Moreover, parental practices that foster children's abilities to accept and experience emotion, but also to regulate emotions and their expression as needed, are likely to promote sympathy. Boys whose parents were restrictive about the expression of negative emotions that were not harmful to others displayed more distress physiologically and facially in response to an empathy-inducing stimulus, although they reported lower levels of distress than did other boys. In contrast, parents' emphasis on controlling emotions that were likely to hurt another was related to higher levels of children's sympathy. In addition, parental emphasis on instrumental coping with emotion has been linked to sympathy for boys (Eisenberg *et al.*, 1991a; Eisenberg *et al.*, 2006).

In summary, initial research suggests that there are associations between parents' behaviors and child-rearing practices and individual differences in children's sympathy and personal distress. However, more work is needed to identify the constellation of parental socialization practices related to sympathy versus personal distress, as well as the ways in which culture influences the socialization of empathy-related responding (Eisenberg *et al.*, 2006).

Shame and guilt

Shame and guilt are viewed as "self-conscious" emotions because the individual's own appraisal and evaluation of a situation are key to such emotions. Research on shame and guilt indicates that these emotions are distinct from one another and are associated with different developmental outcomes (Eisenberg, 2000; Tangney *et al.*, 1996). Thus, in our review we discuss the development of shame and guilt separately, and specify how shame and guilt differentially relate to socioemotional outcomes such as adjustment.

Guilt and shame have been defined in a variety of ways in the literature. Most developmental and social psychology researchers agree, however, that guilt typically arises in response to a specific behavior or action. It is seen as a painful or agitated feeling that involves regret over a specific wrongdoing (Eisenberg, 2000). Guilt is seen as enhancing social relationships in that it motivates people to treat one another fairly and equally (Baumeister *et al.*, 1994). In contrast, shame involves a negative evaluation of the self, rather than a focus on a particular wrongdoing (Barrett, 1995; Tangney, 1991). Shame is a more helpless, severe emotion that involves the dejection of the entire self, and causes one to want to avoid others (Eisenberg, 2000; Ferguson & Stegge, 1998). Thus, shame is believed to be more deleterious to the self than is guilt, and guilt is more often associated with more positive developmental outcomes. Moreover, the socialization of shame and guilt likely involve different types of parenting behavior, and early socialization practices appear to be key in understanding the development of shame and guilt.

The development of shame and guilt

Due to the fact that shame and guilt are by nature social emotions, a child must have some sort of understanding of *how* others view him/her, and how one's actions affect others, as well as a basic understanding of the self before *true* shame and guilt are experienced. Moreover, socialization plays a very important role in the development of shame and guilt because of the social properties of such emotions. Indeed, early experiences of shame usually involve another person being present, most often a caregiver.

The development of shame

Around one year of age, an infant can connect a failure with a negative reaction from someone else, usually a caregiver. Toward the end of the second year (18–24 months), as a child begins to establish representations of the self, simple distress begins to resemble shame, because children can now interpret a parent's reactions to failure as disappointment. Around 2½ to 3 years of age, a child can form representations of the self as "bad" or ineffective, as a result of a parent's disappointment (Mascolo & Fischer, 1995).

Shame appears around 3½ to 4 years of age. At this time, a child begins to compare his or her performance on a task to another child's performance, concluding that he or she is either better or worse at that activity/behavior than the other child (Mascolo & Fischer, 1995). As children move into formal schooling, they begin to compare themselves to others more systematically, and social comparisons increase as children move from grade to grade in school (Ruble *et al.*, 1994). In middle childhood and adolescence, general representations about the self in comparison to others become more sophisticated and advanced. For example, around 6 to 8 years, a child tends to compare him/herself to others based on concrete skills, such as athleticism. Around 10–12 years, with the advancement of more abstract thinking, children begin to make abstractions about personality characteristics and traits, and instead of thinking "I am bad at sports and math," a child may think that because he or she performs poorly in math and sports that he or she is an "incompetent person." In mid to late adolescence, with increased abstract mapping skills, a youth may extend an attribution about another person with an identity related to oneself to him or herself. If he or she relates that person's behavior to the self because of a shared racial, ethnic, or cultural background, shame can result (Mascolo & Fischer, 1995). For example, a teen may feel shame if someone of the same race and background is involved in a school shooting in his or her city.

Researchers attempting to understand associations between shame (or guilt) and the development of depression should consider the ways in which cognitions/appraisals of the self and of others' evaluations of the self are formed, and the important role of socialization and caregiver influence. It would also be useful to examine why shame instead of pride is a more dominant emotion in some individuals. Further, the transition into adolescence may be key in understanding why some youth develop negative self-representations in terms of traits and characteristics as a result of shame. This is because self-representations and social comparisons become more advanced and abstract during this developmental period. Indeed, there is evidence that evaluations of the self differ developmentally, and among girls compared with boys, with younger children and males typically having more self-enhancing, positive biases (Ruble *et al.*, 1994).

The development of guilt

In contrast to shame, guilt concerns responsibility for a wrongdoing. We focus on interpersonal guilt, an emotion associated with hurting others, as this conceptualization of guilt is most closely related to moral development and empathy. As young as 7–8 months of age, infants begin to connect their own actions to distress in others (Hoffman, 1982). As infants develop into toddlers, and begin to understand causal relations, these connections become more abstract (Mascolo & Fischer, 1995). A great deal of research indicates that guilt-like behavior emerges by the end of the second year (Barrett *et al.*, 1993; Cole *et al.*, 1992; Kochanska *et al.*, 1994).

As children's cognitive skills continue to develop, situations in which guilt are experienced become more complex. In early childhood, around ages 4 to 5, children can experience guilt in response to not reciprocating another child's prosocial behavior (Mascolo & Fischer, 1995). Around ages 6 to 8, a child can experience guilt due to not fulfilling a promise or agreement, and in late childhood/early adolescence, guilt can be experienced when an individual breaks a general moral rule (e.g. honoring agreements). In adolescence, as thought becomes more abstract, adolescents are able to judge themselves in comparison to others and may experience guilt if they perceive themselves to have upheld a moral rule less well than someone else (Mascolo & Fischer, 1995).

Adolescence may be a particularly important developmental period for examining guilt and its correlates. There is some evidence that gender differences in guilt, with females experiencing more than males, emerge during adolescence (Bybee, 1998). Moreover, as adolescents begin to develop romantic relationships and become more sexual, many teens experience guilt over their sexual activity, particularly if it violates parental or religious expectations (Tangney & Dearing, 2002). As abstract thinking, maturity demands, and responsibilities increase, there are more opportunities for adolescents to experience guilt, and expectations for males versus females may play some role in the amount of guilt experienced. Thus, high levels of guilt may play an important role in adjustment difficulties experienced by many adolescents.

Obviously, guilt is closely linked to empathy and perspective taking (Hoffman, 2000). There is some evidence that individuals high in guilt are actually better at perspective taking, compared to individuals high in shame who are also high in personal distress (Leith & Baumeister, 1998). In order to experience guilt, an individual must be aware of upsetting another person. However, unlike empathy, an individual does not have to experience the same emotion as the other person. Nonetheless, empathy may often be the basis of guilt in that it alerts children to the effects of their behavior on others. In fact, guilt and empathy are positively related (Tangney, 1991). Guilt and shame also are closely linked, and it is likely that too much guilt may result in the feeling of shame, causing more negative attributions of the self. Moreover, when guilt is based on irrational assessments of the self, rather than on awareness of hurting another person, it is likely to be more serious and maladaptive (Eisenberg, 2000). More research is needed on when guilt *becomes* shame, because it is likely that high levels of guilt over wrongdoings will eventually lead to more harmful feelings about the self. In addition, guilt and shame often co-occur, especially in children (Ferguson *et al.*, 1999). Despite links between guilt and shame, these emotions do appear to be distinct constructs, and research indicates that they are linked to different developmental outcomes (see Barrett, 1995).

Correlates of shame and guilt

Most researchers now agree that differences in shame and guilt are due primarily to degrees of difference in the focus on the self (Eisenberg, 2000; Tangney, 1998). When a person experiences shame, the entire self is affected, feeling exposed and vulnerable. Adults report that shame experiences are more intense and painful than guilt experiences, and that shame is accompanied with a preoccupation regarding the opinions of others. In contrast, guilt is less painful and is viewed as a feeling experienced in response to a behavior rather than in response to a short-coming in oneself (Ferguson *et al.*, 1991; Tangney, 1998). Guilt involves feelings of regret and remorse and does not affect one's identity (Eisenberg, 2000). Shame, and not guilt, is associated with a desire to change the self (Niedenthal *et al.*, 1994), and has been found to be related to discrepancies between the ideal self and the true self (Tangney *et al.*, 1998).

Shame and guilt both involve a sense of responsibility and the idea that one has violated a moral standard (Eisenberg, 2000). Guilt appears to be the more "moral" emotion because shame often involves concern about others' evaluations, rather than concern over harming another person (Tangney, 1992). Guilt is more likely to result in someone trying to rectify a wrongdoing, whereas shame is more likely to cause a person to withdraw (Tangney,

1998). Moreover, guilt is more strongly associated with empathy, compared to shame (see Tangney, 1991), whereas high shame sometimes has been more closely linked to aggression than is high guilt (Tangney, 1992; Tangney *et al.*, 1996; see Eisenberg, 2002, for a review). Low levels of guilt, however, are also likely to be associated with externalizing and antisocial behavior (Frick & Morris, 2004).

Negative emotionality and regulation

Dispositional negative emotionality and emotion regulation are likely correlates of shame and guilt proneness (Eisenberg, 2000). Indeed, guilt and shame have been linked to fear, sadness, anxiety, and hostility in adulthood (Forgas, 1994; Watson & Clark, 1992) and childhood (Zahn-Waxler & Robinson, 1995). Associations between guilt and shame and negative emotionality may vary due to the measures used. Some researchers have found few differences between guilt and shame and negative emotionality, particularly among toddlers (usually assessed behaviorally; e.g. Zahn-Waxler & Robinson, 1995). In contrast, in a study examining associations between shame and guilt and the "Big 5" personality dimensions, shame and anxious guilt were associated with negative emotionality (neuroticism) whereas situational guilt was not (Einstein & Lanning, 1998). Some research suggests that more situationally based guilt is not associated with negative emotions when shame is controlled for in analyses, whereas shame is associated with anxiety and anger, even when guilt is controlled for (Tangney *et al.*, 1996), again highlighting that shame is the more deleterious emotion.

During early childhood, there are some sex differences in the association between negative emotions and guilt or shame (Kochanska *et al.*, 1994). One study found that fear is associated with guilt in boys and not girls (Zahn-Waxler & Robinson, 1995), but another study found that fear is associated with guilt across both sexes even though girls display higher levels of guilt overall compared with boys (Kochanska *et al.*, 2002). There is some evidence that girls show more shame compared with boys, but it is not clear if there are sex differences in guilt beyond early childhood (Ferguson & Eyre, 1999). As was stated previously, it may be the case that in young children shame and guilt often co-occur.

There is some evidence that guilt and shame are specifically associated with depression and anxiety (see Gilbert and Irons, Chapter 11, this volume). For example, using self-report measures, Jones & Kugler (1993) found that state and trait guilt were associated with higher levels of depression, anxiety, shyness, and loneliness. Moreover, Zahn-Waxler *et al.* (1990) found that children of depressed mothers showed maladaptive guilt patterns (assessed via vignettes about interpersonal conflict and distress) compared with children of non-depressed mothers. Zahn-Waxler *et al.*'s findings suggest that children of depressed parents have acute sensitivity to the problems and distress of others, and that this likely results in an over-involvement in their parents' distress. Depressed parents may even create a socialization environment that is more guilt-inducing than the norm, which likely puts children at risk for developing depression themselves.

There are few studies examining links of shame and guilt with self-regulation. There is some evidence that effortful control (i.e. temperamentally based regulation grounded in executive attention) is linked with higher levels of guilt and shame (Rothbart et al., 1994), and that behavioral regulation is associated with higher levels of affective discomfort after a wrongdoing, although the latter was only found among girls (Kochanska et al., 1994). It may be that well-regulated children are able to control their distress responses from guilt and shame more easily than dysregulated children, and that regulation is an important buffer between emotional distress due to guilt and shame and adjustment (Eisenberg, 2000). However, more research is needed to confirm such thoughts.

Relations with parenting (socialization)

Because parents are an important source of information about rules, social roles, and expectations, and because they are key in teaching children what is *right and wrong*, their responses to misbehavior are an important part of socialization (Barrett, 1995). For example, parents can use a child's wrong-doing as a time to teach children about emotions. When a child misbehaves, or violates a parental expectation, shame can result if a parent's own standards and goals for a child are unattainable (e.g. not developmentally appropriate) or if a child perceives love and acceptance from a parent as contingent on his or her behavior/performance. Moreover, disciplinary techniques that degrade a child and/or are overly emotional in nature likely result in shame. In contrast, if a parent focuses more on the act of wrongdoing, and how that behavior affects others, rather than degrading the child, guilt and empathy are more likely to result (see Hoffman, 1970; Tangney & Dearing, 2002). Similarly, responsive parenting, a focus on the consequences of children's actions, and the use of reasoning rather than punitive responses to a wrongdoing, are less likely to result in shame and/or guilty feelings.

For example, Kochanska and her colleagues have found that a mother–child mutually responsive orientation (which reflects a relationship characterized by responsiveness, positivity, and openness to each other's influence; Kochanska et al., 2005) is associated with children's moral emotion (guilt), suggesting that more responsive, authoritative parenting results in higher guilt proneness among children. Similarly, maternal power assertion (assessed via self-report and observation) has been found to be associated with lower levels of guilt in children, indicating that more democratic, child-centered types of control enhance the development of guilt (Kochanska et al., 2002). Guilt has also been associated with the development of the self at 18 months, and to the moral self and compliance at 56 months (Kochanska *et al.*, 2002), suggesting that guilt may be one mechanism through which parenting impacts the development of the self and adjustment. However, it should be noted that child temperament, specifically proneness to fear, may play a role in associations between power assertion and adjustment. For example, Kochanska (1991) found that mothers who de-emphasized power assertion techniques had children with higher levels of internalized conscience (including guilt feelings) 6 years later (assessed from children's narratives), but this was only found among children high in fearful arousal.

Another parental control technique that is likely to be strongly related to the development of shame and guilt is parental psychological control. Psychological control is related to several constructs in the psychology literature (e.g. over-protectiveness, enmeshment) and has been operationalized in various ways (e.g. absence of autonomy granting, emotional manipulation, intrusiveness; Barber, 1996). Barber (1996) defines psychological control as a type of intrusive parental control in which parents attempt to manipulate their children's behavior, identity, and psychological development. Psychologically controlling parents typically use strategies such as excessive criticism, contingent affection, guilt induction, restrictive communication, and invalidation of feelings in an attempt to control their children (Morris *et al.*, 2002).

One way that parents exert psychological control over children is via parents' control and manipulation of children's emotions, and this component of psychological control is most likely linked to shame and guilt. Parents exert this type of psychological control through love withdrawal, guilt induction, and invalidating feelings. Early research on love withdrawal suggests that it may be less harmful than other forms of emotional manipulation if it is in combination with parental warmth and responsiveness (Becker, 1964). However, if a child perceives parental love and acceptance to be contingent on his or her behavior, this is likely to result in maladjustment. Indeed, research indicates that psychological control is related to internalizing and externalizing problems in children and adolescents (Barber, 1996; Hart *et al.*, 1998; Mills & Rubin, 1998).

Specifically, psychological control may be linked to anxiety and depression in middle childhood and adolescence. Research indicates that children and adolescents diagnosed with an anxiety and/or depressive disorder report that their parents are less democratic and lower in autonomy granting, acceptance, and warmth, and more enmeshed and psychologically controlling, compared with children and adolescents not diagnosed with anxiety and/or depression (Messer & Beidel, 1994; Siqueland *et al.*, 1996; Stark *et al.*, 1993). It is likely that children and adolescents suffering from anxiety and/or depression are high in shame, and it may be that the precursors to these adjustment difficulties stem from parents who are high in psychological control and low in autonomy granting. However, more research is needed to examine the role that shame and guilt play in such maladaptive socialization processes, and longitudinal studies examining the effects of these socialization processes early in life are key in understanding the development of psychopathology.

Conclusions

In summary, empathy-related responding, especially sympathy, and guilt have been linked to an array of important socioemotional outcomes. In contrast, shame often has been associated with maladjustment. In addition, there is evidence that these moral emotions develop in early childhood and into middle childhood. Although theorists have argued that moral emotions develop into adolescence, there is a dearth of data documenting these trends. More research is needed, not only documenting developmental changes in moral emotions in adolescence, but also identifying the role of these moral emotions in changes in social and moral cognitions and emotions in adolescence.

Although the research on the relation of moral emotions to parenting is correlational, it suggests that moral emotions are influenced by socialization in the family. However, most of the relevant research has been conducted with young children or elementary school children. Relatively little is known about the role of parenting in the emergence and experience of moral emotions in adolescence, and if there are any unique parenting effects on moral emotions in adolescence. Empirical and theoretical work on the relation of depression in adolescence to maladaptive self-related emotions may provide insight into vulnerabilities uniquely related to adolescence (see Gilbert and Irons, Chapter 11, this volume), as well as parental behaviors that contribute to these vulnerabilities. However, increased attention should be focused on the role of cognitive and social changes in adolescence, including changes in parent–child relationships, which might affect the degree to which adolescents experience moral emotions and their relations to their social and moral behavior and adjustment.

REFERENCES

Bandura, A., Caprara, G.V., Barbaranelli, C., Gerbino, M., & Pastorelli, C. (2003). Role of affective self-regulatory efficacy in diverse sphere of psychosocial functioning. *Child Development*, **74**, 769–782.

Barber, B.K. (1996). Parental psychological control: revisiting a neglected construct. *Child Development*, **67**, 3296–3319.

Barrett, K.C. (1995). A functionalist approach to shame and guilt. In J.P. Tangney & K.W. Fischer (Eds.), *Self-conscious Emotions* (pp. 25–63). New York: Guilford Press.

Barrett, K.C., Zahn-Waxler, C., & Cole, P.M. (1993). Avoiders versus amenders: implications for the investigation of guilt and shame during toddlerhood? *Cognition and Emotion*, 7, 481–505.

Batson, C.D. (1991). *The Altruism Question: Toward a Social-Psychological Answer*. Hillsdale, NJ: Lawrence Erlbaum.

Baumeister, R.F., Stillwell, A.M., & Heatherton, T.F. (1994). Guilt and interpersonal approach. *Psychological Bulletin*, 115, 243–267.

Becker, W.C. (1964). Consequences of different kinds of parental discipline. In M.L. Hoffman & W.W. Hoffman (Eds.), *Review of Child Development Research, Vol. 1* (pp. 169–208). New York: Russell Sage Foundation.

Bengtsson, H. (2003). Children's cognitive appraisal of others' distressful and positive experiences. *International Journal of Behavioral Development*, 27, 457–466.

Bengtsson, H., & Johnson, L. (1987). Cognitions related to empathy in five- to eleven-year old children. *Child Development*, 58, 1001–1012.

Bengtsson, H., & Johnson, L. (1992). Perspective taking, empathy, and prosocial behavior in late childhood. *Child Study Journal*, 22, 11–22.

Bybee, J. (1998). The emergence of gender differences in guilt during adolescence. In J. Bybee (Ed.), *Guilt and Children* (1st edn, pp. 114–122). San Diego: Academic Press.

Carlo, G., & Randall, B.A. (2002). The development of a measure of prosocial behaviors for late adolescents. *Journal of Youth and Adolescence*, 31, 31–44.

Cole, P.M., Barett, K.C., & Zahn-Waxler, C. (1992). Emotion displays in two-year olds during mishaps. *Child Development*, 63, 314–324.

Coleman, P.K., & Byrd, C.P. (2003). Interpersonal correlates of peer victimization among young adolescents. *Journal of Youth and Adolescence*, 32, 301–314.

Davis, M.H., & Franzoi, S.L. (1991). Stability and change in adolescent self-consciousness and empathy. *Journal of Research in Personality*, 25, 70–87.

Del Barrio, V., Aluja, A., & Garcia, L. (2004). Relationship between empathy and the big five personality traits in a sample of Spanish adolescents. *Social Behavior and Personality*, 32, 677–682.

Denham, S.A. (1998). *Emotional Development in Young Children*. New York: Guilford Press.

Einstein, D., & Lanning, K. (1998). Shame, guilt, ego development, and the five-factor model of personality. *Journal of Personality*, 66, 555–582.

Eisenberg, N. (2000). Emotion, regulation, and moral development. *Annual Review of Psychology*, 51, 665–697.

Eisenberg, N., & Fabes, R.A. (1998). Prosocial development. In W. Damon (Series Ed.) & N. Eisenberg (Vol. Ed.), *The Handbook of Child Psychology, Vol. 3. Social, Emotional, and Personality Development* (5th edn, pp. 701–778). New York, NY: John Wiley.

Eisenberg, N., & Lennon, J. (1983). Sex differences in empathy and related capacities. *Psychological Bulletin*, 94, 100–131.

Eisenberg, N., & McNally, S. (1993). Socialization and mothers' and adolescents' empathy-related characteristics. *Journal of Research on Adolescence*, 3, 171–191.

Eisenberg, N., & Morris, A.S. (2002). Children's emotion-related regulation. In R. Kail & H. Reese (Eds.), *Advances in Child Development and Behavior, Vol. 30* (pp. 189–229). San Diego, CA: Academic Press.

Eisenberg, N., Fabes, R.A., Schaller, M., Carlo, G., & Miller, P.A. (1991a). The relations of parental characteristics and practices to children's vicarious emotional responding. *Child Development*, 62, 1393–1408.

Eisenberg, N., Miller, P.A., Shell, R., McNally, S., & Shea, C. (1991b). Prosocial development in adolescence: a longitudinal study. *Developmental Psychology*, **27**, 849–857.

Eisenberg, N., Shea, C.L., Carlo, G., & Knight, G.P. (1991c). Empathy-related responding and cognition: A "child and the egg" dilemma. In W.M. Kurtines & J.L. Gewirtz (Eds.), *Handbook of Moral Behavior and Development, Vol. 2: Research* (pp. 63–88). Hillsdale, NJ: Lawrence Erlbaum.

Eisenberg, N., Fabes, R.A., Murphy, B. *et al.* (1996). The relations of children's dispositional empathy-related responding to their emotionality, regulation, and social functioning. *Developmental Psychology*, **32**, 195–209.

Eisenberg, N., Fabes, R.A., Shepard, S.A. *et al.* (1998). Contemporaneous and longitudinal prediction of children's sympathy from dispositional regulation and emotionality. *Developmental Psychology*, **34**, 910–924.

Eisenberg, N., Zhou, Q., & Koller, S. (2001). Brazilian adolescents' prosocial moral judgment and behavior: relations to sympathy, perspective taking, gender-role orientation, and demographic characteristics. *Child Development*, **72**, 518–534.

Eisenberg, N., Valiente, C., & Champion, C. (2004). Empathy-related responding: moral, social, and socialization correlates. In A.G. Miller (Ed.), *The Social Psychology of Good and Evil* (pp. 386–415). New York: Guilford Press.

Eisenberg, N., Cumberland, A., Guthrie, I.K., Murphy, B.C., & Shepard, S.A. (2005). Age changes in prosocial responding and moral reasoning in adolescence and early adulthood. *Journal of Research on Adolescence*, **15**, 235–260.

Eisenberg, N., Fabes, R.A., & Spinrad, T.L. (2006). Prosocial development. In W. Damon (Series Ed.) & N. Eisenberg (Vol. Ed.), *The Handbook of Child Psychology, Vol. 3. Social, Emotional, and Personality Development* (6th edn, pp. 646–718). New York, NY: John Wiley.

Estrada, P. (1995). Adolescents' self-reports of prosocial responses to friends and acquaintances: the role of sympathy-related cognitive, affective, and motivational processes. *Journal of Research on Adolescence*, **5**, 173–200.

Fabes, R.A., Eisenberg, N., Karbon, M. *et al.* (1994). Socialization of children's vicarious emotional responding and prosocial behavior: relations with mothers' perceptions of children's emotional reactivity. *Developmental Psychology*, **30**, 44–55.

Ferguson, T.J., & Eyre, H.L. (1999). Engendering gender difference in shame and guilt: stereotypes, socialization, and situational pressures. In A. Fischer (Ed.), *Gender and Emotion* (pp. 254–276). Cambridge, UK: Cambridge University Press.

Ferguson, T.J., & Stegge, H. (1998). Measuring guilt in children: a rose by any other name still has thorns. In J. Bybee (Ed.), *Guilt and Children* (pp. 19–74). San Diego, CA: Academic Press.

Ferguson, T.J., Stegge, H., & Damhuis, I. (1991). Children's understanding of guilt and shame. *Child Development*, **62**, 827–839.

Ferguson, T.J., Stegge, H., Miller, E.R., & Olsen, M.E. (1999). Guilt, shame, and symptoms in children. *Developmental Psychology*, **35**, 347–357.

Feshbach, N.D. (1978). Studies of empathic behavior in children. In B.A. Maher (Ed.), *Progress in Experimental Personality Research* (Vol. 8, pp. 1–47). New York, NY: Academic Press.

Forgas, J.P. (1994). Sad and guilty? Affective influences on the explanation of conflict in close relationships. *Journal of Personality and Social Psychology*, **66**, 56–68.

Frick, P.J., & Morris, A.S. (2004). Temperament and developmental pathways to severe conduct problems. *Journal of Clinical Child and Adolescent Psychology, 33*, 54–68.

Hanson, R.A., & Mullis, R.L. (1985). Age and gender differences in empathy and moral reasoning among adolescents. *Child Study Journal, 15*, 181–187.

Hart, C.H., Nelson, D.A., Robinson, C.C., Olsen, S.F., & McNeilly-Choque, M.K. (1998). Overt and relational aggression in Russian nursery-school-age children: parenting style and marital linkages. *Developmental Psychology, 34*, 687–697.

Harter, S. (2006). The self. In N. Eisenberg (Vol. Ed.), W. Damon, & R.M. Lerner (Series Eds.), *The Handbook of Child Psychology, Vol. 3. Social, Emotional, and Personality Development* (6th edn, pp. 505–570). New York, NY: Wiley.

Hoffman, M.L. (1970). Conscience, personality, and socialization techniques. *Human Development, 13*, 90–126.

Hoffman, M.L. (1982). Development of prosocial motivation: empathy and guilt. In N. Eisenberg (Ed.), *The Development of Prosocial Behavior* (pp. 281–313). New York, NY: Academic Press.

Hoffman, M.L. (2000). *Empathy and Moral Development: Implications for Caring and Justice*. New York, NY: Cambridge University Press.

Hughes, C., White, A., Sharpen, J., & Dunn, J. (2000). Antisocial, angry, and unsympathetic: "Hard-to-manage" preschoolers' peer problems and possible cognitive influences. *Journal of Child Psychology and Psychiatry and Allied Disciplines, 41*, 169–179.

Jenkins, J.M., & Ball, S. (2000). Distinguishing between negative emotions: children's understanding of the social-regulatory aspects of emotion. *Cognition and Emotion, 14*, 261–282.

Jones, W.H., & Kugler, K. (1993). Interpersonal correlates of the guilt inventory. *Journal of Personality Assessment, 61*, 246–258.

Karniol, R. (1995). Developmental and individual differences in predicting others' thoughts and feelings: applying the transformation rule model. In N. Eisenberg (Ed.), *Review of Personality and Social Psychology, Vol. 15. Social Development* (pp. 27–48). Thousand Oaks, CA: Sage.

Karniol, R., & Shomroni, D. (1999). What being empathic means: applying the transformation rule approach to individual differences in predicting thoughts and feelings of prototypic and nonprototypic others. *European Journal of Social Psychology, 29*, 147–160.

Karniol, R., Gabay, R., Ochion, Y., & Harari, Y. (1998). Is gender or gender-role orientation a better predictor of empathy in adolescence. *Sex Roles, 39*, 45–59.

Kestenbaum, R., Farber, E.A., & Sroufe, L.A. (1989). Individual differences in empathy among preschoolers: relation to attachment history. *New Directions in Child Development, 44*, 51–64.

Kochanska, G. (1991). Socialization and temperament in the development of guilt and conscience. *Child Development, 62*, 1379–1392.

Kochanska, G., DeVet, K., Goldman, M., Murray, K., & Putnam, S.P. (1994). Maternal reports of conscience development and temperament in young children. *Child Development, 65*, 852–868.

Kochanska, G., Gross, J.N., Link, M., & Nichols, K.E. (2002). Guilt in young children: development, determinants, and relations with a broader system of standards. *Child Development, 73*, 461–482.

Kochanska, G., Forman, D.R., Aksan, N., & Dunbar, S.B. (2005). Pathways to conscience: early mother-child mutually responsive orientation and children's moral emotion, conduct, and cognition. *Journal of Child Psychology and Psychiatry,* **46**, 19–34.

Krevans, J., & Gibbs, J.C. (1996). Parents' use of inductive discipline: relations to children's empathy and prosocial behavior. *Child Development,* **67**, 3263–3277.

Laible, D.J., Carlo, G., & Raffaelli, M. (2000). The differential relations of parent and peer attachment to adolescent adjustment. *Journal of Youth and Adolescence,* **29**, 45–59.

Leith, K.P., & Baumeister, R.F. (1998). Empathy, shame, guilt, and narratives of interpersonal conflicts: guilt-prone people are better at perspective taking. *Journal of Personality,* **66**, 2–37.

Litvak-Miller, W., & McDougall, D. (1997). The structure of empathy during middle childhood and its relationship to prosocial behavior. *Genetic, Social, and General Psychology Monographs,* **123**, 303–325.

Mascolo, M.F., & Fischer, K.W. (1995). Developmental transformations in appraisals for pride, shame, and guilt. In J.P. Tangney & K.W. Fischer (Eds.), *Self-conscious Emotions* (pp. 64–113). New York, NY: Guilford Press.

McWhirter, B.T., Besett-Alesch, T.M., Horibata, J., & Gat, I. (2002). Loneliness in high risk adolescents: the role of coping, self-esteem, and empathy. *Journal of Youth Studies,* **5**, 69–84.

Messer, S.C., & Beidel, D.C. (1994). Psychosocial correlates of childhood anxiety disorders. *Journal of the American Academy of Child and Adolescent Psychiatry,* **33**, 975–983.

Mills, R.S.L., & Rubin, K.H. (1998). Are behavioural and psychological control both differentially associated with childhood aggression and social withdrawal? *Canadian Journal of Behavioural Sciences,* **30**, 132–136.

Morris, A.S., Steinberg, L., Sessa, F.M. *et al.* (2002). Measuring children's perceptions of psychological control: developmental and conceptual considerations. In B.K. Barber (Ed.), *Intrusive Parenting: How Psychological Control Affects Children and Adolescents* (pp. 125–159). Washington, DC: Psychological Association Press.

Murphy, B.C., Shepard, S.A., Eisenberg, N., Fabes, R.A., & Guthrie, I.K. (1999). Contemporaneous and longitudinal relations of dispositional sympathy to emotionality, regulation, and social functioning. *Journal of Early Adolescence,* **19**, 66–97.

Nelson, E.E., Leibenluft, E., McClure, E.B., & Pine, D.A. (2005). The social re-orientation of adolescence: a neuroscience perspective on the process and its relation to pathology. *Psychological Medicine,* **35**, 163–174.

Niedenthal, P.M., Tangney, J.P., & Gavanski, I. (1994). "If only I weren't" versus "If only I hadn't"; distinguishing shame and guilt in counterfactual thinking. *Journal of Personality and Social Psychology,* **67**, 584–595.

Olweus, D., & Endresen, I.M. (1998). The importance of sex-of-stimulus object: age trends and sex differences in empathic responsiveness. *Social Development,* **7**, 370–388.

Oswald, P.A. (2002). The interactive effects of affective demeanor, cognitive processes, and perspective-taking focus on helping behavior. *Journal of Social Psychology,* **142**, 120–132.

Rothbart, M.K., Ahadi, S.A., & Hershey, K.L. (1994). Temperament and social behavior in childhood. *Merrill Palmer Quarterly,* **40**, 21–39.

Ruble, D.N., Eisenberg, R., & Higgins, E.T. (1994). Developmental changes in achievement evaluation: motivational implications of self-other differences. *Child Development,* **65**, 1095–1110.

Selman, R.L. (1980). *The Growth of Interpersonal Understanding: Developmental and Clinical Analysis.* New York, NY: Academic Press.

Siqueland, L., Kendall, P.C., & Steinberg, L. (1996). Anxiety in children: perceived family environments and observed family interaction. *Journal of Clinical Child Psychology,* **25**, 225–237.

Stark, K.D., Humphrey, L.L., Laurent, J., Livingston, R., & Christopher, J. (1993). Cognitive, behavioral, and family factors in the differentiation of depressive and anxiety disorders during childhood. *Journal of Consulting and Clinical Psychology,* **61**, 878–886.

Steinberg, L., & Morris, A.S. (2001). Adolescent development. *Annual Review of Psychology,* **52**, 83–110.

Strayer, J. (1980). A naturalistic study of empathic behaviors and their relation to affective states and perspective-taking skills in preschool children. *Child Development,* **51**, 815–822.

Strayer, J. (1993). Children's concordant emotions and cognitions in response to observed emotions. *Child Development,* **64**, 188–201.

Strayer, J., & Roberts, W. (1997). Facial and verbal measures of children's emotions and empathy. *International Journal of Behavioral Development,* **20**, 627–649.

Tangney, J.P. (1991). Moral affect: the good, the bad, and the ugly. *Journal of Personality and Social Personality,* **61**, 598–607.

Tangney, J.P. (1992). Situational determinants of shame and guilt in young adulthood. *Personality and Social Psychology Bulletin,* **18**, 199–206.

Tangney, J.P. (1998). How does guilt differ from shame? In J. Bybee (Ed.), *Guilt and Children* (pp. 1–17). San Diego, CA: Academic Press.

Tangney, J.P., & Dearing, R.L. (2002). *Shame and Guilt.* New York, NY: Guilford Press.

Tangney, J.P., Miller, R.S., Flicker, L., & Barlow, D.H. (1996). Are shame, guilt, and embarrassment distinct emotions? *Journal of Personality and Social Psychology,* **70**, 1256–1269.

Tangney, J.P., Niedentahl, P.M., Covert, M.V., & Barlow, D.H. (1998). Are shame and guilt related to distinct self-discrepancies? A test of Higgin's (1987) hypotheses. *Journal of Personality and Social Psychology,* **75**, 256–268.

Trommsdorff, G., & Friedlmeier, W. (1999). Motivational conflict and prosocial behaviour of kindergarten children. *International Journal of Behavioral Development,* **23**, 413–429.

Valiente, C., Eisenberg, N., Fabes, R.A. *et al.* (2004). Prediction of children's empathy-related responding from their effortful control and parents' expressivity. *Developmental Psychology,* **40**, 911–926.

Waters, E., Hay, D., & Richters, J. (1986). Infant-parent attachment and the origins of prosocial and antisocial behavior. In D. Olweus, J. Block, & M. Radke-Yarrow (Eds.), *Development of Antisocial and Prosocial Behavior: Research, Theories, and Issues* (pp. 97–125). Orlando, FL: Academic Press.

Watson, D., & Clark, L.A. (1992). Affects separable and inseparable: on the hierarchical arrangement of the negative affects. *Journal of Personality and Social Psychology,* **62**, 489–505.

Zahn-Waxler, C., & Robinson, J. (1995). Empathy and guilt: early origins of feelings of responsibility. In J.P. Tangney & K.W. Fischer (Eds.), *Self-conscious Emotions: The Psychology of Shame, Guilt, Embarrassment, and Pride* (pp. 143–173). New York, NY: Guilford.

Zahn-Waxler, C., Kochanska, G., Krupnick, J., & McKnew, D. (1990). Patterns of guilt in children of depressed and well mothers. *Developmental Psychology*, **26**, 51–59.

Zhou, Q., Eisenberg, N., Losoya, S.H. *et al.* (2002). The relations of parental warmth and positive expressiveness to children's empathy-related responding and social functioning: a longitudinal study. *Child Development*, **73**, 893–915.

11

Shame, self-criticism, and self-compassion in adolescence

Paul Gilbert and Chris Irons

The transition from childhood to adolescence is a time of rapid maturation of neurophysiological systems which regulate affect and self-identity (Schore, 1994). In addition, this transition is accompanied by an elevated focus on peer-group relationships, sense of belonging, and acceptance. The outcome of these changes clearly impact on mental health. It is estimated that in any 12-month period approximately 1% of pre-pubertal children, rising to 3% of post-pubertal adolescents, suffer from depression, with gender differences in rates beginning to emerge post-puberty (Angold & Costello, 2001). In a major review, Hankin (2006) notes that 20–50% of adolescents report sub-syndromal symptoms of depression. In addition, there is a major increase in the rate of depression from mid- to late adolescence.

There are many processes that can underpin affective disorders, but one critical group of processes relate to the emerging sense of self and self-to-self relating (e.g. self-criticism). Shame and self-criticism are associated with a range of psychological difficulties, including various forms of depression, substance misuse, eating disorder, social anxiety, and psychosis (see Gilbert & Irons, 2005; Zuroff et al., 2005 for review). These disorders have in common shame, self-criticism, feelings of inferiority (unfavorable social comparison), and submissive behavior. This chapter will explore these processes in relation to mood, and in particular, the way they are linked to children's and adolescents' experience of social place and acceptance.

Shame and its relationship to self-criticism

Humans are a highly social species, whose survival and reproductive opportunities depend on how they relate to others and how others relate to the self.

Adolescent Emotional Development and the Emergence of Depressive Disorders, ed. Nicholas B. Allen and Lisa B. Sheeber. Published by Cambridge University Press. © Cambridge University Press 2009.

As we grow, social relationships influence the way our brain matures (Schore, 1994, 2001) and the regulation of stress and immune functions conducive to health (Cacioppo *et al.*, 2000). Social relationships are key to joy and happiness (Argyle, 1987), depression and anxiety (Gilbert, 1992), resilience to life stressors (Masten, 2001), and self-evaluations (Baldwin & Dandeneau, 2005).

As we mature, a suite of evolved, social motivational systems come on line that will guide us to forming certain types of social roles and to understand and think about the nature of our relationships with self and others. These include seeking and responding to attachment to carers (Bowlby, 1969; Cassidy & Shaver, 1999) and groups (Baumeister & Leary, 1995), and concern with our relative social place (Gilbert, 1992, 2000a, 2000b). In addition, there are unfolding competencies for social understanding (such as theory of mind; Byrne, 1995) and self-conscious awareness (Lewis, 2003; Tracy & Robins, 2004). All of these make us very sensitive, focused, and responsive to "what others think and feel about us." Conscious and non-conscious processing systems monitor self-in-relationship-to-others, influencing both social behavior and self-evaluation (Baldwin, 2005).

One of the important social needs that link to a felt sense of security in relationships is the need to create positive affect in the mind of others. It has been suggested that with maturation, it is the knowledge that we are valued and seen as individuals of worth by others that creates a sense of security in the social domain (Gilbert, 1989, 1997, 2005a). This mirroring creates emotional memories of existing positively in the mind of others, contributing to a sense of self as loveable/valued (Leary, 1995).

Various models of shame have evolved from Helen Lewis' original observations (Lewis, 1971). These models are very focused on self-evaluation and self-feeling. In contrast, Gilbert's (1992, 1997, 1998, 2003) model of shame is linked to the work of Cooley (1902), Kohut (1977) and Bowlby (1969) that stresses the co-construction of self, and the importance of the experience of self in the mind of the "other." These theorists stress that humans are innately motivated to seek social acceptance. Relationships conducive to health and prosperity involve eliciting care, developing supportive alliances, and attracting friends and sexual partners. These in turn are dependent on being able to create positive affect about the self (e.g. liking, desire) in the mind of others. Thus, we seek to be liked by our friends, seen as competent and talented by our bosses, and desirable by our lovers. Potential partners in these roles will, in their turn, choose to invest in relationships that are conducive to their own self-interests such that they will (say) form friendships with those who are supportive of them, and seek out sexual partners who are desirable. Thus, social competition is often about competing to be seen as *attractive in the minds* of another so that they will choose in our favor (Etcoff, 1999; Gilbert, 1997, 2002, 2003). Social relationships can therefore be *competitive* for social place, and people may at times attempt to undermine the perceived attractiveness of others (e.g. spreading rumors or shaming) or even attack potential competitors in various social rivalries. The experiences of shame have therefore been likened to the experience of threat or loss of abilities to create desirable images in the mind of the other so that the other will reject the self (Gilbert, 1998). The depressed child and adolescent often focus on their ability to feel acceptable to, and wanted by, others in their group.

Self-evaluation is derived from evaluation by others

There is increasing evidence that self-evaluation cannot be easily separated from expectations of evaluation by others. Santor & Walker (1999) have shown that having qualities that one thinks *others will value* is especially related to self-esteem. This is more so than having qualities that are only valued by oneself. Leary *et al.* (1995) suggested that self-esteem is a form of internal tracking of one's attractiveness to others and sense of belonging. In other words, it is what one thinks others will value about the self that is often key to self-esteem and confidence (Santor & Walker, 1999). Baldwin & Holmes (1987) found that people who were primed with (asked to think about) a highly evaluative relationship, and who then failed at a laboratory task, showed depressive-like responses of blaming themselves for their failure and drawing broad negative conclusions about their personality (i.e. a typical shame response). Conversely, individuals who were instead primed with a warm, supportive relationship were much less upset by the failure and attributed the negative outcome to situational factors rather than personal shortcomings. People can cope better with failures if they have access to schema of others as warm and supportive. In another study, students were asked to generate research ideas and were then subliminally primed (outside of conscious awareness) with either the approving or disapproving face of the department professor. Those primed with the disapproving face rated their ideas more unfavorably than those primed with the approval face. *Self*-evaluation was non-consciously linked to approval/disapproval of another (see Baldwin & Dandeneau, 2005, for reviews). It appears that the degree to which people are able to access warm and supportive, or condemning and critical, other-to-self and self-to-self-scripts and memories has a central bearing on emotional and social responses to events.

The central focus of "the mind of the other," and how one experiences oneself as existing in the mind of the other, is reflected in a host of evolved cognitive competencies that are specifically designed for these functions. From early childhood onwards through adolescence, humans have evolved a variety of maturating cognitive competencies, which are specifically focused on understanding and working out what is occurring in the mind of others

(Byrne, 1995). Animals can engage in socially avoidant, fearful or approach behavior because they can interpret various social cues (e.g. that the other is sexually receptive or in an aggressive state of mind). However, they may not be able to symbolically understand the reasons for such states. They probably can't appreciate that one can be criticized or rejected because others are making judgments of the self as untrustworthy, stupid, or lazy. Humans, however, have evolved high level cognitive, meta-cognitive and symbolic abilities that can attribute intentions and feelings to others (e.g. I believe that she does not like me *because* she sees me as bad, untrustworthy, or ugly). Suddendorf & Whitten (2001) suggest that these competencies (for theory of mind, symbolic self-other representations, and meta-cognition) make the human mind a "collating mind," capable of building complex models of self, and self in relation to others.

Shame

Shame is typically linked to the experience of having negative aspects of self exposed (Lewis, 1992, 2003); that is to say, to the experience of the other feeling contempt or ridicule for various aspects of the self. Although negative *self*-evaluation is an important feature of shame (Tangney & Dearing, 2002; Tracy & Robins, 2004), the first shame experiences probably begin as a felt sense of how another person is experiencing/reacting to oneself. It is possible that these experiences are linked to motor programs in that a child may automatically find an angry, blank/disinterested, or disgust face aversive. This aversive experience may act as a precursor of shame (Draghi-Lorenz *et al.* 2001; Trevarthen & Aitken 2001).

In terms of *shame responses* in social interactions, these involve changes in non-verbal behaviors, self-evaluations, and self-conscious emotions, many of which can be seen as submissive-like forms of defense (Gilbert & McGuire, 1998). Here, however, we focus on aspects of shame that seem especially relevant to later childhood and adolescence where the competitions for social place become more intense. Looked at in terms of competitions for social attractiveness, shame can be seen to act as an internal warning that one will not, or has not, been able to create positive feelings in others, and that, consequently, they will/do see oneself negatively (e.g. as untalented, boring, or having some positively unattractive qualities). Although shame is commonly seen as a self-focused and self-evaluative experience of being inadequate in some way (Tangney & Dearing, 2002; Tracey & Robins, 2004), the research noted above suggests that self-experiences are related to how we think we exist in the minds of others.

There is a long tradition of distinguishing internally focused (on self) and externally focused (on the other) attention in relation to emotions

(Arndt & Goldenberg, 2004; Duval & Wicklund, 1972). Thus, Gilbert (1997, 1998, 2002, 2003, 2007) suggested that shame can focus on two types of evaluation. *External shame* relates to the way attention and cognitive processing is attuned externally – to what is going on in the minds of others about the self. *Internal shame* relates to the way attention and cognitive processing are attuned inwardly, to our own emotions, personal characteristics, and behavior. However, such a focus is still socially contextualized to the extent that the focus of internal shame relates to social definitions that distinguish the attractive and desirable from the unattractive and undesirable. For example, being quick to use aggression may be treated with respect in one social group (e.g. street gang) but be deeply shaming in another (e.g. a Buddhist monastery).

Although, as discussed shortly, shame can emerge from peer-group relationships, especially those involving bullying, its earliest precursors are in more intimate and family relationships. For example, we can imagine a young child who shows off a new dance or dress to her parents. The parents respond with facial expressions of positive affect and pleasure: "wow that looks wonderful!". These emotions, expressed by the parent, then stimulate positive emotions in the child about herself. It is as a result of stimulating this response in the mind of the other that she is able to feel pleasure and pride in her appearance. If, in contrast, the parent is dismissive or outwardly critical, this will have a detrimental effect on the experience of self, and may even generate a shame response. From a conditioning point of view, negative emotions in the other, which stimulate negative emotions (e.g. shame) in the self, may become associated with the display behavior (Gilbert, 2003). Whenever the child may think about displaying herself in a new dress, the emotional memories will be of creating negative emotions in others and a negative experience of self.

We suggest that such conditioning experiences, which are derived from the need to create positive affect in the mind of the other, can serve as one basis for the emergence of internal shame. In other words, experiences of shame, which operate within an interactional experience, can become the basis for negative self-experience and negative self-evaluation. This process continues into adolescence as youth become more sensitive to the images and emotions they are creating in their peers. The motivation remains the same throughout life (i.e. to be valued and included), but the targets change (e.g. shifting from parents to peers). Generating negative affect in the minds of peers, which may result in being excluded, shamed, or ridiculed, can become associated with the child and adolescent's maturing sense of self (Lewis, 2003). Both in childhood and adolescence therefore, what is key to shame and self-to-self relating is the way in which others are experienced as relating to the self.

Although internal shame has been linked to failing to meet self-standards, the evidence does not support this view unless these "failures" are seen to render one as an unattractive social agent in some way. Indeed, using qualitative methods to explore the idea that shame was about failure to live up to ideals, Lindsay-Hartz *et al.* (1995) reported that:

> To our surprise we found that most of the participants rejected this formulation. Rather, when ashamed, participants talked about being who they did *not* want to be. That is, they experienced themselves as embodying an anti-ideal, rather than simply not being who they wanted to be. The participants said things like "I am fat and ugly," not "I failed to be pretty;" or "I am bad and evil," not "I am not as good as I want to be." This difference in emphasis is not simply semantic. Participants insisted that the distinction was important . . . (p. 277).

It would appear then that internal shame requires a perception of self as actually "unattractive" – not just as failing to reach a standard (Gilbert, 1992, 1997, 2002); that is to say, it is closeness to an undesired and unattractive self rather than distance from a desired self that is at issue (Ogilive, 1987).

Model outline

In this approach to shame it is *external* shame that sits centrally in our orientation to social relationships and self-evaluations. This can be depicted in a simple model as shown in Figure 11.1. The model begins by recognizing our innate motives to form attachments to others and to use attachment objects as a "secure" base with soothing qualities (Bowlby 1969, 1973). In addition, humans have innate needs to be able to stimulate positive affect in the minds of others. This allows us to form supportive bonds both within and outside of family settings. With maturation come various cognitive competencies for self-evaluations and also for "thinking about" what is going on in the minds of others about the self. These motives and cognitive competencies are all attuned for social living and become acutely focused on peers during adolescence.

People's experiences within relationships occur within social and cultural contexts. These contexts can create benign or hostile environments and define what is attractive or acceptable from what is not. Clearly, this has a major implication for ethnic variation. Cultural values and interpersonal styles are located either within the family or in wider social groups. These experiences, arising from specific interactions, indicate whether the individual is regarded as attractive, accepted, belonging or esteemed, in contrast to unattractive and vulnerable to social harm. It is the latter that opens the potential for shame experiences.

At the center of the model is external shame, where we experience ourselves through the minds of others or "how we exist in the mind of others." It is when we feel the other sees us with negative affect, especially contempt with a desire to criticize, exclude, or avoid that external shame can be activated.

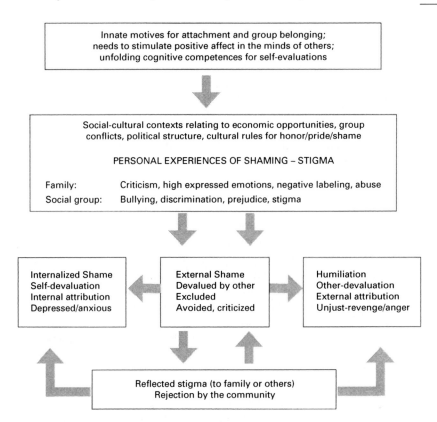

Figure 11.1. An evolutionary and biopsychosocial model for shame (adapted from Gilbert, 2002).

A key component of this model is that this experience of the other, as a threat to self and self-identity, activates different types of defenses. Internalized shame is where there is identification with the mind of the other, such that the person self-devalues. This is much more likely to occur in the context of a powerful other where any counter-attack could be severely put-down. As described elsewhere (Gilbert & McGuire, 1998), shame is related to submissive self-monitoring and internalizing defenses. In contrast, perceiving others as critical or ridiculing could ignite anger with a strong desire to retaliate. When this defensive response is prominent, humiliation is the nature of the experience. Hence, humiliation involves an attribution that the negative image in the mind of the other about the self is because of some flaw or "badness" in the other (Gilbert, 1998). This model therefore distinguishes between internalizing and externalizing defenses to the same threat, namely negative evaluation by others.

From shame to self-criticism

One view of internal shame is that it is based on the experience of self as flawed and inadequate (Tangney & Dearing, 2002), becoming an undesired and unattractive self (Gilbert 1998). These self-focused judgments can be linked to self-criticism. In fact many of the items on a well-known shame measure (the Test of Self-Conscious Affect; TOSCA) developed by Tangney and Dearing focus on self-critical and self-condemning thoughts in specific situations. Gilbert *et al.* (2004) explored how students responded when things went wrong for them. We measured various forms and functions of self-criticism and abilities to be self-reassuring. Self-criticism was associated with depression and shame, but abilities to be self-reassuring, focusing on one's positive attributions, was inversely correlated with shame and depression. Self-criticism and self-attacking may be central to the internal shame response. To put this another way, internal shame and self-criticism are highly fused processes, making self-criticism an internal shaming process. Zuroff *et al.* (2005) review a wealth of research on pathogenic qualities of self-criticism associated with negative affect. Whelton & Greenberg (2005) found that it was the degree of contempt in self-criticism, the shame response of lowered body posture and sadness, and an inability to defend self against self-criticism (e.g. by coming up with counter-arguments) that were especially linked to depression.

Shame can involve a range of experiences including self-conscious feelings of inferiority, a sense of self being flawed, and being self-critical. Gilbert *et al.* (2005) found that the frequency of shame thoughts was related to depression and anger rumination. Cheung *et al.* (2004) found that feelings of shame and inferiority were significantly linked to depression rumination. In other words, people may well tend to ruminate on things they are ashamed of or feel self-critical about.

Striving to compete

The idea that feeling under pressure to earn one's place and avoid inferiority is related to psychopathology (which as we will note below is heightened in adolescence) is not new. Alfred Adler (1870–1937) suggested that such striving could develop to compensate for an inferiority complex. This complex could be the result of sibling rivalry or sibling favoritism. Indeed, Gilbert & Gelsma (1999) found that feeling that siblings were more favored than oneself was strongly associated with shame and depression.

A paradigm linked to competitive motivation is perfectionism, where individuals strive to reach unrealistic standards set either by themselves or by others. Dunkley *et al.* (2006a, 2006b) found that whilst some perfectionism was associated with personal standards, other forms of perfectionism were associated with evaluative concerns, especially being judged negatively by others. It is this perfectionist striving to improve the self, because of fear of others' evaluation that is particularly linked to psychopathology. Dunkley *et al.* (2003) suggest that self-critical perfectionists experience chronic dysphoria "because they experience minor hassles in catastrophic terms and perceive others as condemning, unwilling, or unavailable to help them in times of stress" (p. 235). Thus, the work of Dunkley and colleagues suggests that it is both the self-critical aspects that emerge when individuals fall short of their standards, and worrying about what others expect of them, that is particularly linked to psychopathology. Perfectionism in the absence of self-criticism seems less pathogenic.

Self-criticism and negative views of the self have also been strongly linked to depression in adolescence. Zuroff *et al.* (1994) found that self-criticism at the age of 12 predicted later adjustment and vulnerability to psychopathology. Shahar *et al.* (2003) found that in a large group of adolescents ($n=860$), self-criticism predicted less positive life events. They suggested that self-critical or self-reassuring styles impact upon what one elicits from the social and non-social environment. Self-critics may be less able to develop supportive peer group relations, the absence of which are highly linked to depression vulnerability.

Shame and self-criticism in adolescence

The above has offered a theory and outline for the linkage of shame to a variety of evolved social motives (e.g. to compete for social attractiveness in the minds of others), social evaluative competencies (e.g. theory of mind) and internal self-evaluative styles. We can explore these ideas in relation to the onset and progress through adolescence.

The dawning of adolescence precipitates a series of physiological, relational, and environmental changes including increasingly complex models of self and others, the formation of a new, more independent self-identity, the formation of new peer group identities, concerns with in-group and out-groups, a movement away from the family (and towards the peer group) as the source of self-evaluation and support, and the dialectical conflict between "getting on" and "getting ahead" (Allen & Land, 1999; Steinberg, 2002; Wolfe *et al.*, 1986). Research has suggested that as children progress into early- to mid-adolescence, they rate their peers as equal or greater in value than their parents in a number of domains, such as support and reassurance (Buhrmester, 1996). Steinberg (2002) notes that in adolescence, more than 50% of the day is spent with peers, in comparison to just 15% with parents.

Adolescence precipitates changing dynamics with attachment figures, with strivings for autonomy/distance from the parent and the use of peers for support (Allen & Land, 1999). In effect, the individual is entering a stage of life where they become more orientated towards joining groups of peers and competing for resources/social position. From an evolutionary point of view, adolescence is an entry into the reproductive phase of life and competition for reproduction-securing resources. Such resources are not just about the quality of mate one can attract but also the alliances one can develop to support a range of survival and reproductively linked life tasks. Thus, adolescence sees an invigoration of mutual evaluation and competition with each other for approval, acceptance, and status, as well as developing concern with being attractive to potential sex partners. Adolescence may be the time when the two key concerns of "getting along and getting ahead" come to the fore (Wolfe *et al.*, 1986). Looked at another way, because seeking to develop peer relationships, fit in and be attractive to others becomes so crucial, it also opens the potential for major difficulties with self-presentations, self-consciousness, shame, fear of rejection, and being allocated unwanted low social rank positions. Adolescents begin to compare themselves to others in a variety of domains and with a sense of vulnerability to rejection, exclusion, or bullying if that comparison is unfavorable (Irons & Gilbert, 2005). It is possible that a sense of disappointment and/or frustration with self in these socially competitive arenas can be one source for shame and self-criticism.

Some origins of shame

Carrying a vulnerability to a sense of inferiority can impact on a young person's sense of self, with a need to strive to impress others or make an impact (Leary, 1995). A key question is what the adolescents carry forward from their childhood in terms of internal models of self and others that may increase their need to strive to earn their social place, feelings of social insecurity, styles of social comparison and shame. For example, in what ways do secure and insecure attachment facilitate or interfere with abilities to engage in adolescent social competitions? Gilbert (1992, 2005a) suggested that insecure attachment could lead to a striving for recognition and a competitive orientation to various life tasks and goals. In a group of adolescents, Irons & Gilbert (2005) found that secure attachment was associated with favorable social comparison, whereas both avoidant and ambivalent attachment were associated with making unfavorable comparisons of self to others. In a mediation model it was found that insecure attachment was related to depression through its effect upon social comparison and submissive behavior. In other words, insecure attachment exerts its effect upon depression via vulnerability to unfavorable social comparison and submissive behavior. In comparison, for those adolescents who had secure attachment relationships, social rank variables did not mediate this relationship to depression. So it appears that insecure attachment may make adolescents sensitive to the social competitions of this phase of life, where they tend to experience themselves in relatively low rank and vulnerable positions.

Andrews (1998, 2002) has shown that childhood sexual abuse is associated with heightened shame, especially body shame, and this mediates the link between abusive experiences and depression. Feiring *et al.* (2002) found that in both children and adolescents the ability to adjust to sexual abuse was very much related to attributional style and the person's experience of shame. Their measure of shame does not distinguish between external shame and internalized shame. It is not only traumatizing experiences such as sexual abuse that are linked to shame and subsequent psychopathology (Andrews, 1998; Feiring *et al.*, 2002); other forms of harsh, critical, and abusive parenting have also been linked to shame proneness and vulnerability to psychopathology (Tangney & Dearing, 2002). Stuewig & McCloskey (2005) explored various self-conscious emotions during children's transition to adolescence. They found that harsh parenting in childhood, which involves both verbally and physically abusive experiences, was related to shame prone-ness. This relationship was maintained at 8-year follow up, but was mediated by parental rejection. This term is a slight misnomer, however, because the authors state that "parental rejection was unique to our study and was designed . . . to measure humiliating or shaming tactics used by parents." Teicher *et al.* (2006) explored the depressive and other pathogenic impacts of verbal, physical, and sexual abuse. Although considerable attention has been given to sexual and physical abuse, these researchers found that verbal abuse (being shouted at and called names in hostile emotional tones) was highly linked to subsequent depression and anxiety. Verbal abuse not only makes the other highly threatening but also has a major impact on the sense of self and shame proneness. Thus in effect the data are suggesting that in adolescence the link between harsh parenting and shame is mediated by parental shaming/humiliating. Interestingly, given the fact that shame is often regarded as a pathogenic variable, whereas guilt is a more moral and less pathogenic variable (Gilbert, 2003; Tangney & Dearing, 2002), Stuewig & McCloskey (2005) found that parental warmth was relatively unrelated to shame, but positively associated with guilt. Guilt probably depends on a capacity for empathy and an emotional connectedness and concern for others that shame does not (Gilbert, 1989, 2003).

Developmental consequences

In a major review of the developmental consequences of shame in adoles-cence, Reimer (1996) highlighted the fact that shame proneness has been poorly studied during this developmental phase. He notes that the experience of shame clusters around some key themes that either emerge for the first time in adolescence or begin to take more solid form. These include identity formation and emerging sexualities. As noted above, adolescence is a time when we can no longer rely on an identity formed in a family context but need to create one that will facilitate engagement with increasingly important peer groups. Processes such as stability of the peer group will affect these identities. Although not tested as far as we know, frequent moves of school may make difficulties of "fitting in" and making one's mark more pronounced, thus increasing risk of shame.

A second theme relates to the emergence of sexual feelings and bodily changes. Not only can this bring concerns with bodily changes, such as onset of menstruation, but also with increases in body fat and size, especially for girls. The meaning of these experiences will be contextualized within social arenas. A number of authors have suggested that young women are particularly vulnerable to shame in these domains because many social groups are more controlling of female sexuality. Shame is a common way to regulate social behavior, and women's bodies and behavior are more objectified and open to social comment/judgment (Fredrickson & Roberts, 1997).

The ability to both "display" sexual maturity and to regulate aspects of these changes (e.g. body size) can become an area for intense social competition and some girls, as a result of shame-related feelings, become more vulnerable to depression and eating disorders (Goss & Gilbert, 2002). Shame around sexual feelings, sexual behaviors (such as masturbation and same sex attractions), and conflicts with parental rules (e.g. feeling one's parents would be highly condemning/disgusted of sexual feelings/behaviors) are also heightened in this age period. Same sex attractions can be experienced as especially difficult and shaming for some adolescents.

Adolescence is a time when, in most Western societies, individuals are 'herded' together in large schools with an expectation that they will follow certain rules, apply themselves to certain goals, and achieve certain outcomes. Individuals may struggle to achieve these and be aware of the comparative success of their peers, creating a possible source of shame and envy. Those who are talented may worry about envious and shaming attacks from others.

Peer bullying, especially in adolescence, is well known to increase vulnerability to psychopathology (Hawker & Boulton, 2000). Although aggressive bullying – the use of physical intimidation to control another – is endemic to many animals (Gilbert, 2005b) and occurs in many forms of social relationships (Ireland, 2005; Schuster, 1996), it is probably only humans who use shaming and stigmatizing as a bullying and intimidatory tactic. Such forms of bullying as name calling, ridiculing and excluding, only make sense in social contexts where one is competing for attractiveness in the minds of others, for social places, and for the stress buffering power of positive relationships with others. Public forms of shaming act to try to create negative reputations about the self and affect one's ability to relate to others. For example, some adolescents may worry about forming friendships with those who have been shamed by a bully in case they receive the same treatment from the bully. This relates to the concern of "stigma consciousness" where people worry about being seen as having characteristics that locate them in a stigmatized group (Pinel, 1999). These forms of bullying, shaming, and stigmatizing are deeply problematic for some children, challenging their ability to manage self-identity and elicit social support in such situations (Hawker & Boulton, 2000). Moreover, problems with shame may be an underlying reason for adolescent bullying (Ahmed & Braithwaite, 2004).

Group ecology

There is increasing evidence that self-identities are associated with the social and physical ecologies of groups. For example, in hostile environments male identity tends to focus on "men are strong and fearless, who are able to demonstrate their courage." There may be a need to clearly segregate a male from a female identity. These processes are less pronounced in benign environments where individual and group survival does not depend upon "fearless" males (Gilmore, 1990; Gilbert, 2005a). Adolescent groups are also related to ecology where bullying and aggression are more likely in certain sections of society than others. Wright et al. (1986) discuss the literature on social status in small social groups with a focus on adolescents. They note that, in general, children who are socially competent, pro-social, and cooperative are liked, and win more competitions for acceptance than hostile, withdrawn or socially incompetent children. However, they suggest that aggression "appears not to predict social status as commonly as one might expect" (p. 524). In their view, rejection, acceptance, or even popularity relates more to the distinctiveness between the type of group and the person. They note several mechanisms that may underlie the relationship of status and accept-ance in the dimension of similarity and attraction. These include: (1) shared attitudes and beliefs providing consensual validation and consistency of values; and (2) common interests and goals. Thus, in groups with few aggressive children, aggressive children were likely to be unpopular. However, in groups consisting of many aggressive children it is withdrawn children who are likely to be unpopular. Wright et al. (1986) also note earlier work that shows positive verbal communication may be more predictive of popu-larity for middle-class children than working-class children. Hence, bullying and shame proneness appear to be related to "group fit."

Early background and self-criticism

As noted above, a key element of internal shame is a process of internal shaming that involves self-criticism and self-attacking. A number of studies have explored the relationship between early attachment, parental acceptance and mirroring, and self-critical styles in later childhood or adolescence. Koestner *et al.* (1991) used a longitudinal design to examine how parenting experiences at age 5 related to levels of self-criticism at age 10. They also explored the stability of self-criticism from ages 12 to 31. These data were taken from a study originally commenced in the early 1950s. They found that a restrictive and rejecting maternal style was related to the development of self-criticism, particularly in girls, even controlling for the child's early temperament. For women, self-criticism was stable throughout early adolescence to adulthood, but this was not true for men. These different trajectories for self-criticism in adolescent girls and boys have also been found by Shahar *et al.* (2004). For adolescent girls, self-criticism appears to drive depressive symptoms in a vicious circle, where the more depressed girls became, the more self-critical they became.

Brewin *et al.* (1996) found that self-criticism in young women was related to their perceived criticism from their mothers, but not the mothers' own judgment of criticism. Also, self-criticism regarding appearance was unrelated to parental criticism. Although not tested, this may relate to a more peer-focused domain. Thus it seems that maternal criticism has a powerful impact on self-criticism for adolescents. A number of models of the association between maternal rearing styles and self-criticism have been proposed. For example, Thompson & Zuroff (1999) proposed a model whereby maternal dissatisfaction with general life circumstances, relationships and interactions with their child impacts upon a warmth-coldness dimension of care. This dimension in turn affects the security of a daughter's attachment to her mother, which in turn impacts upon the daughter's self-critical style. In 54 pairs of mother–daughter dyads, where the daughter was 12–15, they found good evidence for this model. Importantly however, the relationship between maternal coldness and daughter self-criticalness was mediated by the degree of insecurity of the daughter's attachment to her mother.

Compassion and self-compassion

Taking all the above together suggests that self-identities and self-to-self relationships emerge in social contexts where we experience how we exist in the minds of the other. Shame and self-criticism are often fused, especially in contexts where externalizing anger at social put down can be dangerous, and safer strategies are those of internalizing and using submissive defenses of self-monitoring, self-blame, and social inhibition (Gilbert & Irons, 2005). Thus, in the model presented, we have suggested that shame and self-criticism often emerge in the context of harsh parenting and/or school bullying. In essence they emerge in contexts of threatening and unsafe environments, and hence shame and its submissive profile can be seen as a defensive strategy (Gilbert & Irons, 2005). In contrast, children and adolescents who grow up in a loving, caring, supportive and safe environment seem far less likely to adapt these strategies.

Another way to think of some of these difficulties is that people who suffer from them may be limited in their ability to be self-soothing and reassuring. This may partly be because they do not have many internalized emotional memories of others being kind and warm to them. The pathogenic qualities of self-criticism have been linked to two key processes. First is the degree of self-directed hostility, contempt, and self-loathing that permeates self-criticism (Gilbert, 2000a; Whelton & Greenberg, 2005; Zuroff *et al.*, 2005). Second is the relative inability to generate feelings of self-directed warmth, reassurance, soothing, and self-liking (Gilbert, 2000a; Gilbert *et al.*, 2004; Whelton & Greenberg, 2005). Even if one can help people reduce self-criticism, this may not activate self-soothing and self-compassionate abilities.

A number of therapies are now focusing on the importance of helping people develop inner compassion and self-soothing abilities. This is especially noted in Dialectical Behavior Therapy (Linehan, 1993). The cognitive therapists McKay & Fanning (1992), who developed a self-esteem program, see self-compassion as a key antidote to self-criticism. They view compassion as consisting of understanding, acceptance, and forgiveness. Gilbert's (2000a, 2005a; Gilbert & Irons, 2005) model of compassion and compassion training was developed specifically to help people with high levels of shame and self-criticism (Gilbert, 2000a; Gilbert & Irons, 2005). It links concepts related to the evolution of caring behavior to new research in the neuroscience of socially focused positive affects (Depue & Morrone-Strupinsky, 2005). It addresses the elements of: developing genuine concern for one's well-being (not just achievements); being able to be sensitive and sympathetic to one's distress; becoming distress tolerant (including tolerance of one's limitations rather than hating oneself for them); developing empathy and deep understanding for one's feelings and states of mind; cultivating a non-judgmental approach to self; and fostering feeling of warmth and acceptance of self. Research is currently exploring the extent to which therapeutic interventions that target these processes can be helpful (Gilbert & Procter, 2006), and we hope to extend this research to an adolescent population.

Conclusion

Adolescence is a time of major physical, psychological, and social change as youth prepare to focus their social lives less on parents in favor of peers. This is a phase of life which sees an invigoration of competition for resources conducive to well-being and reproductive trajectory. It is a time of making and breaking friendships and alliances, as well as of concerns with in-group and out-group, social presentation, fitting in, and being accepted and valued.

How adolescents engage and navigate through these competitive arenas is dependent on a range of factors related to the stability and ecology of groups and what adolescents bring to their relationships as a result of temperament and early history. This chapter has suggested that a number of psychological processes are linked together in regard to social competition. These include proneness to feelings of shame, a heightened focus on social comparison (and one's relative social place), submissive behavior, and internal self-regulation that is linked to self-criticism or self-reassuring.

The shame constellation of emotions includes self-evaluations that emerge more commonly when social environments are hostile, resources are relatively few, and mutually supportive and caring behavior is not highly reinforced. Certainly it would seem that proneness to these feelings and evaluations are linked to early childhood experiences. If adolescence is a time of increased vulnerability to psychopathology, we can focus on the competitive dynamics of adolescence and ponder how certain environments invigorate competitive behavior in both helpful and unhelpful ways.

REFERENCES

Ahmed E., & Braithwaite, V. (2004). "What, me ashamed?" Shame management and school bullying. *Journal of Research in Crime and Delinquency,* **41**, 269–294.

Allen, J.P., & Land, D. (1999). Attachment in adolescence. In J. Cassidy & P. Shaver (Eds.), *Handbook of Attachment: Theory, Research and Clinical Applications* (pp. 319–335). New York, NY: Guilford Press.

Andrews, B. (1998). Shame and childhood abuse. In P. Gilbert & B. Andrews (Eds.), *Shame: Interpersonal Behavior, Psychopathology and Culture* (pp. 176–190). New York, NY: Oxford University Press.

Andrews, B. (2002). Body shame and abuse in childhood. In P. Gilbert and J. Miles (Eds.), *Body Shame: Conceptualisation, Research and Treatment* (pp. 256–266). London: Routledge.

Angold, A., & Costello, E.J. (2001). The epidemiology of depression in children and adolescents. In I.M. Goodyer (Ed.), *The Depressed Child and Adolescent* (2nd edn, pp. 143–178). Cambridge, UK: Cambridge University Press.

Argyle, M. (1987). *The Psychology of Happiness.* London: Routledge.

Arndt, J., & Goldenberg, J.L. (2004). From self-awareness to shame proneness: evidence of causal sequence amongst women. *Self and Identity,* **3**, 27–37.

Baldwin, M.W. (Ed.). (2005). *Interpersonal Cognition.* New York, NY: Guilford Press.

Baldwin, M.W., & Dandeneau, S.D. (2005). Understanding and modifying the relational schemas underlying insecurity. In M.W. Baldwin (Ed.), *Interpersonal Cognition* (pp. 33–61). New York, NY: Guilford Press.

Baldwin, M.W., & Holmes, J.G. (1987). Salient private audiences and awareness of the self. *Journal of Personality and Social Psychology,* **52**, 1087–1098.

Baumeister, R.F., & Leary, M.R. (1995). The need to belong: desire for interpersonal attachments as a fundamental human motivation. *Psychological Bulletin,* **117**, 497–529.

Bowlby, J. (1969). *Attachment and Loss.* New York: Basic Books.

Bowlby, J. (1973). *Attachment and Loss, Vol. II. Separation.* New York: Basic Books.

Brewin, C.R., Andrews, B., & Furnham, A. (1996). Self-critical attitudes and parental criticism in young women. *British Journal of Medical Psychology,* **69,** 69–78.

Buhrmester, D. (1996). Need fulfillment, interpersonal competence, and developmental contexts of early adolescent friendships. In W.M. Bukowski, A.F. Newcomb, & W.W. Hartup (Eds.), *The Company they Keep: Friendship in Childhood and Adolescence* (pp. 158–185). New York: Cambridge University Press.

Byrne, R.W. (1995). *The Thinking Ape.* Oxford, UK: Oxford University Press.

Cacioppo, J.T., Berston, G.G., Sheridan, J.F., & McClintock, M.K. (2000). Multilevel integrative analysis of human behavior: social neuroscience and the complementing nature of social and biological approaches. *Psychological Bulletin,* **126,** 829–843.

Cassidy, J., & Shaver, P.R. (Eds.) (1999). *Handbook of Attachment: Theory, Research and Clinical Applications* (pp. 115–140). New York, NY: Guilford Press.

Cheung, M.S.P., Gilbert, P., & Irons, C. (2004). An exploration of shame, social rank and rumination in relation to depression. *Personality and Individual Differences,* **36,** 1143–1153.

Cooley, C.H. (1902). *Human Nature and the Social Order.* New York, NY: Scribner's.

Depue, R.A., & Morrone-Strupinsky, J.V. (2005). A neurobehavioral model of affiliative bonding. *Behavioral and Brain Sciences,* **28,** 313–395.

Draghi-Lorenz, R., Reddy, V., & Costall, A. (2001). Rethinking the development of "nonbasic" emotions: a critical review of existing theories. *Developmental Psychology,* **21,** 263–304.

Dunkley, D.M., Zuroff, D.C., & Blankstein, K.R. (2003). Self-critical perfectionism and daily affect: dispositional and situational influences on stress and coping. *Journal of Personality and Social Psychology,* **84,** 234–252.

Dunkley, D.M., Blankstein, K.R., Zuroff, D.C., Lecce, S., & Hui, D. (2006a). Self-critical and personal standards factors of perfectionism located within the five-factor model of personality. *Personality and Individual Differences,* **40,** 409–420.

Dunkley, D.M., Zuroff, D.C., & Blankstein, K.R. (2006b). Specific perfectionism components versus self-criticism in predicting maladjustment. *Personality and Individual Differences,* **40,** 665–676.

Duval, S., & Wickland, R.A. (1972). *A Theory of Objective Self-Awareness.* New York: Academic Press.

Etcoff, N. (1999). *Survival of the Prettiest: The Science of Beauty.* New York, NY: Doubleday.

Feiring, C., Taska, L., & Lewis. M. (2002). Adjustment following sexual abuse discovery: the role of shame and attributional style. *Developmental Psychology,* **38,** 79–92.

Fredrickson, B.L., & Roberts, T.A. (1997). Objectification theory: toward understanding women's lived experiences and mental health risks. *Psychology of Women Quarterly,* **21,** 173–206.

Gilbert, P. (1989). *Human Nature and Suffering.* Hove, UK: Lawrence Erlbaum.

Gilbert, P. (1992). *Depression: The Evolution of Powerlessness.* New York: Guilford Press.

Gilbert, P. (1997). The evolution of social attractiveness and its role in shame, humiliation, guilt and therapy. *British Journal of Medical Psychology,* **70,** 113–147.

Gilbert, P. (1998). What is shame? Some core issues and controversies. In P. Gilbert & B. Andrews (Eds.), *Shame: Interpersonal Behavior, Psychopathology and Culture* (pp. 3–38). New York, NY: Oxford University Press.

Gilbert, P. (2000a). Social mentalities: internal 'social' conflicts and the role of inner warmth and compassion in cognitive therapy. In P. Gilbert & K.G. Bailey (Eds.), *Genes on the Couch: Explorations in Evolutionary Psychotherapy* (pp. 118–150). Philadelphia: Brunner-Routledge.

Gilbert, P. (2000b). The relationship of shame, social anxiety and depression: the role of the evaluation of social rank. *Clinical Psychology and Psychotherapy*, **7**, 174–189.

Gilbert, P. (2002). Body shame: a biopsychosocial conceptualisation and overview, with treatment implications. In P. Gilbert & J.N.V. Miles (Eds.), *Body Shame: Conceptualisation, Research and Treatment* (pp. 3–54). Hove, East Sussex: Brunner-Routledge.

Gilbert, P. (2003). Evolution, social roles, and differences in shame and guilt. *Social Research: An International Quarterly of the Social Sciences*, **70**, 1205–1230.

Gilbert, P. (2005a). Compassion and cruelty: a biopsychosocial approach. In P. Gilbert (Ed.), *Compassion: Conceptualisations, Research and Use in Psychotherapy* (pp. 9–74). London, UK: Routledge.

Gilbert, P. (2005b). Bullying in prisons: an evolutionary and biopsychosocial approach. In J.L. Ireland (Ed.), *Bullying among Prisoners: Innovations in Theory and Research*. Cullompton, UK: Willan.

Gilbert, P. (2007). The evolution of shame as marker for relationship security: a biopsychosocial approach. In J. Tracy, R. Robins, & J. Tangney (Eds.), *The Self-conscious Emotions: Theory and Research* (pp. 283–309). New York, NY: Guilford Press.

Gilbert, P., & Gelsma, C. (1999). Recall of favouritism in relation to psychopathology. *British Journal of Clinical Psychology*, **38**, 357–373.

Gilbert P., & Irons C. (2005). Focused therapies and compassionate mind training for shame and self attacking. In P. Gilbert (Ed.), *Compassion: Conceptualisations, Research and Use in Psychotherapy* (pp. 263–325). London, UK: Routledge.

Gilbert, P., & McGuire, M. (1998). Shame, social roles and status: the psychobiological continuum from monkey to human. In P. Gilbert & B. Andrews (Eds.), *Shame: Interpersonal Behavior, Psychopathology and Culture* (pp. 99–125). New York, NY: Oxford University Press.

Gilbert, P., & Procter S. (2006). Compassionate mind training for people with high shame and self-criticism: a pilot study of a group therapy approach. *Clinical Psychology and Psychotherapy*, **13**, 353–379.

Gilbert, P., Clarke, M., Hempel, S., Miles, J.N.V., & Irons, C. (2004). Criticising and reassuring oneself: an exploration of forms, styles and reasons in female students. *British Journal of Clinical Psychology*, **43**, 31–50.

Gilbert, P., Cheung, M., Irons, C., & McEwan, K. (2005). An exploration into depression focused and anger focused rumination in relation to depression in a student population. *Behavioural and Cognitive Psychotherapy*, **33**, 1–11.

Gilmore, D.D. (1990). *Manhood in the Making: Cultural Concepts of Masculinity*. New Haven, CT: Yale University Press.

Goss, K., & Gilbert, P. (2002). Eating disorders, shame and pride: a cognitive–behavioural functional analysis. In P. Gilbert & J. Miles (Eds.), *Body Shame: Conceptualisation, Research and Treatment* (pp. 219–255). London, UK: Brunner-Routledge.

Hankin, B.L. (2006). Adolescent depression: description, causes and interventions. *Epilepsy and Behaviour*, **8**, 102–114.

Hawker, D.S., & Boulton, M.J. (2000). Twenty years' research on peer victimisation and psychosocial maltreatment: a meta-analytic review of cross sectional studies. *Journal of Child Psychology and Psychiatry and Allied Disciplines*, **41**, 441–455.

Ireland, J.L. (Ed.). (2005). *Bullying among Prisoners: Innovations in Theory and Research*. Cullompton, UK: Willan.

Irons, C., & Gilbert, P. (2005). Evolved mechanisms in adolescent anxiety and depression symptoms: the role of the attachment and social rank systems. *Journal of Adolescence*, **28**, 325–341.

Koestner, R., Zuroff, D.C., & Powers, T.A. (1991). Family origins of adolescent self-criticism and its continuity into adulthood. *Journal of Abnormal Psychology*, **100**, 191–197.

Kohut, H. (1977). *The Restoration of the Self*. New York, NY: International Universities Press.

Leary, M.R. (1995). *Self-presentation: Impression Management and Interpersonal Behavior*. Madison, WI: Brown & Benchmark's.

Leary, M.R., Tambor, E.S., Terdal, S.K., & Downs, D.L. (1995). Self-esteem as an interpersonal monitor: the sociometer hypothesis. *Journal of Personality and Social Psychology*, **68**, 519–530.

Lewis, H.B. (1971). *Shame and Guilt in Neurosis*. New York, NY: International University Press.

Lewis, M. (1992). *Shame: The Exposed Self*. New York, NY: The Free Press.

Lewis, M. (2003). The role of the self in shame. *Social Research, An International Quarterly of the Social Sciences*, **70**, 1181–1204.

Lindsay-Hartz, J., de Rivera, J., & Mascolo, M.F. (1995). Differentiating guilt and shame and their effects on motivations. In J.P. Tangney & K.W. Fischer (Eds.), *Self-conscious Emotions. The Psychology of Shame, Guilt, Embarrassment and Pride* (pp. 274–300). New York, NY: Guilford Press.

Linehan, M. (1993). *Cognitive Behavioral Treatment of Borderline Personality Disorder*. New York, NY: Guilford Press.

Masten, A.S. (2001). Ordinary magic: Resilience processes in development. *American Psychologist*, **56**, 227–238.

McKay, M., & Fanning, P. (1992). *Self-esteem: A Proven Program of Cognitive Techniques for Assessing, Improving, and Maintaining your Self-esteem* (2nd edn). Oakland, CA: New Harbinger Publishers.

Pinel, E.C. (1999). Stigma consciousness: the psychological legacy of social stereotypes. *Journal of Personality and Social Psychology*, **76**, 114–128.

Reimer, M.S. (1996). Sinking into the ground: the development and consequences of shame in adolescence. *Developmental Review*, **16**, 321–363.

Ogilive, D.M. (1987). The undesired self: a neglected variable in personality research. *Journal of Personality and Social Psychology*, **52**, 379–388.

Santor, D., & Walker, J. (1999). Garnering the interests of others: mediating the effects among physical attractiveness, self-worth and dominance. *British Journal of Social Psychology*, **38**, 461–477.

Schore, A.N. (1994). *Affect Regulation and the Origin of the Self: The Neurobiology of Emotional Development*. Hillsdale, NJ: Lawrence Erlbaum.

Schore, A.N. (2001). The effects of early relational trauma on right brain development, affect regulation, and infant mental health. *Infant Mental Health Journal*, **22**, 201–269.

Schuster, B. (1996). Rejection, exclusion, and harassment at work and in schools. *European Psychologist*, 1, 293–317.

Shahar, G., Henrich, C.C., Blatt, S.J., Ryan, R., & Little, T.D. (2003). Interpersonal relatedness, self-definition and their motivational orientation during adolescence: a theoretical and empirical integration. *Developmental Psychology*, **39**, 470–483.

Shahar, G., Blatt, S.J., Zuroff, D.C., Kupermine, G.P., & Leadbeater, B.J. (2004). Reciprocal relationship between depressive symptoms and self-criticism (but not dependency) among early adolescent girls (but not boys). *Cognitive Therapy and Research*, **28**, 85–103.

Steinberg, L. (2002). *Adolescence*. Boston, MA: McGraw Hill.

Stuewig, J., & McCloskey, L.A. (2005). The relation of child maltreatment to shame and guilt among adolescents: psychological routes to depression and delinquency. *Child Maltreatment*, **10**, 324–336.

Suddendorf, T., & Whitten, A. (2001). Mental evolutions and development: evidence for secondary representation in children, great apes and other animals. *Psychological Bulletin*, **127**, 629–650.

Tangney, J.P., & Dearing, R.L. (2002). *Shame and Guilt*. New York, NY: Guilford Press.

Teicher, M.H., Samson, J.A., Polcari, A., & McGreenery, C.E. (2006). Sticks and stones and hurtful words: relative effects of various forms of childhood maltreatment. *American Journal of Psychiatry*, **163**, 993–1000.

Thompson, R., & Zuroff, D.C. (1999). Development of self-criticism in adolescent girls: roles of maternal dissatisfaction, maternal coldness, and insecure attachment. *Journal of Youth and Adolescence*, **28**, 197–210.

Tracy, J.L., & Robins, R.W. (2004). Putting the self into self-conscious emotions: a theoretical model. *Psychological Inquiry*, **15**, 103–125.

Trevarthen, C., & Aitken, K. (2001). Infant intersubjectivity: research, theory, and clinical applications. *Journal of Child Psychology and Psychiatry*, **42**, 3–48.

Whelton, W.J., & Greenberg, L.S. (2005). Emotion in self-criticism. *Personality and Individual Differences*, **38**, 1583–1595.

Wolfe, R.N., Lennox, R.D., & Cutler, B.L. (1986). Getting along and getting ahead: empirical support for a theory of protective and acquisitive self-presentation. *Journal of Social and Personality Psychology*, **50**, 356–361.

Wright, J.C., Giammarino, M., & Parad, H.W. (1986). Social status in small groups: individual-group similarity and social "misfit." *Journal of Personality and Social Psychology*, **50**, 523–536.

Zuroff, D.C., Koestner, R., & Powers, T.A. (1994). Self-criticism at age 12: a longitudinal study of adjustment. *Cognitive Therapy and Research*, **18**, 367–385.

Zuroff, D.C., Santor, D., & Mongrain, M. (2005). Dependency, self-criticism, and maladjustment. In S.J. Blatt, J.S. Auerbach, K.N. Levy, & C.E. Schaffer (Eds.), *Relatedness, Self-definition, and Mental Representation: Essays in Honor of Sidney J. Blatt.* (pp. 75–90) London: Routledge.

12

Temperament in early adolescence

Ann V. Sanson, Primrose Letcher, and Diana Smart

Introduction – Why study temperament in the context of early adolescent development?

The publication of the report by Thomas, Chess and colleagues on the New York Longitudinal Study (Thomas *et al.*, 1963) reflected the start of a paradigm shift from a predominantly environmentalistic, unidirectional perspective on child development, to one which acknowledged the child's own active part in the developmental process. They demonstrated clear differences between children in such qualities as their responsiveness to stimulation and capacity to regulate their emotions and attention that impacted upon their subsequent socio-emotional development. While notions of temperament predated Thomas and Chess by two millennia (at least from the time of Galen, 131–201 AD), the modern interest in *child* temperament can largely be dated to this publication.

While there has always been interest in the connections between early temperament and adolescent functioning, interest in adolescent temperament itself is more recent and less advanced. However, there is increasing evidence of the role of temperament-based individual differences in explaining socio-emotional functioning in adolescence. This chapter seeks to provide an account of current understanding and empirical findings regarding the nature of adolescent temperament, its connections with child temperament and adolescent/adult personality, and its associations with various aspects of socio-emotional functioning.

Adolescent Emotional Development and the Emergence of Depressive Disorders, ed. Nicholas B. Allen and Lisa B. Sheeber. Published by Cambridge University Press. © Cambridge University Press 2009.

Theoretical models of temperament

Theoretical models of temperament in infancy and childhood

Emerging out of long-standing debate is a consensus that the term "temperament" refers to constitutionally based differences in reactivity and regulation that are visible from the child's earliest years. More specifically, temperament is commonly defined as individual differences in emotional, motor, and attentional reactivity to stimulation, and in patterns of emotional, behavioral, and attentional self-regulation (Rothbart & Bates, 2006; Sanson *et al.*, 2004).

In their seminal work, Thomas, Chess and colleagues identified nine dimensions of temperament, namely approach-withdrawal, adaptability, quality of mood, intensity of reaction, distractibility, persistence or attention span, rhythmicity, threshold of responsiveness, and activity level (Thomas *et al.*, 1963). Various other models of child temperament have been proposed, some of which emphasize biological bases for temperament. For example, Posner & Rothbart (1998) point to the role of the anterior cingulate in the effortful regulation of attention, and Kagan and colleagues posit a role for threshold to arousal in the amygdala (Kagan & Fox, 2006).

Despite these differing views, three broad aspects of child temperament are gaining wide acceptance: *Reactivity or Negative Emotionality*, referring to irritability, negative mood and high-intensity negative reactions, which can be differentiated into distress to limitations (irritability, anger) and distress to novelty (fearfulness); *Self-Regulation*, which has three subcomponents – the effortful control of attention (e.g. persistence, non-distractibility), of emotions (e.g. self-soothing), and of behavior (e.g. delay of gratification); and a dimension variously labeled *Approach-Withdrawal, Inhibition,* or *Sociability,* which describes the tendency to approach novel situations and people or conversely to withdraw and be wary, and includes aspects of positive emotionality. *Surgency,* a factor in Rothbart's model (Rothbart *et al.*, 2000), incorporates these aspects of approach with other facets such as activity.

Theoretical models of temperament in adolescence

There are three issues to consider concerning the relationship of adolescent temperament to infant and child temperament: possible changes in the underlying structure of temperament (its major dimensions); changes in mean levels or expression of temperament traits (i.e. normative trends for decreases or increases); and the across-time stability of temperament over this period (i.e. changes in temperament for individuals). Adolescence is characterized by major biological, cognitive, and social changes, in which new behaviors are expressed and there is increasing capacity to modulate the expression of underlying propensities. During adolescence, temperament traits also continue to be shaped by experience and the environment. Hence some variation in both the structure and the expression of temperament from childhood to adolescence could be expected. This section addresses the issue of structural continuity; changes in mean levels and individual rank-order stability are taken up in the following section.

Models of temperament in the adolescent period have received limited theoretical and empirical attention, and conclusions are constrained by several factors. First, most researchers have focused on temperament in childhood, even when they have assessed its influence on outcomes in adolescence. Second, different measures of temperament have been employed at different ages, in part a necessity for tapping age-appropriate expressions of temperament, but restricting across-age comparisons. Many researchers have simply modified child temperament measures for use with adolescent samples (see McClowry et al., 2003), while others have applied adult personality or temperament models to adolescence (e.g. Lonigan et al., 2003; Putnam et al., 2001; Wills et al., 1998). Finally, there are a limited number of longitudinal studies following representative samples from early childhood through adolescence.

One of the few studies which have gathered detailed information on temperament from infancy to early adulthood is the Australian Temperament Project (ATP) which has followed a representative sample of children from the Australian state of Victoria from infancy to young adulthood, with temperament reported primarily by parent report (see Prior et al., 2000a). McClowry's School-Age Temperament Inventory (SATI; McClowry, 1995) has been used in the ATP from 12 to 18 years of age. Besides showing clear parallels to the temperament factors identified at earlier ages, the temperament dimensions in the SATI (negative reactivity, approach/shyness, persistence, and activity) emerged consistently in factor analyses of the data from 12 to 18 years (Prior et al., 2000a), confirming stability in structure of temperament from late childhood to late adolescence.

Rothbart and colleagues (Putnam et al., 2001) used their model of adult temperament to develop the parent- and self-report Revised Early Adolescent Temperament Questionnaire (REATQ), which contains eight temperament dimensions – high-intensity pleasure, shyness, fear, frustration, activation control, attention control, inhibitory control, and affiliation. These eight scales reflect the three broad dimensions also included in their childhood model (Surgency, Negative Affectivity, and Effortful Control), plus a fourth dimension, Affiliation. Thus, their findings suggest substantial structural continuity from childhood. In a study of 1978 Dutch pre-adolescents using parent reports, Oldehinkel et al. (2004) found some cross-national support for this structure. Five of the eight finer-grained dimensions emerged; Attention Control and Activation Control combined as one dimension of Effortful Control, and fear had high loadings on both the higher-order Surgency and Negative Affectivity dimensions.

Windle & Lerner's (1986) Dimensions of Temperament Survey (DOTS-R) is designed to cover the age range from early childhood to early adulthood with similar items across age, thus sacrificing some developmental sensitivity for across-age comparability. It is based on Thomas and Chess' 9-factor model of temperament, and includes 10 factors which are not identical in content across ages but show substantial similarities. A confirmatory factor analysis of adolescent data identified three higher-order dimensions: Adaptability/Positive Affect, General Rhythmicity, and Attentional Focus (Windle, 1992).

Some researchers have focused exclusively on positive and negative emotionality as temperament dimensions in adolescence, specifically in regard to their role as predictors of depression and anxiety (e.g. Lonigan et al., 2003). Support for these two relatively independent dimensions is growing, and they are partially reflected in broad-band factors in more comprehensive models of temperament, e.g. Rothbart's Surgency and Negative Affectivity, and the ATP's Approach and Reactivity factors.

Further longitudinal work with multiple informants across childhood and adolescence may assist in clarifying temperament structure in these developmental periods. However, on existing evidence, there appears to be considerable continuity in structure of temperament from childhood into adolescence. As with child temperament, and despite minor differences in emphasis and content of scales, the factors of Negative Reactivity or Emotionality, Self Regulation (especially effortful control of attention), and Approach/Inhibition or the broader construct of Surgency appear robust and salient aspects of adolescent temperament.

Stability and change in temperament from childhood to adolescence

Individual rank-order stability

The fact that there is at least moderate stability of temperament and personality traits across time is well-established. For example, inter-correlations in the ATP indicate substantial rank-order consistency in trait dimensions from late childhood (12 years) to late adolescence (18 years), with an average inter-correlation across the four time points of 0.66. Roberts & DelVecchio (2000) conducted a meta-analysis of longitudinal studies of temperament and personality traits, and concluded that consistency tends to increase with age from infancy to middle age. Stability tends to be relatively low prior to age 3 (an average rank-order consistency coefficient of 0.35), and moderate over childhood and adolescence, averaging 0.48. The ATP analyses (Pedlow et al., 1993) showed that stability coefficients increased considerably once measurement error was taken into account (being around 0.7–0.8 from 3 to 8 years).

There is also some evidence that children with more extreme temperamental traits are more likely to show stability of these traits than those with more moderate profiles (Kagan *et al.*, 1988; Sanson *et al.*, 1996).

Even these relatively high stability coefficients imply a considerable amount of change in an individual's temperament over time (a correlation coefficient of 0.70 implying less than 50% shared variance between two temperament assessments). At present, the bases for changes in temperament are poorly understood (Putnam *et al.*, 2002). A variety of reactive, evocative, and pro-active transactions between the child and the environment may either maintain, or change, a temperament profile (Caspi, 2000; Sanson *et al.*, 1996). For example, labeling a child as "shy" or "cheerful," by parents or others, may become a self-fulfilling prophecy as those around the child respond in accord with the label; and active niche-picking (e.g. of solitary or sociable pursuits) may exacerbate pre-existing temperamental tendencies towards withdrawal or approach.

The fact that temperament can be modified by environmental experiences is becoming increasingly apparent. Intervention studies have shown that changes in parental behavior can lead to changes in child negative reactivity (Rapee, 2002; van den Boom, 1995). Eisenberg *et al.* (2005), in a 3-wave longitudinal study in early adolescence, showed that positive parenting led to increases in effortful control. The ATP data showed that children who were at risk of antisocial behavior at 12 years but who showed resilience against developing antisocial behavior throughout adolescence, became less reactive and more persistent over the adolescent years, and concurrently their relationships with parents and teachers improved (Smart *et al.*, 2003). While this study cannot determine the mechanisms involved in modifying temperament traits, it does suggest that social relationships may be important in instigating change.

Normative developmental changes in temperament

The above findings refer to an individual's status on a temperament measure across time, relative to the rest of the sample. As noted above, given the substantial cognitive and other changes that occur with the onset of adolescence, it would be reasonable to suppose that there may also be normative developmental changes in temperament. Given the requirement for longitudinal data with comparable assessments over time, very few datasets have been able to examine this question.

The developmental course of self-regulation was investigated in a cohort of 646 children from the National Longitudinal Survey of Youth (Raffaelli *et al.*, 2005). They found an increase in self-regulation from early childhood (4–5 years) to middle childhood (8–9 years), as expected, but no change from middle childhood to adolescence (12–13 years). In the ATP study, there was evidence for normative changes in temperament traits over time, according to parent reports. There were clear normative trends for a decrease in negative reactivity and an increase in persistence from late childhood to mid-adolescence, suggesting that adolescents' increasing capacity to modulate their emotional reactions and control attention may support normative changes in temperamental expression. Levels of shyness tended to slightly increase across this time-span, perhaps reflecting the increasing complexity and importance of social relationships in adolescence. Across-time trends for activity were less clear-cut.

Thus the scant data available suggest that with maturation, self-regulatory capacities do increase. However, there is a clear need for further longitudinal research to advance understanding of the developmental course of temperament traits.

Relationship of child and adolescent temperament to personality

A pertinent issue when considering adolescent temperament is the relationship between temperament and personality, both of which refer to basic facets of individual differences. Clarification of these connections opens the door to consolidation of two often disparate areas of enquiry (Diener, 2000). Although the constructs of temperament and personality overlap considerably, temperament is generally thought to have a stronger biological basis, while personality is considered to develop later and be influenced more by learning, experience, and cognitive development (Eisenberg *et al.*, 2000; Hagekull & Bohlin, 1998).

Attempts to study the relationship between temperament and personality have been hindered by problems including the lack of an integrated literature on individual differences spanning childhood and adulthood, and measurement issues (e.g. different terms are often used to describe similar constructs, and the same term is sometimes used to refer to quite different constructs). Furthermore, child temperament tends to be assessed by parent report or observation, whereas personality is almost always assessed by self-report. Diener (2000) noted that "data that shed a bright light on the transition from childhood to adult personality have been hard to obtain and are scarce" (p. 120). Nevertheless, there is a growing literature on the nature and strength of the developmental connections between temperament and personality factors.

Several studies have documented associations between temperament and the Five Factor model of personality (comprising Extraversion, Neuroticism or Emotional Stability, Agreeableness, Conscientiousness, and Intellect or Openness to Experience). Despite difficulties comparing studies due to the differing measurement instruments, some consistent trends are emerging (Hagekull & Bohlin, 1998; Prior *et al.*, 2000a; Rothbart *et al.*, 2000; Shiner & Caspi, 2003). Extraversion has been linked to Surgency, including dimensions such as activity, inhibition/approach, and positive emotionality. Neuroticism is closely related to negative reactivity and affectivity, as well as approach. Conscientiousness is related to effortful control and persistence, as well as reactivity. Intellect/openness has been linked to inhibition/approach, and weakly to reactivity and persistence. In the ATP, the personality trait of Agreeableness was associated with lower negative reactivity and higher persistence.

These linkages are apparent not only concurrently but also prospectively. The ATP data, for instance, indicate that temperament at 11–14 years predicts substantial amounts of variance in personality at 16 years, with earlier Persistence (or effortful control) having particularly strong predictive relationships with Agreeableness, Extraversion, and Conscientiousness (Prior *et al.*, 2000a).

There thus seem strong grounds for considering temperament dispositions as forming the core of developing personality (Rothbart *et al.*, 2000). However, the processes by which early temperament may shape or become elaborated into later personality structures have received little attention to date. In addition to genetic influences (see Saudino, 2005), Shiner & Caspi (2003) discussed various developmental processes that may be involved, similar to those discussed earlier for the maintenance of temperamental stability. For example, temperament may shape older children's choices about their environment and reinforce and sustain certain characteristics. Thus, a child high in inhibition/shyness may seek to minimize social interaction, which serves to shape introversion. As consensus grows regarding the structure of temperament and personality, our understanding of developmental processes will hopefully improve. It may be that the impact of early temperament on later social and emotional adjustment is through its influence on personality development; alternatively, temperament may continue to have relatively direct effects on adolescent development. Unraveling this issue is an important area for future research.

Measuring the relation of temperament to socio-emotional functioning

A challenging conceptual and methodological issue in temperament research is the overlap between temperament and socio-emotional development constructs. While it is generally assumed that empirical associations between temperament and development are due to the contribution of temperament to developmental outcomes, they may also be due to developmental continuity between early temperament and later child characteristics (i.e. they are in essence the same construct as manifested at different ages), conceptual fuzziness (the concept of socio-emotional development includes aspects of temperament), and/or methodological overlap (measures of temperament blur over into measures of social development). Such issues are especially pertinent if the same informant has been used for both constructs.

Apparent methodological overlap between the indicators used for temperament dimensions and socio-emotional outcomes can be found in many studies in this area. For example, fearfulness is commonly used as an indicator of temperamental inhibition, and excessive fear as a symptom of anxiety. Sanson *et al.* (1990) first drew attention to this issue by showing that child development experts often regarded items taken from standard temperament questionnaires as better measures of behavior problems, and vice versa. This was especially true for items designed to assess internalizing problems which were often regarded as better measures of temperament. Several more recent studies have suggested that the effects of such confounding do not invalidate conclusions regarding the influence of temperament on social development. For example, when confounding items have been removed from temperament and behavior problem questionnaires, temperament-adjustment relations have still been evident (Lemery *et al.*, 2002; Lengua *et al.*, 1998). Sheeber's (1995) intervention study found that parental ratings of child temperament remained stable after treatment whereas their ratings of behavior problems improved, suggesting a significant differentiation between temperament attributes and behavior problems. Oldehinkel *et al.* (2004), factor-analyzing parent reports on over 2000 pre-adolescents, found substantial numbers of cross-loading items from the REATQ and the Child Behavior Checklist, but removal of these items had little effect on associations between the two constructs.

Despite these somewhat reassuring results, the issue of overlap in indicators is clearly a complex one. The problem is not limited to socio-emotional development: Lahey (2004) recently drew attention to the "vexing conceptual and methodologic roadblocks" (p. 88) which need to be overcome to distinguish between temperament and psychopathology constructs. Some careful theoretical and empirical unpacking remains to be done in future studies to better understand, and circumvent, this problem. At this point in time, readers should carefully examine measures used in published studies to check if measurement choices avoid conceptual confounding.

How does temperament affect social and emotional functioning?

Early socialization research focused on environmental effects on development and assumed a unidirectional transmission from adult to child (see Schaffer, 1999). Temperament research has its focus explicitly on individuals' own contribution to their development, but ironically has often erred on the other side and underplayed the influence of the environment. Most studies have adopted a correlational methodology, and interpreted associations between temperament and socio-emotional development as evidence of unidirectional effects of temperament.

Various models have been posited to explain the developmental processes through which temperament exerts its effects on socio-emotional development. The review of the literature below is organized around three broad models, and is illustrative rather than comprehensive (Klein, Dougherty, Laptook, and Olino, see Chapter 13, this volume for a discussion of models). To give more confidence in causal explanations of associations, we rely mostly on longitudinal studies in which temperament is measured prior to later outcomes. Given Klein's chapter on links between temperament and mood disorders, our goal is to examine temperament links with socio-emotional functioning considered as a continuum. Where we do examine poor socio-emotional functioning, our emphasis is on internalizing problems (see Sanson & Prior, 1999 for review of associations between temperament and externalizing problems). We also focus mostly on outcomes in late childhood or early adolescence.

Direct effects

A unidirectional view is that temperament has direct linear effects on development. Thus, a finding that very high inhibition is related to anxiety disorder may be interpreted to mean that the extreme end of this temperament dimension is equivalent to the disorder, or that inhibition serves as a predisposition or vulnerability to the disorder and plays a direct causal role. Most research to date has been framed so as to detect only such direct effects, and there are numerous examples of both concurrent and prospective linkages. Some examples follow.

A large body of research shows that temperament directly affects children's social relationships, particularly with peers. Two influential sets of studies on social withdrawal in early childhood have been conducted by Kagan and colleagues, generally implying direct effects, and Rubin and colleagues, who adopt a mediational model (reviewed in the following section). Both sets of work are characterized by careful laboratory observations, in particular the use of the "behavioral inhibition paradigm" in which children's reactions to novel events are coded for indicators of inhibition, such as proximity to mother and latency to approach a strange person or object.

The studies by Kagan and colleagues imply a direct continuity between temperament and social relationships. Their work has largely focused on "high reactive" infants who show distress (crying and fretting) and vigorous motor activity in response to stimuli. Following children from infancy into adolescence (e.g. Biederman et al., 2001; Kagan & Snidman, 1999), this body of work suggests that temperament (particularly reactivity and inhibition) is associated with internalizing problems, especially anxiety. As toddlers, high-reactive infants showed more fear and inhibition to unfamiliar events than low-reactive infants; were more likely to be inhibited and withdrawn at 4 years, and more had developed anxiety symptoms at 7 years (45% versus 15%). In adolescence, 61% of adolescents who had been classified as inhibited toddlers displayed social anxiety symptoms, compared with 27% of adolescents who were uninhibited toddlers (Schwartz *et al.*, 1999).

Other researchers have found only modest associations between early reactivity and inhibition and later anxiety when examined across childhood and adolescence. For example, early high reactivity was not found to increase the risk for anxiety in adolescence in the ATP (Prior *et al.*, 2000b). Shyness in infancy and toddlerhood were modest risk factors for later anxiety. Stronger associations were found when shyness persisted over time, with 42% of children who were rated shy at multiple time points between infancy and late childhood exhibiting anxiety problems in adolescence. Looking back in time, only one fifth of adolescents with anxiety problems had been persistently shy, suggesting that temperamental shyness or inhibition was only one of a number of risk factors for the development of anxiety in adolescence. Caspi (2000), following the group of children identified as "inhibited" at 3 years in the Dunedin longitudinal study, found 28% had a depression diagnosis at 21 years (in comparison to the base rate of 18%), and more were unassertive and had made suicide attempts. Little work has been done to identify the characteristics distinguishing those inhibited children who do and do not continue to show difficulties in adolescence, an essential task if at-risk children are to be targeted for early intervention.

The tripartite model of anxiety and depression (Clark & Watson, 1991) can be seen as an example of a direct effects model in which the temperament traits of positive affect (PA) and negative affect (NA) are vulnerability or predisposing factors for the development of these disorders. For example, Lonigan *et al.*'s (2003) longitudinal study of 4th to 11th grade children found that NA predicted changes in symptoms of anxiety and depression, whereas PA predicted changes in symptoms of depression only. Although this study was constrained by a limited temporal window (7 months) and reliance on self-report, findings suggest the value of pursuing such associations in larger-scale, longitudinal, multi-informant studies. Cross-cultural support for the model is also growing (Austin & Chorpita, 2004; Compas *et al.*, 2004).

Among research on the contribution of temperament to positive social functioning, the series of studies by Eisenberg and colleagues has highlighted the importance of emotionality and self-regulation for prosocial behavior, as well as gender differences in these relationships. For example, Eisenberg *et al.* (1993) showed that self-regulation capacities and negative emotionality were powerfully related to social skills as assessed by parents, teachers, and observers, with self-regulation appearing most salient. High negative emotionality was a risk factor for poor social skills for both boys and girls, whereas low negative emotionality was protective only for boys. Similarly, Murphy *et al.* (2004) examined the social adjustment of 10–12-year-olds and found that, compared with young adolescents with poor social functioning, those with high social competence and low levels of behavioral problems had displayed lower emotionality and higher self-regulation up to 6 years earlier.

Consistent with North American studies, ATP analyses have identified attentional self-regulation, sociability and negative reactivity as important predictors of social skills at 11–12 years assessed concurrently by parent, teacher, and child report, explaining almost half of the variance. Longitudinal predictors of social skills were task orientation and flexibility (attentional and emotional self-regulation) at 5–6 and 7–8 years, explaining 16–20% of the variance (Prior *et al.*, 2000a).

Indirect effects

A second model posits indirect, mediated effects. Mediational models suggest that temperament impacts on developmental outcomes through the influence of a third variable, or temperament itself may be the mediator. Researchers are increasingly investigating such models. For example, Katainen *et al.* (1999) examined predictors of depressive tendencies over 9 years among 389 Finnish children, and found that maternal perceptions of child temperamental "difficultness" and low maternal role satisfaction at 6 years led to more hostile child-rearing at 9 years, which in turn led to more depressive symptoms in adolescence.

As noted earlier, Rubin and colleagues propose a mediational model linking inhibition with social relationships (e.g. Rubin & Stewart, 1996). In this model, infant inhibition is considered a potential stressor to which, in the context of other family stressors, parents may react negatively (i.e. with insensitivity, overprotection, and/or overcontrol), resulting in insecure parent–child attachment. Insecure children may then withdraw from the social environment, and eventually be rejected by peers. Inhibition also gives the child fewer opportunities to interact with others, and hence fewer chances to learn how to interact effectively with peers. Here temperament is seen as a risk factor whose effect is largely mediated by the parental behavior elicited by it. Other aspects of temperament (e.g. reactivity, self-regulation) are not specifically addressed in this model.

A series of studies by Wills and colleagues investigating connections between temperament and adolescent substance use also consistently found indirect linkages through other individual characteristics and environmental factors (Wills *et al.*, 1995, 1998). Temperament dimensions such as activity, mood, negative emotionality, and sociability were mediated in their effects on substance use by other aspects of functioning such as self-control, maladaptive coping styles, novelty seeking, and academic competence; and by environmental factors such as negative life events and deviant peer affiliations. Compas *et al.* (2004) have also proposed that the relationship between temperament and depression may be mediated by coping styles. (They further suggest that temperament may moderate, and be moderated by, stress responses and coping in their effects on depression.)

Interactional effects

Finally there are interactional models, also referred to as moderational, transactional, or diathesis-stress models. Thomas & Chess (1977) argued that temperament affects development primarily through its "goodness of fit," or match, with the child's environment. Thus, compatibility between temperament capacities and contextual requirements facilitates healthy development, whereas a mismatch compromises development. Interactional influences imply multiplicative effects (i.e. the co-occurrence of particular temperamental and environmental variables exert an effect beyond their separate contributions). Moderational models suggest that the impact of temperament on outcomes is exacerbated or diminished by a third variable such as parenting; or temperament may be the moderator (Klein *et al.*, 1993; Letcher *et al.*, 2004).

Much of the research in this area has focused on interactions between temperament and parenting (e.g. Morris *et al.*, 2002; Paterson & Sanson, 1999; for review see Putnam *et al.*, 2002). For example, Morris *et al.* (2002) found that child-reported maternal psychological control interacted with temperamental irritable distress in the prediction of teacher-rated internalizing but not externalizing problems (at mean age 7 years); psychological control predicted internalizing problems among children high but not low in irritable distress.

Kochanska's body of research (Kochanska, 1995, 1997) shows that temperamental fearfulness can have both direct (main) and interactive effects on children's developing internalization of moral rules. Children high in fearfulness respond strongly to gentle discipline which elicits sufficient arousal to allow the child to internalize the parents' goals. Such parenting is ineffective for more fearless children, who are more strongly motivated by reward and respond to parenting efforts based on positive anticipation.

Another example of temperament conceptualized as a moderator of environmental factors is Davies & Windle's (2001) study of 360 adolescents which found that early difficult temperament characteristics of dysrhythmicity and poor task orientation (attentional control, persistence) potentiated effects of marital discord on adolescent trajectories of depression and delinquency over 2 years.

Parenting was conceptualized as a moderator of temperament effects in a cross-sectional investigation of 13–14-year-olds in the ATP (Letcher et al., 2004). Here, interactive effects of specific temperament features and parenting styles were examined in the prediction of a range of behavior problems, assessed via composites of parent and adolescent reports. Amongst several significant interactions between temperament and parenting, the interactions of parental warmth with the temperament dimensions of shyness and negative reactivity predicted adolescent depression. The prevalence of depression was low among those with low temperamental shyness or low negative reactivity regardless of the level of parental warmth. Adolescents who were high in shyness or negative reactivity were at elevated risk of depression, and those who also experienced low warmth were at even greater risk. Thus, lower warmth in the parent–adolescent relationship appeared to have a particularly strong moderating role on those at greater temperamental risk.

Hudson & Rapee (2004), in noting that temperamental high arousal, emotionality, and inhibition are likely to place a child at risk for later anxiety problems, also noted the likely interaction of temperament with parental overprotection and attachment style. They found that preschoolers with high inhibition and avoidant attachments were more likely to develop anxiety symptoms.

Some temperament-by-temperament interactions have also been found. For example, the previously mentioned research by Eisenberg et al. (1993) found that children who were both highly emotional and poorly regulated had the lowest levels of social skills and peer sociometric status.

The role of temperament in resilience is an example of the moderation of risk by temperament. Perhaps the most well-known study of resilience is the Kauai Longitudinal Study, which followed the 1955 birth cohort of 698 children from Kauai with multiple data collections from childhood to adulthood (Werner & Smith, 1992). Within the sample, one third of those who were identified as high-risk became competent, confident, and caring adults. Especially for girls, an active, outgoing temperamental disposition was an important predictor of resilience. The authors argued that an easy disposition facilitated at-risk children and adolescents gaining better access to support and having better relationships with parents. For boys, external supports (such as mentors) were more protective than temperament. The ATP analyses of resilience against antisocial behavior (Smart et al., 2003) also indicated an important role for temperament in resilience. In this case, changes in temperament over adolescence appeared to have a protective effect.

More elaborated, transactional models are increasingly accepted (e.g. Cicchetti & Toth, 1998). These posit that understanding the process of development requires analysis of the ongoing interaction among intrinsic child characteristics and aspects of the environment. Thus, a child's characteristics, such as temperament, health status and cognitive capacities, together with parent and family circumstances and the wider sociocultural context, all interconnect to explain and predict developmental pathways. In such models, temperament is often seen as a risk or protective factor. For example, Windle & Mason's (2004) multifactorial study of 10–11th graders found lower levels of approach-withdrawal, general rhythmicity, and flexibility (assessed by self-reports on the DOTS-R) contributed, along with stressful life events and low family support, to higher levels of depression a year later. Similarly, path analysis was used to investigate inter-relationships between child and early adolescent temperament, early behavior problems, school, family, and peer adjustment in pathways to depression in mid-adolescence in the ATP sample (Smart *et al.*, 1999). Anxiety and low family and school attachment explained approximately 30% of variance in depression. Anxiety was itself predicted by temperamental approach/inhibition and negative reactivity; thus connections between temperament and depression were mediated through anxiety.

Culture as a moderator of temperament effects

While temperament may be biologically based, its social acceptance and impact on individual functioning and development may be moderated by societal and cultural conditions and expectations. Although research on temperament has predominantly been conducted in Western, industrialized countries, cultural differences have been noted in the expression, but less in the structure, of temperament (see, for example, Prior *et al.*, 2000a).

While a "difficult" temperament style is often associated with adjustment problems (Sanson & Prior, 1999), it can be an asset in some environments. A notable and often-quoted finding is the relationship between difficult temperament and lower infant mortality among the Masai of East Africa during a famine (DeVries, 1984). Difficult temperament was thought to increase chances of survival because infants who displayed greater fussing and crying were more likely to gain attention and be fed, suggesting that difficult temperament was a good "fit" with this extreme environment. Providing further evidence of the impact of culture, temperamental inhibition was associated with positive developmental outcomes in China, and poor outcomes in North America (Chen *et al.*, 1995). Chinese children identified by their peers as inhibited were also more accepted by peers and rated more positively by teachers and peers on "honorship" and leadership than were average or aggressive children. Further, inhibition was positively related to maternal acceptance and encouragement of achievement in this sample. However, shyness was consistently associated with negative outcomes for a Canadian sample (Chen *et al.*, 1998). Together, these results suggested that inhibition is more highly valued in Chinese culture compared with Canadian culture. Interestingly, more recent work (Chen *et al.*, 2005) comparing relationships between shyness and adjustment in China in 1990, 1998, and 2002 suggests that these cultural differences are weakening, with 2002 data being comparable to North American findings. The authors interpret these findings in the light of social and economic reforms in China which have led to assertiveness, competitiveness, and independence becoming valued over traditional Chinese values of restraint. Overall, these culturally informed studies point to the cultural relativity of the impact of temperament on social development.

A closer examination of culture-specific attitudes, expectations, and beliefs about temperament and their impact on parenting practices may further extend our understanding of how temperament works in a broader social context. For example, if temperamental shyness is a valued trait, it may elicit parental warmth rather than overprotectiveness and disapproval, and may lead to later self-confidence and social competence. Reactivity may be seen as a sign of alertness or intelligence in one culture, and hence elicit parental approval, whereas in another it may be regarded as difficult and non-compliant and lead to parental rejection and punitiveness. Similarly, cultures may vary in their beliefs about the extent to which a child can control or moderate the expression of their temperament proclivities, and hence influence responses to and strategies for managing the child.

Gender as a moderator of temperament effects

Existing findings suggest temperament has the same underlying structure for boys and girls, but that, regardless of age, girls often have a stronger ability to regulate or allocate attention and control inappropriate responses, whereas boys are often more active and derive more pleasure from high-intensity activity (Else-Quest et al., 2006). There is increasing interest in the possibility that gender may moderate associations between temperament and social adjustment, although little consistency has emerged to date in the nature of such gender effects. For instance, as noted above, Werner & Smith (1992) found temperament predicted resilience for girls only, whereas Eisenberg et al. (1993) found that low negative emotionality was protective against the development of poor social skills for boys only. In a sample of toddlers and preschoolers, Kochanska et al. (1994) found different relationships between temperament and two components of conscience (Affective Discomfort and Moral Regulation/Vigilance) for boys and girls. For girls, Affective Discomfort was predicted by higher reactivity and focus/effortful control (i.e. attentional regulation), whereas no temperament dimensions were predictive for boys. High reactivity was a prominent predictor of low Moral Regulation/Vigilance, whereas impulsivity and sensation seeking were important for boys. Further investigation, grounded in theory, appears to be needed on the role of gender in temperament-adjustment relations.

Multiple pathways between temperament and socio-emotional functioning

The three different pathways identified above (direct, indirect, and interactional) are not necessarily mutually exclusive, and it is indeed unlikely that any one model can account for all pathways between temperament and socio-emotional functioning. Several studies find evidence for two or more types of association. For example, Lengua and colleagues investigated direct, mediated and moderated effects of temperament among children of divorcing parents. Direct temperament effects were indicated by Lengua & Long (2002) who found negative emotionality was related to threat appraisals, avoidance coping, and higher internalizing and externalizing problems. Interactional effects were found by Lengua *et al.* (2000) where positive emotionality interacted with parental rejection in predicting depressive symptoms – if children were low in positive emotionality, parental rejection led to an increase in depressive symptoms; if they were high in positive emotionality, they were protected from adverse effects of rejection. The link between inconsistent discipline and symptoms was strongest for those with poor attentional control.

The growth in longitudinal studies and recent advances in statistical modeling have allowed for more developmentally sensitive investigations of relations between predictors and outcomes. Predictors of changes in socio-emotional functioning can be studied using hierarchical or latent growth curve analysis, in order to describe normative developmental patterns (that is, whether overall levels increase, decrease, or remain stable over time). As an illustration, the Leve *et al.* (2005) study of children from 5 to 17 years found that temperamental fear/shyness at age 5 significantly and uniquely predicted age-17 internalizing problems but temperament did not significantly predict change over time. Maternal depression assessed at age 5 also predicted age-17 internalizing problems in both sexes, and girls whose mothers reported higher levels of depression and had lower family incomes showed increases in internalizing behavior over time. Such studies provide a more dynamic picture of how temperament and other psychosocial factors contribute to shifts in socio-emotional adjustment over time.

Growth mixture models for longitudinal data (see e.g. Nagin, 1999) allow for heterogeneity in developmental trajectories, by examining whether qualitatively distinct subgroups of individuals can be identified for a given outcome. Brendgen *et al.* (2005) identified four trajectories of self-reported depression in adolescents from Quebec, assessed annually over 11–14 years. Maternally reported temperamental reactivity at 6–7 years increased the risk of following a depression trajectory that was either consistently high or increasing over 11–14 years. Adolescent-reported problems in relationships with parents also predicted elevated depression trajectories. Interactions were also investigated; while there was no evidence for a diathesis-stress model of temperament and parenting-adolescent relationships, rejection by same-sex peers (assessed using peer nominations) increased the risk of following an increasing depression trajectory only in reactive girls. This finding points to a possible reason for increased levels of depression in girls from early adolescence onwards, suggesting that problems in peer relations may have greater significance for highly reactive adolescent girls than boys.

Conclusions

Despite limited research or theorizing specifically focusing on temperament in adolescence, the available evidence suggests that it plays a significant role in the development of adolescent socio-emotional functioning. In this section we briefly summarize the main conclusions arising from this review, and point to directions for further research.

There appears to be substantial continuity in the structure of temperament from childhood through adolescence, with key temperament dimensions across these epochs being reactivity (or emotionality), self-regulation (with attentional, emotional, and behavioral components) and inhibition/approach. There are clear and substantial links between temperament and emerging personality, supporting the notion that early temperament is a building block for later personality. Hence the extensive literature on the impact of personality on adolescent and adult socio-emotional functioning also provides support for the significance of earlier temperament. Little progress has been made on understanding mechanisms underlying these linkages, which is a fruitful area for further research.

The literature clearly indicates that individuals tend to show moderate stability in temperament from childhood to adolescence. However, this stability is far from absolute and some level of change is the norm. The scant data available also suggest there may be some normative changes in temperament over this period, with a decrease in negative reactivity and an increase in self-regulation. Reasons for changes in temperament are not well understood, but may involve both environmental mechanisms (e.g. through parents' behavior), and the individual's own moderation of the expression of their temperamental proclivities. Both intervention and longitudinal studies suggest the importance of parents (and others in the child's world) taking their children's temperament into account when choosing strategies to soothe, control, stimulate, and guide their child (Putnam et al., 2002). There is a clear role for further well-designed and well-evaluated temperament-based parenting interventions to understand how parental responses can modify "difficult" temperament characteristics, and also for temperament-focused interventions with children, assisting them to moderate their own predispositions and to learn effective coping styles (see McClowry et al., 2005).

While most models of development would predict relatively complex relations between early temperament and later adjustment, most research has explored only direct linear linkages. This body of research clearly demonstrates that temperament is an important predictor of psychosocial adjustment, both in childhood and adolescence. In particular, temperamental contributions to the broad domains of social competence, internalizing and externalizing problems, and more specific aspects of development such as social withdrawal, anxiety, parent–child relations, and school adjustment are well-documented. Inhibition and negative reactivity are consistent predictors of internalizing problems, and high reactivity and poor self-regulation are typically predictive of externalizing problems (Eisenberg *et al.*, 2000; Sanson *et al.*, 2004).

Far more attention has been given to role of temperament in the development of socio-emotional maladjustment than to its role in facilitating healthy development. Similarly, there has been much emphasis on negative emotionality and the absence of positive affect, but little on the presence of positive affect and other "positive" aspects of temperament such as low reactivity and high self-regulation. Nevertheless, there is some evidence that such characteristics are associated with resilience, prosocial behavior, and social competence (Sanson *et al.*, 2004). Further work on pathways to positive adolescent and adult development will be welcome.

Much past research has not been theoretically grounded. We conclude that it is timely to move from merely identifying direct links between some facet/s of temperament and some facet/s of socio-emotional functioning, to examining more complex pathways. The recent research which is trying to better understand the nature of temperament-development linkages by testing more complex models positing mediational or interactional relationships, often using large longitudinal samples and sophisticated statistical modeling techniques, provides a model for future work.

Overall, on present evidence, we conclude that temperament continues to have important, but perhaps increasingly indirect, influences on socio-emotional functioning as development progresses. These include its role as a building block for personality, and as a continuing source of resilience or vulnerability in complex multidimensional pathways to socio-emotional adjustment and maladjustment.

REFERENCES

Austin, A. A., & Chorpita, B. F. (2004). Temperament, anxiety, and depression: comparisons across five ethnic groups of children. *Journal of Clinical Child and Adolescent Psychology*, **33**, 216–226.

Biederman, J., Hirshfeld-Becker, D. R., Rosenbaum, J. F. *et al.* (2001). Further evidence of association between behavioral inhibition and social anxiety in children. *American Journal of Psychiatry*, **158**, 1673–1679.

Brendgen, M., Wanner, G., Morin, A.J.S., & Vitaro, F. (2005). Relations with parents and with peers, temperament, and trajectories of depressed mood during early adolescence. *Journal of Abnormal Child Psychology*, **33**, 579–594.

Caspi, A. (2000). The child is father of the man: personality continuities from childhood to adulthood. *Journal of Personality and Social Psychology*, **78**, 158–172.

Chen, X., Rubin, K.H., & Li, B. (1995). Social and school adjustment of shy and aggressive children in China. *Development and Psychopathology*, **7**, 337–349.

Chen, X., Hastings, P.D., Rubin, K.H. *et al.* (1998). Child-rearing attitudes and behavioral inhibition in Chinese and Canadian toddlers: a cross-cultural study. *Developmental Psychology*, **34**, 677–686.

Chen, X., Cen, G., Li, D., & He, Y. (2005). Social functioning and adjustment in Chinese children: the imprint of historical time. *Child Development*, **76**, 182–195.

Cicchetti, D., & Toth, S.L. (1998). The development of depression in children and adolescents. *American Psychologist*, **53**, 221–241.

Clark, L.A., & Watson, D. (1991). Tripartite model of anxiety and depression: psychometric evidence and taxonomic implications. *Journal of Abnormal Psychology*, **100**, 316–336.

Compas, B.E., Connor-Smith, J., & Jaser, S.S. (2004). Temperament, stress reactivity, and coping: implications for depression in childhood and adolescence. *Journal of Clinical Child and Adolescent Psychology*, **33**, 21–31.

Davies, P., & Windle, M. (2001). Interparental discord and adolescent adjustment trajectories: the potentiating and protective role of intrapersonal attributes. *Child Development*, **72**, 1163–1178.

DeVries, M. (1984). Temperament and infant mortality among the Masai of East Africa. *American Journal of Psychiatry*, **141**, 1189–1194.

Diener, E. (2000). Introduction to the special section on personality development. *Journal of Personality and Social Psychology*, **78**, 120–121.

Eisenberg, N., Fabes, R.A., Bernzweig, J. *et al.* (1993). The relations of emotionality and regulation to preschoolers' social skills and sociometric status. *Child Development*, **64**, 1418–1438.

Eisenberg, N., Fabes, R.A., Guthrie, I.K., & Reiser, N. (2000). Dispositional emotionality and regulation: their role in predicting quality of social functioning. *Journal of Personality and Social Psychology*, **78**, 136–157.

Eisenberg, N., Zhou, Q., Spinrad, T.L. *et al.* (2005). Relations among positive parenting, children's effortful control, and externalizing problems: a three-wave longitudinal study. *Child Development*, **76**, 1055–1071.

Else-Quest, N.M., Shibley-Hyde, J., Goldsmith, H.H., & van Hulle, C.A. (2006). Gender differences in temperament: a meta-analysis. *Psychological Bulletin*, **132**, 33–72.

Hagekull, B., & Bohlin, G. (1998). Preschool temperament and environmental factors related to the five-factor model of personality in middle childhood. *Merrill-Palmer Quarterly*, **44**, 194–215.

Hudson, J.L., & Rapee, R.M. (2004). From anxious temperament to disorder: an etiological model of generalized anxiety disorder. In R.G. Heimberg, C.L. Turk, & D.S. Mennin (Eds.), *Generalized Anxiety Disorder: Advances in Research and Practice* (pp. 51–74). New York: Guilford Press.

Kagan, J., & Fox, N.A. (2006). Biology, culture, and temperamental biases. In N. Eisenberg, W. Damon, & R.M. Lerner (Eds.), *Handbook of Child Psychology, Vol 3: Social, Emotional and Personality Development* (6th edn, pp. 167–225). New York: Wiley.

Kagan, J., & Snidman, N. (1999). Early childhood predictors of adult anxiety disorders. *Biological Psychiatry*, **46**, 1536–1541.

Kagan, J., Reznick, J., & Snidman, N. (1988). Biological bases of childhood shyness. *Science*, **240**, 167–171.

Katainen, S., Räikkönen, K., Keskivaara, P., & Keltikangas-Järvinen, L. (1999). Maternal child-rearing attitudes and role satisfaction and children's temperament as antecedents of adolescent depressive tendencies: follow-up study of 6- to 15-year-olds. *Journal of Youth and Adolescence*, **28**, 139–163.

Klein, M.H., Wonderlich, S., & Shea, M.T. (1993). Models of relationships between personality and depression: toward a framework for theory and research. In M.H. Klein, S. Wonderlich, & M.T. Shea (Eds.), *Personality and Depression: A Current View* (pp. 1–54). New York: Guilford Press.

Kochanska, G. (1995). Children's temperament, mother's discipline, and security of attachment: multiple pathways to emerging internalization. *Child Development*, **66**, 597–615.

Kochanska, G. (1997). Multiple pathways to conscience for children with different temperaments: from toddlerhood to age 5. *Developmental Psychology*, **33**, 228–240.

Kochanska, G., DeVet, K., Goldman, M., Murray, K., & Putnam, S.P. (1994). Maternal reports of conscience development and temperament in young children. *Child Development*, **65**, 852–868.

Lahey, B.B. (2004). Commentary: role of temperament in developmental models of psychopathology. *Journal of Clinical Child and Adolescent Psychology*, **33**, 88–93.

Lemery, K.S., Essex, M.J., & Smider, N.A. (2002). Revealing the relation between temperament and behavior problem symptoms by eliminating measurement confounding: expert ratings and factor analyses. *Child Development*, **73**, 867–882.

Lengua, L.J., & Long, A.C. (2002). The role of emotionality and self-regulation in the appraisal-coping process: tests of direct and moderating effects. *Journal of Applied Developmental Psychology*, **23**, 471–493.

Lengua, L.J., West, S.G., & Sandler, I.N. (1998). Temperament as a predictor of symptomatology in children: addressing contamination of measures. *Child Development*, **69**, 164–181.

Lengua, L.J., Wolchik, S.A., Sandler, I.N., & West, S.G. (2000). The additive and interactive effects of parenting and temperament in predicting adjustment problems of children of divorce. *Journal of Clinical Child Psychology*, **29**, 232–244.

Letcher, P., Toumbourou, J., Sanson, A. *et al.* (2004). Parenting style as a moderator of the effect of temperament on adolescent externalising and internalising behaviour problems. *Australian Educational and Developmental Psychologist*, **19–20**, 5–34.

Leve, L.D., Kim, H.K., & Pears, K.C. (2005). Childhood temperament and family environment as predictors of internalizing and externalizing trajectories from ages 5 to 17. *Journal of Abnormal Child Psychology*, **33**, 505–520.

Lonigan, C.J., Phillips, B.M., & Hooe, E.S. (2003). Relations of positive and negative affectivity to anxiety and depression in children: evidence from a latent variable longitudinal study. *Journal of Consulting and Clinical Psychology*, **71**, 465–481.

McClowry, S., Snow, D.L., & Tamis-LeMonda, C.S. (2005). An evaluation of the effects of INSIGHTS on the behavior of inner city primary school children. *Journal of Primary Prevention*, **26**, 567–584.

McClowry, S.G. (1995). The development of the school-age temperament inventory. *Merrill-Palmer Quarterly*, **41**, 233–252.

McClowry, S.G., Halverson, C.F., & Sanson, A. (2003). A re-examination of the validity and reliability of the School-Age Temperament Inventory. *Nursing Research*, **52**, 176–182.

Morris, A.S., Silk, J.S., Steinberg, L. *et al.* (2002). Temperamental vulnerability and negative parenting as interacting predictors of child adjustment. *Journal of Marriage and Family*, **64**, 461–471.

Murphy, B.C., Shepard, S., Eisenberg, N., & Fabes, R.A. (2004). Concurrent and across time prediction of young adolescents' social functioning: the role of emotionality and regulation. *Social Development*, **13**, 56–86.

Nagin, D.S. (1999). Analysing developmental trajectories: a semiparametric, group-based approach. *Psychological Methods*, **4**, 139–157.

Oldehinkel, A.J., Hartman, C.A., De Winter, A.F., Veenstra, R., & Ormel, J. (2004). Temperament profiles associated with internalizing and externalizing problems in preadolescence. *Development and Psychopathology*, **16**, 421–440.

Paterson, G., & Sanson, A. (1999). The association of behavioural adjustment to temperament, parenting and family characteristics among 5 year-old children. *Social Development*, **8**, 293–309.

Pedlow, R., Sanson, A., Prior, M., & Oberklaid, F. (1993). Stability of maternally reported temperament from infancy to 8 years. *Developmental Psychology*, **29**, 998–1007.

Posner, M.I., & Rothbart, M.K. (1998). Attention, self regulation and consciousness. *Philosophical Transactions of the Royal Society of London B*, **353**, 1915–1927.

Prior, M., Sanson, A., Smart, D., & Oberklaid, F. (2000a). *Pathways from Infancy to Adolescence: Australian Temperament Project: 1983–2000*. Melbourne, Australia: Australian Institute of Family Studies.

Prior, M., Smart, D., Sanson, S., & Oberklaid, F. (2000b). Does shy-inhibited temperament in childhood lead to anxiety disorder in adolescence? *Journal of the American Academy of Child and Adolescent Psychiatry*, **39**, 461–468.

Putnam, S.P., Ellis, L.K., & Rothbart, M.K. (2001). The structure of temperament from infancy through adolescence. In A. Eliasz & A. Angleitner (Eds.), *Advances in Research on Temperament* (pp. 165–182). Germany: Pabst Science.

Putnam, S.P., Sanson, A., & Rothbart, M.K. (2002). Child temperament and parenting. In M. Bornstein (Ed.), *Handbook of Parenting* (2nd edn, pp. 255–277). Mahwah, NJ: Lawrence Erlbaum.

Raffaelli, M., Crockett, L.J., & Shen, Y. (2005). Developmental stability and change in self-regulation from childhood to adolescence. *Journal of Genetic Psychology*, **166**, 54–75.

Rapee, R.M. (2002). The development and modification of temperamental risk for anxiety disorders: prevention of a lifetime of anxiety? *Biological Psychiatry*, **52**, 947–957.

Roberts, B.W., & DelVecchio, W.F. (2000). The rank-order consistency of personality traits from childhood to old age: a quantitative review of longitudinal studies. *Psychological Bulletin*, **126**, 3–25.

Rothbart, M.K., & Bates, J.E. (2006). Temperament. In N. Eisenberg, W. Damon, & R.M. Lerner (Eds.), *Handbook of Child Psychology, Vol 3: Social, Emotional and Personality Development* (6th edn, pp. 99–166). New York: Wiley.

Rothbart, M.K., Ahadi, S.A., & Evans, D.E. (2000). Temperament and personality: origins and outcomes. *Journal of Personality and Social Psychology*, **78**, 122–135.

Rubin, K.H., & Stewart, S.L. (1996). Social withdrawal. In E.J. Mash & R.A. Barkley (Eds.), *Child Psychopathology* (pp. 277–307). New York, NY: Guilford Press.

Sanson, A., & Prior, M. (1999). Temperament and behavioural precursors to oppositional defiant disorder and conduct disorder. In H.C. Quay & A.E. Hogan (Eds.), *Handbook of Disruptive Behaviour Disorders* (pp. 397–417). New York: Kluwer Academic/Plenum Publishers.

Sanson, A., Prior, M., & Kyrios, M. (1990). Contamination of measures in temperament research. *Merrill-Palmer Quarterly*, **36**, 179–192.

Sanson, A., Pedlow, R., Cann, W., Prior, M., & Oberklaid, F. (1996). Shyness ratings: stability and correlates in early childhood. *International Journal of Behavioral Development*, **19**, 705–724.

Sanson, A., Hemphill, S.A., & Smart, D. (2004). Connections between temperament and social development: a review. *Social Development*, **13**, 142–170.

Saudino, K.J. (2005). Behavioral genetics and child temperament. *Journal of Developmental and Behavioral Pediatrics*, **26**, 214–223.

Schaffer, H.R. (1999). Understanding socialization: from unidirectional to bidirectional connections. In M. Bennett (Ed.), *Developmental Psychology: Achievements and Prospects* (pp. 272–288). Philadelphia, PA: Psychology Press.

Schwartz, C.E., Snidman, N., & Kagan, J. (1999). Adolescent social anxiety as an outcome of inhibited temperament in childhood. *Journal of the American Academy of Child and Adolescent Psychiatry*, **38**, 1008–1015.

Sheeber, L.B. (1995). Empirical dissociations between temperament and behavior problems: a response to the Sanson, Prior, and Kyrios study. *Merrill-Palmer Quarterly*, **41**, 554–561.

Shiner, R., & Caspi, A. (2003). Personality differences in childhood and adolescence: measurement, development and consequences. *Journal of Child Psychology and Psychiatry*, **44**, 2–32.

Smart, D., Sanson, A., Toumbourou, J., Prior, M., & Oberklaid, F. (1999, September). *Longitudinal Pathways to Adolescent Antisocial Behaviour and Depression*. Paper presented at the Life History Research Society Conference, Kauai, Hawaii.

Smart, D., Vassallo, S., Sanson, A. et al. (2003). *Patterns and Precursors of Adolescent Antisocial Behaviour: Types, Resiliency and Environmental Influences.* Second report. Melbourne, Victoria, Australia: Crime Prevention Victoria.

Thomas, A., & Chess, S. (1977). *Temperament and Development.* New York: Bruner/Mazel.

Thomas, A., Chess, S., Birch, H.G., Hertzig, M.E., & Korn, S. (1963). *Behavioural Individuality in Early Childhood.* New York, NY: New York University Press.

van den Boom, D.C. (1995). Do first-year intervention effects endure? Follow-up during toddlerhood of a sample of Dutch irritable infants. *Child Development*, **66**, 1798–1816.

Werner, E.E., & Smith, R.S. (1992). *Overcoming the Odds. High Risk Children from Birth to Adulthood.* Ithaca, NY: Cornell University Press.

Wills, T.A., DuHamel, K., & Vaccaro, D. (1995). Activity and mood temperament as predictors of adolescent substance use: tests of a self-regulation mediational model. *Journal of Personality and Social Psychology*, **68**, 901–916.

Wills, T.A., Windle, M., & Cleary, S.D. (1998). Temperament and novelty seeking in adolescent substance use: convergence of dimensions of temperament with constructs from Cloninger's theory. *Journal of Personality and Social Psychology,* **74**, 387–406.

Windle, M. (1992). Revised Dimensions of Temperament Survey (DOTS-R): Simultaneous group confirmatory factor analysis for adolescent gender groups. *Psychological Assessment,* **4**, 228–234.

Windle, M., & Lerner, R.M. (1986). Reassessing the dimensions of temperament individuality across the lifespan: the Revised Dimensions of Temperament Survey (DOTS-R). *Journal of Adolescent Research,* **1**, 213–230.

Windle, M., & Mason, W.A. (2004). General and specific predictors of behavioral and emotional problems among adolescents. *Journal of Emotional and Behavioral Disorders,* **12**, 49–61.

13

Temperament and risk for mood disorders in adolescents

Daniel N. Klein, Lea R. Dougherty, Rebecca S. Laptook, and Thomas M. Olino

There has been longstanding interest in the role of temperament in the etiology and development of mood disorders (Akiskal *et al.*, 1983; Klein *et al.*, 2002). Work in this area is important for at least five reasons. First, the mood disorders are moderately heritable (McGuffin *et al.*, 2003). Rather than coding directly for mood disorders, however, genes probably code for intermediate phenotypes that increase risk. Temperament traits associated with emotional experience, expression, and regulation may be intermediate phenotypes that are more tractable targets for genetic research than clinical disorders (Silberg & Rutter, 2002).

Second, if temperament is associated with risk for mood disorders, tracing the pathways between temperament and mood disorder phenotypes can help elucidate more proximal processes involved in the development of these conditions. Third, temperament may provide a means to identify at-risk youth who could benefit from prevention and early intervention efforts. Fourth, temperament may be useful in identifying more homogenous subgroups of mood disorders and mapping the different developmental pathways that lead to mood disorder outcomes.

Finally, there is substantial comorbidity between mood disorders and other forms of psychopathology, particularly anxiety disorders. Some temperament traits, such as negative emotionality (NE)/neuroticism (N), are associated with multiple psychiatric disorders. Thus, temperament could help explain patterns of comorbidity between classes of disorders and point toward more etiologically relevant classification systems (Clark, 2005; Khan *et al.*, 2005).

The incidence of mood disorders increases sharply in early adolescence, and the lifetime prevalence of mood disorders approaches adult levels by late

Adolescent Emotional Development and the Emergence of Depressive Disorders, ed. Nicholas B. Allen and Lisa B. Sheeber. Published by Cambridge University Press. © Cambridge University Press 2009.

adolescence (Nolen-Hoeksema, 2002). This suggests that if temperament is a risk factor for mood disorders, it may be activated or amplified by the complex psychosocial and biological changes associated with puberty and the transition to adolescence. This is consistent with the suggestion that individual differences in personality are most clearly expressed, and have the greatest impact, during major developmental transitions (Caspi & Moffitt, 1993). Moreover, temperament and personality appear to play a stronger role in juvenile-onset than adult-onset mood disorders (Klein *et al.*, 2002). Hence, adolescence may provide a critical window for understanding the role of temperament in the pathogenesis of mood disorders.

Nature of the relation between temperament and mood disorders

Numerous studies have documented an association between mood disorders and temperament traits such as NE/N and positive emotionality (PE)/extraversion (E). However, this association can be explained in a variety of ways (Klein *et al.*, 1993). These models are not mutually exclusive, and different models may apply to different subgroups.

The common cause model views temperament and mood disorders as arising from the same, or at least an overlapping, set of processes. In other words, temperament and mood disorders are both expressions of a common set of etiological factors. For example, there is evidence linking the temperament/personality trait of NE/N with major depressive disorder (MDD), both NE/N and MDD are heritable, and the genes contributing to NE/N and MDD overlap (Kendler *et al.*, 1993).

The precursor model views temperament as an early manifestation of mood disorder. Like the common cause model, temperament and mood disorders are caused by similar etiological factors. However, the precursor model assumes a developmental sequence, with the temperamental manifestations temporally preceding the onset of clinical mood disorders. This perspective also tends to assume that there is some phenomenological similarity, or homotypic continuity, between the temperament traits and mood disorder symptoms.

The predisposition model is similar to the precursor model in that temperament features are assumed to precede the onset of mood disorders. However, in the predisposition model, the processes that underlie temperament are presumed to differ from those that lead to mood disorders. Temperament is conceptualized as increasing the risk of developing mood disorders (e.g. by increasing sensitivity to stress).

Multivariate twin studies, prospective longitudinal studies of persons prior to the onset of mood disorders, and studies of populations at increased risk for mood disorders can be used to test the common cause, precursor, and predisposition models. Multivariate twin studies demonstrating that the same genes predispose to both temperament and mood disorders would support both the common cause and precursor models. Prospective longitudinal studies of persons with no prior history of mood disorder showing that particular temperament traits predict the onset of mood disorders would support both the precursor and predisposition models. Studies demonstrating temperament differences between children and adolescents at high and low risk for developing mood disorders can provide additional, albeit less direct, evidence for the precursor and predisposition models. Though no single design can distinguish between all three models, the combination of designs can. Finding substantial common genetic variance in twin studies, but no evidence of developmental sequencing in longitudinal and high risk studies, would support the common cause model; substantial common genetic variance and developmental sequencing would support the precursor model (particularly if the temperament trait was also phenomenologically similar to the mood disorder); and developmental sequencing but little common genetic variance would support the predisposition model.

The pathoplasticity model is similar to the predisposition model in that temperament is viewed as having a causal impact on mood disorders. However, rather than increasing the risk of mood disorders, temperament influences the expression of the disorder. This can take the form of temperament affecting the severity or pattern of symptomatology, response to treatment, or the course of the mood disorder. The pathoplasticity model can be evaluated in studies of persons with mood disorders by examining the associations between temperament traits and clinical features. However, it is difficult to rule out the possibility that the temperament trait is a marker for a more severe, chronic, or etiologically distinct subgroup, rather than having a causal influence on the expression of the disorder.

The final two models reverse the direction of temporal sequencing. The idea that mood disorders influence temperament may seem odd, given that temperament is generally presumed to be an early emerging and stable source of individual differences. However, as discussed below, contemporary temperament theorists recognize that temperament can be modified by maturational and environmental influences (Caspi & Shiner, 2006; Rothbart & Bates, 2006).

In the concomitants (or state-dependent) model, individuals' reports of temperament or observations of their temperament-relevant behavior are influenced by their current mood state. This model implies that the measures of temperament traits return to baseline levels after recovery from the episode, and raise questions about whether the measures truly reflect temperament. The concomitants model can be tested in cross-sectional studies comparing persons who have recovered from episodes of mood disorder to healthy controls, or even better, with longitudinal studies assessing individuals when they are in an episode and again after they have recovered. If temperamental abnormalities are present in remission, it would suggest that they are trait-markers, rather than concomitants of mood episodes.

Finally, the complications (or scar) model holds that mood disorder has an enduring effect on temperament, such that changes in temperament persist after recovery. This model can be evaluated by assessing persons before and after a mood disorder episode. If temperamental abnormalities are not evident before the episode, but appear after the episode, it would support the complications model.

Conceptualizations of temperament

As a thorough review of current models and conceptualizations of temperament is beyond the scope of this chapter, we limit our discussion of these issues to five points. First, although temperament has traditionally been distinguished from personality, which is presumed to be a broader construct, the distinction appears increasingly arbitrary (Caspi & Shiner, 2006). Hence, we will draw on relevant constructs from both literatures in this chapter. Second, while temperament traits are presumed to be rooted in early-emerging biological systems and relatively stable over time, their behavioral manifestations can vary as a function of maturation, and they can be modified by environmental factors (Fox *et al.*, 2005; Rothbart & Bates, 2006). Thus, as we discuss below, it is important to consider factors that moderate the temperament–mood disorder relationship.

Third, most current models conceptualize temperament and personality as being organized hierarchically, with a small number of "superfactors" (typically three to five) at the upper tier, each of which is divisible into a larger number of narrower traits or "facets" (Caspi & Shiner, 2006). For example, all major models include higher-order factors related to PE/E or surgency, NE/N, and effortful control/constraint. Lower-order traits subsumed under PE/E/surgency include positive affect, sociability, and approach/appetitive behavior; NE/N includes sadness, fear, anxiety, and anger; self-regulation/constraint includes attention, inhibitory control, persistence, and self-regulation.

Finally, while the literature emphasizes multidimensional quantitative models, Jerome Kagan and other theorists have proposed qualitatively distinct temperament traits. The most widely studied example is behavioral inhibition (BI), which refers to fear, reticence, and restraint in unfamiliar situations (Fox *et al.*, 2005). From a dimensional perspective, BI can be viewed as a combination of low PE, high NE, and high constraint.

Methodological issues

At least two methodological issues must be considered in discussing the relationship between temperament and mood disorders: the heterogeneity of mood disorders and assessment of temperament.

Heterogeneity of mood disorders

The mood disorders are clinically, and probably etiologically, heterogenous, reflecting the convergence of multiple developmental pathways. Thus, it is important to consider whether the role of temperament varies as a function of the specific form of mood disorder (e.g. bipolar disorder versus MDD), subtype of mood disorder (e.g. psychotic, melancholic, atypical), and key clinical characteristics such as age of onset, recurrence, and chronicity. Failure to take heterogeneity into account may obscure important temperament-mood disorder associations. Conversely, temperament may provide a basis for identifying more homogenous subgroups within the mood disorders.

Assessment of temperament

Temperament can be assessed using a variety of methods, including informant (e.g. parent, teacher) reports, self-report, and observations in naturalistic settings (e.g. home, school) or using structured laboratory tasks. Each approach has strengths and weaknesses, and their relative utility and validity may vary according to the temperament dimension, characteristics of the informant or observational context, and criterion examined. From the standpoint of studying the relationship between child temperament and psychopathology, however, parents' reports warrant special concern. As parents' reports may be influenced by their own psychopathology and mood state (Youngstrom et al., 1999), it can create spurious associations between child temperament and indices of familial risk for psychopathology.

A second issue concerns the overlap between many temperament and psychopathology constructs (e.g. NE/N with depression and anxiety), and the fact that many items in widely used temperament and psychopathology measures are similar (see Chapter 12, this volume). This is a significant problem, because in order to evaluate the associations between temperament and psychopathology, the two domains must be defined and assessed independently. Several recent studies have demonstrated that child temperament–psychopathology associations remain after removing overlapping items (Lemery et al., 2002; Lengua et al., 1998). Nonetheless, the conceptual overlap between the two domains raises the problem of circularity (Lahey, 2004). Hence, it is critical that studies of temperament and psychopathology employ independent measures and data sources, use longitudinal designs, and ensure that participants do not already have diagnosable psychopathology when temperament is assessed.

Temperament and risk for mood disorders

Though there are a number of possible relationships between temperament and mood disorders, we believe that the most heuristically valuable models view temperament as increasing the risk for mood disorders. In this section, we briefly discuss the literature on temperament/personality and mood disorders in adults in order to provide a context for the work on adolescent mood disorders, and then review high-risk and prospective studies of children and adolescents. We emphasize the two temperament superfactors NE/N and PE/E and Kagan's concept of BI as they have received the greatest attention in the literature on temperament and mood disorders. In addition, among the various forms of mood disorder, we emphasize MDD for the same reason.

Temperament and mood disorders in adults

Numerous cross-sectional studies have reported that depressed adults exhibit elevated levels of NE/N on self-report inventories (Klein *et al.*, 2002). These differences are not specific to MDD, as most forms of psychopathology are associated with elevated NE (Clark *et al.*, 1994). This lack of specificity suggests that broad temperament dimensions underlie a variety of forms of psychopathology and may contribute to the high rates of comorbidity that are consistently observed in clinical and community samples (Khan *et al.*, 2005).

There is relatively strong support for the precursor and predisposition models of NE/N in adults (Klein *et al.*, 2002). A number of prospective studies have reported that NE/N or related traits predict the first onset of MDD (Kendler *et al.*, 1993; Ormel *et al.*, 2004). Biometric analyses of twin data indicate that the majority (55%) of the liability to MDD is shared with N, primarily due to overlapping genes (Kendler *et al.*, 1993). Together with the phenomenological overlap between NE/N and depressive symptoms, the evidence seems to favor the precursor and common cause models over the predisposition model. However, NE/N could serve as both a precursor *and* a predisposition, as N can generate stressful life events that then interact with personality in producing symptoms.

Cross-sectional studies also report that depressed adults exhibit lower levels of PE/E than non-depressed controls. Unlike NE/N, low PE/E is relatively specific to depression, although it is also evident in some other disorders, such as schizophrenia, anorexia, and social phobia (Klein *et al.*, 2002).

A number of studies have reported that levels of PE/E are similar before, during, and after depressive episodes (Kendler *et al.*, 1993; Shea *et al.*, 1996). Even after recovery, persons with a history of depression report lower levels of PE/E than non-depressed controls or published norms (Klein *et al.*, 2002). This suggests that PE/E may be a trait marker, providing indirect support for the precursor and predisposition models. However, direct evidence from prospective studies of non-depressed individuals has been less supportive. One study reported that asthenia (or low energy), which can be regarded as a facet of PE, predicted a first lifetime episode of depression in males, but not females (Rorsman *et al.*, 1993). In contrast, three studies found that PE/E did not predict the first onset of depression (Hirschfeld *et al.*, 1989; Kendler *et al.*, 1993; Roberts & Kendler, 1999).

Temperament and mood disorders in youths

A number of retrospective studies have reported that adults with a juvenile onset of mood disorder exhibit greater personality dysfunction than those with an adult onset (Ramklint & Ekselius, 2003). This suggests that temperament may play a greater role in adolescent mood disorders. Unfortunately, the literature directly addressing the association between temperament and adolescent mood disorders is limited. Similar to the adult literature, studies of children and adolescents have reported contemporaneous associations between depressive symptoms and self-report of high NE/N, low PE/E, and high BI (Cheng & Furnham, 2003; Muris *et al.*, 2003). For example, Anthony *et al.* (2002) assessed self-reported temperament and depressive symptoms in a large sample of 10–17-year-old youths. High NE was significantly associated with both depressive and anxiety symptoms, while low PE was associated only with depressive symptoms.

A few studies have also reported prospective associations between high NE/N and low PE/E, and subsequent depressive symptoms in community samples of adolescents (Katainen *et al.*, 1999; Lonigan *et al.*, 2003). Unfortunately, in studies of depressive symptoms in community samples, it is unclear whether the symptoms are clinically significant, and the onset of mood disorder cannot be distinguished from maintenance and recurrence, confounding the predisposition and precursor models with pathoplasticity. Hence, the most relevant evidence for the role of temperament in the development of mood disorders is provided by family-genetic high-risk studies and prospective studies that start with participants who are young enough that they are unlikely to already have mood disorders by the time of the initial temperament assessment.

High risk studies

Offspring of depressed parents have an approximately two-fold greater risk for developing depressive disorders than offspring of non-depressed parents

(Klein *et al.*, 2005). Moreover, the onset of MDD is earlier among individuals with depressed parents (Weissman *et al.*, 1997). Hence, studies of temperament in the offspring of depressed parents may provide important information about the association between temperament and risk for early-onset mood disorders. However, these studies have several limitations. First, it is important to establish that the offspring do not already have mood disorders by the time temperament is assessed. Second, families with a depressed parent often differ from other families on a number of variables besides parental depression, such as other forms of psychopathology, marital discord, quality of parenting, and stress (Downey & Coyne, 1990) that could influence comparisons on temperament. Finally, cross-sectional comparisons between high- and low-risk groups provide only indirect information; it is necessary to follow offspring over time to determine whether temperament actually predicts the onset of mood disorders.

Several studies have used observational measures of temperament in young children of depressed parents. These studies have used standard laboratory paradigms, in which children interact with stimuli designed to elicit various emotional reactions. It is important to distinguish these studies from observations of interactions between the depressed parent and the child, which may be more informative about the dyadic relationship than broader temperamental dispositions.

Durbin *et al.* (2005) examined the association between a history of maternal depressive disorders and laboratory observation measures of PE, NE, and BI in a sample of 3-year-old children. Child low PE was significantly associated with maternal history of depressive disorder. Interestingly, this relationship was evident for the affective and motivational, but not social, components of PE. The association was particularly strong for early-onset and recurrent forms of maternal depression. Moreover, the child low PE-maternal depression association remained significant after controlling for current maternal depressive symptoms, maternal depression during the child's lifetime, comorbid psychopathology, marital discord, socioeconomic status, and home observation measures of parenting. Neither child NE nor BI were related to maternal depression. However, a measure of child NE in situations in which it was inappropriate to the context (e.g. fear in a situation that normally elicits positive affect) was associated with maternal depression, suggesting that it is not NE in general, but a failure to respond and/or regulate negative emotions in accord with the situational context, that may be related to risk. This sample was followed up at ages 5 and 7. Low PE at age 3 predicted EEG asymmetries at age 5 that have been found in depressed adults and adolescents (Shankman *et al.*, 2005), and helplessness and depressotypic memory biases at age 7 (Hayden *et al.*, 2006), providing further support for a link between low PE and risk for depression.

Kochanska (1991) examined BI using laboratory tasks in toddlers of mothers with histories of MDD, bipolar disorder, or no mood disorder.

The children of mothers with MDD exhibited significantly greater BI than the children of mothers with bipolar disorder; however neither group differed from the children of mothers with no history of mood disorder.

Rosenbaum *et al.* (2000) also assessed BI using laboratory measures in 2–6-year-old children of parents with a history of major depressive episodes and/or panic disorder and parents with no history of mood or anxiety disorders. The children of patients with histories of both panic disorder and major depressive episodes exhibited a significantly higher rate of BI than children of parents with no history of mood or anxiety disorder. Children of parents with major depressive episodes alone had an intermediate rate of BI that did not differ significantly from children of parents in the other groups.

These investigators recently reported secondary analyses exploring whether the small subgroup of offspring of parents with both a history of major depressive and manic/hypomanic episodes in the sample were characterized by the opposite of BI, behavioral disinhibition. Indeed, they found that although the offspring of bipolar and non-bipolar parents did not differ on BI, the former group exhibited a significantly higher rate of behavioral disinhibition (Hirshfeld-Becker *et al.*, 2006). Behavioral disinhibition is not specific to bipolar disorder, however, as it is also characteristic of children with externalizing disorders.

Several studies have examined parent and/or self-reports of temperament in older children and adolescents of parents with mood disorders. Unfortunately, most of these studies did not distinguish offspring who had and had not developed mood disorders by the time of the temperament assessment (Merikangas *et al.*, 1998; Mufson *et al.*, 2002). However, Ouimette *et al.* (1992) compared the 14–22-year-old offspring of depressed parents and non-depressed controls on a battery of self-report measures of personality. After excluding offspring with a history of mood disorder, there were no differences on NE/N or PE/E. A limitation of studying adolescent offspring, however, is that many vulnerable participants may have already developed a mood disorder and been excluded from the analyses.

Prospective studies of non-depressed children and adolescents

There are only a handful of prospective studies examining the role of NE/N, PE/E, and related traits to the subsequent onset of mood disorders. Krueger (1999) studied a New Zealand birth cohort that had been assessed for personality and psychopathology at age 18 and followed up at age 21. After controlling for mood disorder in the year prior to the initial assessment, higher self-reported NE and lower well-being (a subscale of PE) predicted the presence of a mood disorder at age 21. Negative emotionality at age 18 also predicted anxiety disorders, substance dependence, and antisocial personality at age 21. Unfortunately, this study did not control for mood-disorder episodes prior to age 17.

Several studies have examined parent and teacher reports of temperament and behavior in younger children as predictors of depression in adolescence. Kasen *et al.* (1996) examined the association between mother-reported temperament in children aged 1–10 and MDD 8 years later. Maternal reports of NE-like traits such as affective problems and anxiety did not predict the subsequent development of MDD. Similarly, Reinhertz *et al.* (1993) did not find an association between maternal ratings of BI-like traits such as fear of new things and shyness at age 5 and the onset of MDD by age 18. However, maternal ratings of dependence (which is often conceptualized as falling within the NE/N domain) at age 5 predicted depression at age 18 for males, but not females. In a subsequent paper from the same study, Reinhertz *et al.* (2000) reported that teacher ratings of anxious/depressed behavior in kindergarten predicted a lifetime diagnosis of MDD by age 21.

Three studies have examined the association between temperament-related variables in childhood and later MDD in large birth cohorts. Caspi and colleagues (Caspi, 2000; Caspi *et al.*, 1996) applied cluster analysis to examiners' ratings of child behavior at age 3. One cluster, labeled "inhibited," was characterized by a combination of low PE and high NE/BI behaviors, including sluggishness, low approach, social reticence, and fearfulness. Children in this cluster had significantly higher levels of parent-rated internalizing behavior problems at ages 13 and 15 (Caspi, 2000). Most importantly, children in the inhibited cluster had elevated rates of interview-assessed depressive disorders and suicide attempts, but not anxiety disorders, alcoholism, or antisocial behavior, in young adulthood (Caspi *et al.*, 1996). In a subsequent report from this study, Jaffee *et al.* (2002) found that among participants with major depression at age 26, those with an onset in childhood or adolescence were significantly more likely to have been rated as inhibited at age 3 than those with an adult onset.

In a large British birth cohort, van Os *et al.* (1997) found that physicians' ratings of behavioral apathy during childhood predicted teacher-reported depression at ages 13 and 15. Finally, Goodwin *et al.* (2004) found that a composite of parent and teacher ratings of anxious and withdrawn behaviors at age 8 predicted MDD at ages 16–18. This association persisted after controlling for a number of confounding variables.

In conclusion, although the data are limited, high-risk and prospective longitudinal studies suggest that low PE/E and at least some forms of high NE/N in youths are associated with risk for MDD, and particularly juvenile-onset MDD. However, these findings may apply only to some facets of PE/E and NE/N, and the effects appear to be weaker for parent reports than other methods. Hence, it is important that future studies employ multiple data sources and conduct analyses at the facet level.

The literature on BI is inconclusive. Offspring of parents with comorbid depression and anxiety disorders exhibit elevated BI, however the findings in offspring of depressed but non-anxious parents are weaker. Finally, there are few data on temperament and risk for bipolar disorder, although a recent study reporting increased behavioral disinhibition in the offspring of parents with bipolar disorder is intriguing (Hirshfeld-Becker et al., 2006). It will be important to examine the behavioral disinhibition construct more closely to determine whether there are components that distinguish risk for bipolar disorder from risk for externalizing disorders.

Mediators of the temperament-depression relationship

To the extent that temperament contributes to the development of mood disorders in adolescence, the effects occur over a relatively long time span, suggesting that more proximal processes mediate the relationship (Caspi & Shiner, 2006). In this section we briefly discuss four sets of variables that may play a particularly important mediating role.

Interpersonal deficits and difficulties

Adolescent depression is characterized by interpersonal deficits and problems in relationships with family members, peers, and romantic partners (Lewinsohn et al., 1994). Moreover, longitudinal studies suggest that interpersonal problems may influence subsequent depressive symptoms. For example, in a longitudinal study of a community sample of adolescents, Davila et al. (1995) found that poor interpersonal problem-solving predicted higher levels of interpersonal stress, which in turn predicted increased levels of depressive symptoms.

There is also a growing literature documenting the association between temperament and social competence in children. In general, children who are lower on PE/E, Agreeableness, and Constraint, and children who are higher on NE/N have more interpersonal problems (Caspi & Shiner, 2006). For example, Newman et al. (1997) examined the relationship between observations of temperament at age 3 and interpersonal functioning at age 21 in the Dunedin sample. They found that children who were rated as being inhibited or undercontrolled at age 3 had lower levels of interpersonal adjustment and greater interpersonal conflict in young adulthood.

This literature suggests that children with high NE/N, and possibly low PE/E, lack the skills to handle interpersonally challenging encounters in an adaptive fashion, fail to respond appropriately in certain interpersonal situations, and elicit negative interpersonal responses from others. This could produce a vicious cycle in which these children do not have as many opportunities to engage in peer interactions and may avoid them, leading to developmental lags in the acquisition of social skills. This, in turn, could lead to greater interpersonal problems, culminating in an increased risk for depression. Interpersonal deficits and difficulties may play a particularly critical role in risk for depression in adolescence, when relationships with peers and romantic partners assume increasing significance.

Depressotypic cognitions

Major depressive disorder is associated with a variety of cognitive styles and information processing biases, including dysfunctional attitudes and attributions, rumination, and attentional and memory biases for emotionally valenced self-relevant information (Christensen et al., 2006). Moreover, there is evidence that these features may contribute to the onset of depressive episodes (Alloy et al., 2006).

Negative emotionality/neuroticism has been associated with many of the same cognitive styles and biases that have been implicated in depression. For example, NE/N is associated with rumination (Muris et al., 2005; Nolan et al., 1998) and better recall of negative, and poorer recall of positive, information, particularly when it is relevant to the self (Ruiz-Caballero & Bermúdez, 2001; Rusting, 1999). Thus, the association between NE/N and the subsequent onset of depressive disorders may be mediated by the development of depressive cognitive styles and biases (Martin, 1985). Indeed, several studies have reported evidence suggesting that rumination mediates the association between NE/N and depression (Muris et al., 2005; Nolan et al., 1998).

Cognitive variables may also play a role in the association between low PE/E and depressive disorders (Collins & Depue, 1992; Davidson et al., 2002). High PE is associated with a broader attentional focus and greater cognitive flexibility, while low PE is associated with a narrow and inflexible style of information processing that limits coping and problem-solving (Ashby et al., 1999; Fredrickson, 2001). Hamburg (1998) hypothesized that deficits in PE hinder the development of mastery and competence in children and lead to the development of negative outcome expectancies and low perceived control over future events. Consistent with this hypothesis, Hayden et al. (2006) found that low PE in 3-year-old children predicted helpless behavior and depressotypic memory biases at age 7.

Maladaptive coping

A number of studies have indicated that adolescents and adults with MDD are more likely to employ emotion-focused and avoidant coping strategies, as opposed to problem-solving coping to deal with stressful situations than non-depressed individuals (e.g. Holahan et al., 2005). Individual differences in temperament may influence coping, and thereby affect risk for depression (Compas et al., 2001). For example, several studies have reported that children and adolescents with higher levels of NE/N are more likely to use avoidant coping than those with lower NE/N (Kardum & Krapić, 2001; Lengua & Long, 2002). In contrast, children and adolescents with higher levels of PE are more likely to use problem-solving coping (Kardum & Krapić, 2001). Of course, coping also influences mood, so that over time there may be reciprocal effects between temperament and coping.

Neuroendocrine stress reactivity

A fourth pathway by which temperament could lead to depression is through neuroendocrine responses to stress. Some personality traits appear to be associated with individual differences in physiological reactivity to stressors which, in turn, could increase susceptibility to depression. It should be noted, however, that the direction of the relationship between temperament and neuroendocrine stress reactivity may be difficult to discern, and it is conceivable that temperament and physiological stress reactivity reflect similar processes at different levels of analysis.

Depression in adults, adolescents, and children has been associated with dysregulation of the hypothalamic-pituitary-adrenal (HPA) axis, the major physiological stress response system hypothesized to play a role in the development of mood disorders (Gold et al., 1988). Recent prospective studies have reported that morning cortisol hypersecretion is a risk factor for the onset of MDD in adolescents of both sexes and adult women (Goodyer et al., 2000; Harris et al., 2000). Importantly, these findings were independent of psychosocial adversities and self-reported depressive symptoms, raising the possibility that HPA dysregulation is influenced by more distal factors such as temperament.

A number of studies have examined the relation between child temperament and biological indices of stress response system function. For example, BI and NE are associated with elevated levels of cortisol (Ahnert et al., 2004; Buss et al., 2003). Moreover, early individual differences in stress reactivity may be amplified in adolescence. Thus, cross-sectional and longitudinal studies of salivary and urinary cortisol find an increase with age during adolescence, with the most significant rise occurring at 13 years (Walker & Bollini, 2002). These changes are also evident at the behavioral level, as the strength of the relationship between negative life events and dysphoric mood also increases during adolescence (Rice et al., 2003).

Temperament and sex differences in the rate of depressive disorders

Depressive disorders are approximately twice as common in females compared to males, with this difference emerging in early adolescence (Nolen-Hoeksema,

2002). There are two ways in which temperament could play a role in the sex differences in depression: (1) male–female differences in levels of depression-relevant temperament traits; (2) sex differences in the strength of the association between temperament and depression.

A number of studies have compared levels of various temperament traits in males and females. Else-Quest *et al.* (2006) recently reported a meta-analysis of sex differences in child temperament and found that girls tended to exhibit greater fear than boys, but found little evidence for sex differences in other forms of NE. In contrast, among adults, women tend to experience higher levels of NE/N than men (Costa *et al.*, 2001; Lynn & Martin, 1997). Interestingly, this difference first emerges after age 13 (Canals *et al.*, 2005), paralleling the increase in rates of depression among females. This raises several important questions, including (1) what factors account for the increase in NE/N in adolescent girls and (2) does this increase precede, and therefore potentially explain, the growing rate of depression in girls at this time, or is it a concomitant or consequence of the increase in depression? One possibility is that childhood fearfulness leads to a generalized increase in NE in early adolescence, and subsequently to the development of depressive disorders. This is consistent with evidence that childhood anxiety is a major pathway to adolescent and adult depression (Silberg *et al.*, 2001). Alternatively, there may be sex differences in the expression of NE/N and psychopathology that emerge in adolescence. Thus, childhood NE may lead to withdrawal-related negative affects (sadness, fear, anxiety) and internalizing disorders in adolescent girls, and approach-related negative affects (anger) and externalizing disorders in adolescent boys (Else-Quest *et al.*, 2006).

In their meta-analysis, Else-Quest *et al.* (2006) reported significant sex differences in several components of PE in children. Boys exhibited higher levels of surgency and high-intensity pleasure, whereas girls experienced more low-intensity pleasure. These findings are interesting in light of recent evidence that high- and low-intensity positive affect may reflect different processes (Rothbart & Bates, 2006), and that a lack of high-intensity positive affect is significantly related to risk for depression (as indexed by maternal history of mood disorders) while low-intensity positive affect is not related to depression risk (Olino, Klein, Durbin, & Hayden, unpublished manuscript). The literature on sex differences in PE/E in adult personality suggests that males continue to exhibit higher levels of PE/E in adulthood (Lynn & Martin, 1997), although consistent with the child temperament literature, this depends on which facets are examined (Costa *et al.*, 2001). Thus, it is conceivable that the lower levels of high-intensity pleasure and surgency in young girls render them more vulnerable to developing depressive disorders when they encounter the demands and challenges of adolescence.

The literature on whether sex moderates the relation between temperament and adjustment is inconsistent, and does not afford any conclusions

(Rothbart & Bates, 2006). More specifically, there are surprisingly few data on whether the association between temperament and depression differs between males and females. In one of the few studies to address this question, Goodwin & Gotlib (2004) suggested that there was a stronger relationship between NE/N and MDD in women than men in a large epidemiological sample. However, their analyses demonstrated that sex and NE/N had additive effects on MDD; the results of the sex by personality trait interaction that is necessary to demonstrate moderation were not presented.

Moderators of the temperament–psychopathology relationship

It is unlikely that high NE/N and BI and low PE/E always result in mood disorders, or that all persons suffering from mood disorders exhibit elevated levels of these traits. In order to explain divergent developmental pathways between temperament and mood disorders, it is important to consider possible moderating variables. We touched on the role of sex as a moderator above. In this final section, we briefly consider four additional variables that could potentially moderate the association between temperament and the development of mood disorders in adolescence.

Life stress and the psychosocial challenges of adolescence

Adolescence is characterized by a number of potentially stressful transitions and challenges (Steinberg & Morris, 2001). These include physical changes, such as puberty; entering new school environments and expectations of mastering more complex academic skills; expectations for increasing independence from their families; and increasing importance of peer relationships, commencement of dating and romantic relationships, and peer pressures regarding alcohol, drugs, and sex (Steinberg & Morris, 2001). Thus, it is not surprising that rates of stressful life events increase during adolescence, and are associated with increases in depressive symptoms and disorders (Ge et al., 2006; Silberg et al., 1999).

The stress of the transitions and challenges of adolescence may amplify the psychosocial difficulties of children with high NE/N, high BI and/or low PE/E, and increase the risk of depressive disorders. For example, adolescents with high NE/N may be more reactive to, and less able to cope with, the new interpersonal and academic stressors that they experience. In a prospective study of a large community sample of early adolescents, Brendgen et al. (2005) found that girls with a high level of NE/N who also experienced a high level of peer rejection were more likely to experience a trajectory of increasing levels of depressive symptoms over time than girls with high NE/N or high peer rejection alone. More speculatively, adolescents with high BI may have difficulty dealing with the novel environments and interpersonal situations that they face. Similarly, adolescents with low PE/E may lack the initiative to pursue new roles and develop new relationships, and fall behind academically and/or socially.

Neurobiological and neurocognitive changes associated with adolescence

The temperament–depression association may also be moderated by the significant neurodevelopmental changes that occur during adolescence. These changes include increasing connectivity among different brain regions through the myelination of nerve fibers, and synaptic pruning, especially in frontal areas that are crucial to executive functioning (Blakemore & Choudhury, 2006; Casey et al., 2005). It is likely that these changes in connectivity between regions of the prefrontal cortex and the limbic system affect the interplay between cognition and emotion and influence the ways in which individuals evaluate and respond to risk and reward (Steinberg, 2005). Importantly, the surges in arousal and motivation brought on by puberty precede these changes in neurodevelopment, creating a discontinuity between the adolescent's affective experience and his or her ability to regulate arousal and motivation. This developmental lag between emotion, cognition, and behavior may help to explain why adolescence is such a period of heightened risk for psychopathology (Nelson et al., 2004; Steinberg, 2005), particularly for individuals with preexisting temperamental vulnerabilities. For example, emotionally reactive (high NE/N) children may have particular difficulty in regulating newly emergent and highly motivated behavior in an appropriate manner, increasing the risk for emotional and behavioral problems (Nelson et al., 2004). Thus, the association between temperament and depression may increase during adolescence as the emotional processes linking them may be more intense and less likely to be managed by developing regulatory systems.

Interactions between temperament dimensions

Other temperament dimensions may also moderate the temperament-adolescent mood disorder relationship. For example, PE may buffer the effects of stress on depression and anxiety (Meehl, 1975). Thus, Tugade & Fredrickson (2004) reported that the experience of positive emotions was associated with accelerated cardiovascular recovery from negative emotional arousal, suggesting that positive emotions may undo the lingering effects of stress. This suggests that the combination of high NE/N or BI and low PE/E may increase risk over and above the effects of either factor alone. Indeed, in a prospective study of a large sample of college freshmen, Gershuny & Sher

(1998) found that after controlling for depressive symptoms at baseline, the interaction between N and E significantly predicted depressive symptomatology 3 years later.

As suggested in the previous section on neurobiological development, effortful control/constraint may also moderate the effects of NE/N and PE/E on the risk for depression. For example, children who are high in attentional control may be better able to use voluntary strategies, including distraction and controlled shifting of attention, to reduce emotional distress (Compas *et al.*, 2001). A number of studies have reported that youths with both high NE/N and low self-regulation exhibit particularly poor social functioning and greater internalizing and externalizing behavior problems (Eisenberg *et al.*, 2000; Rothbart & Bates, 2006). Moreover, Lonigan *et al.* (2004) recently summarized data indicating that effortful control moderated the effects of high NE and low PE on depressive symptoms in adolescents.

Parenting

Finally, there is growing evidence that parenting moderates the effects of NE and BI on later adjustment (Rothbart & Bates, 2006). For example, Rubin *et al.* (2002) reported that 2-year-old children with a high level of BI were more likely to exhibit social reticence with unfamiliar peers 2 years later if their mothers were derisive or overly intrusive and controlling. Data on PE are more limited, however, Lengua *et al.* (2000) found that parental rejection moderated the association between child PE and behavior problems after divorce, with parental rejection having the greatest adverse impact on children with low PE. It is reasonable to speculate that maladaptive parenting could increase risk in temperamentally vulnerable youth.

Conclusions and future directions

Available research suggests that low PE/E, high NE/N, and possibly high BI may be precursors or predisposing factors for the development of depressive disorders in adolescents. In addition, these studies indicate that some aspects of PE and NE may be more related to risk than others. However, the existing evidence is only suggestive, as no studies have directly demonstrated that temperament, assessed prior to the onset of mood disorders, predicts diagnosable mood disorders in adolescents. Hence, there is a need for prospective studies that use multiple methods to assess key temperament constructs in youths with no history of mood disorder, and follow the participants through adolescence using semi-structured diagnostic interviews to identify first-onset cases of mood disorder. The literature on temperament and adolescent bipolar disorder is even more limited, so there is a pressing need for work in this area. In addition, it is likely that temperament is more strongly associated with risk for some forms of mood disorder than others, so it is important for future studies to take this heterogeneity into account. Finally, although there is a fairly large literature on cultural and racial/ethnic differences in temperament and personality (see Chapter 12, this volume), there is almost no research considering cultural or racial/ethnic differences in the relationship between temperament and mood disorder (for a noteworthy exception see Austin & Chorpita, 2004). Hence, this is an important question for future studies.

In addition to confirming the association between temperament and adolescent mood disorders, it will be important to use genetically informative designs, which together with longitudinal studies, can tease apart precursor, predisposition, and common cause models. As temperament is a relatively distal influence on adolescent mood disorders, it is also critical to develop and test mediational models that explore the processes through which temperament leads to the development of mood disorders.

Finally, the most consistent finding in the epidemiology of depression is the rising incidence in early adolescence, particularly among girls. Thus, it is important to continue to identify factors that interact with temperament to account for the sharp increase in the rate of mood, and to explore whether and how temperament plays a role in the gender disparity that emerges at this time.

In conclusion, individual differences in personality may have the greatest impact during major developmental transitions, such as from childhood to adolescence (Caspi & Moffitt, 1993). Retrospective studies of adults with mood disorders and prospective studies of children who later developed mood disorders suggest that temperament plays a greater role in juvenile-onset than adult-onset mood disorders (Klein *et al.*, 2002; van Os *et al.*, 1997). Hence, research on temperament is likely to play an important role in understanding the development of mood disorders in adolescence.

REFERENCES

Ahnert, L., Gunnar, M.R., Lamb, M.E., & Barthel, M. (2004). Transition to childcare: associations with infant-mother attachment, infant negative emotion and cortisol elevations. *Child Development*, **75**, 639–650.

Akiskal, H.S., Hirschfeld, R.M.A., & Yerevanian, B.I. (1983). The relationship of personality to affective disorders: a critical review. *Archives of General Psychiatry*, **40**, 801–810.

Alloy, L.B., Abramson, L.Y., Whitehouse, W.G. *et al.* (2006). Prospective incidence of first onsets and recurrences of depression in individuals at high and low cognitive risk for depression. *Journal of Abnormal Psychology*, **115**, 145–156.

Anthony, J.L., Lonigan, C.J., Hooe, E.S., & Phillips, B.M. (2002). An affect-based, hierarchical model of temperament and its relations with internalizing symptomatology. *Journal of Clinical Child and Adolescent Psychology*, **31**, 480–490.

Ashby, F.G., Isen, A.M., & Turken, A.U. (1999). A neuropsychological theory of positive affect and its influence on cognition. *Psychological Review*, **106**, 529–550.

Austin, A., & Chorpita, B.F. (2004). Temperament, anxiety, and depression: comparisons across five ethnic groups of children. *Journal of Clinical Child and Adolescent Psychology*, **33**, 216–226.

Blakemore, S.J., & Choudhury, S. (2006). Development of the adolescent brain: implications for executive function and social cognition. *Journal of Child Psychology and Psychiatry*, **47**, 296–312.

Brendgen, M., Wanner, B., Morin, A.J.S., & Vitaro, F. (2005). Relations with parents and with peers, temperament, and trajectories of depressed mood during early adolescence. *Journal of Abnormal Child Psychology*, **33**, 579–594.

Buss, K.A., Schumacher, J.R.M., Dolski, I. *et al.* (2003). Right frontal brain activity, cortisol, and withdrawal behavior in 6-month-old infants. *Behavioral Neuroscience*, **117**, 11–20.

Canals, J., Vigenl-Colet, A., Chico, E., & Marti-Henneberg, C. (2005). Personality changes during adolescence: the role of gender and pubertal development. *Personality and Individual Differences*, **39**, 179–188.

Casey, B.J., Tottenham, N., Liston, C., & Durston, S. (2005). Imaging the developing brain: what have we learned about cognitive development? *Trends in Cognitive Science*, **9**, 104–110.

Caspi, A. (2000). The child is father of the man: personality continuities from childhood to adulthood. *Journal of Personality and Social Psychology*, **78**, 158–172.

Caspi, A., & Moffitt, T.E. (1993). When do individual differences matter? A paradoxical theory of personality coherence. *Psychological Inquiry*, **4**, 247–271.

Caspi, A., & Shiner, R.L. (2006). Personality development. In W. Damon, R. Lerner, & N. Eisenberg (Eds.), *Handbook of Child Psychology, Sixth Edition: Social, Emotional, and Personality Development* (Vol. 3, pp. 300–365). New York: Wiley.

Caspi, A., Moffitt, T.E., Newman, D.L., & Silva, P.A. (1996). Behavioral observations at age 3 years predict adult psychiatric disorders. *Archives of General Psychiatry*, **53**, 1033–1039.

Cheng, H., & Furnham, A. (2003). Personality, self-esteem, and demographic predictors of happiness and depression. *Personality and Individual Differences*, **34**, 921–942.

Christensen, B.K., Carney, C.E., & Segal, Z.V. (2006). Cognitive processing models of depression. In D.J. Stein, D.J. Kupfer, & A.F. Schatzberg (Eds.), *The American Psychiatric Publishing Textbook of Mood Disorders* (pp. 131–144). Washington, DC: American Psychiatric Publishing.

Clark, L.A. (2005). Temperament as a unifying basis for personality and psychopathology. *Journal of Abnormal Psychology*, **114**, 505–521.

Clark, L.A., Watson, D., & Mineka, S. (1994). Temperament, personality, and the mood and anxiety disorders. *Journal of Abnormal Psychology*, **103**, 103–116.

Collins, P.F., & Depue, R.A. (1992). A neurobehavioral systems approach to developmental psychopathology: implications for disorders of affect. In D. Cicchetti & S.L. Toth (Eds.), *Developmental Perspectives on Depression. Rochester Symposium on Developmental Psychopathology* (Vol. 4, pp. 29–101). Rochester, NY: University of Rochester Press.

Compas, B.E., Connor-Smith, J.K., Saltzman, H., Thomsen, A.H., & Wadsworth, M.E. (2001). Coping with stress during childhood and adolescence: problems, progress, and potential in theory and research. *Psychological Bulletin*, **127**, 87–127.

Costa, P. Jr., Terracciano, A., & McCrae, R.R. (2001). Gender differences in traits across cultures: robust and surprising findings. *Journal of Personality and Social Psychology*, **81**, 322–331.

Davidson, R.J., Lewis, D.A., Alloy, L.B. *et al.* (2002). Neural and behavioral substrates of mood and mood regulation. *Biological Psychiatry*, **52**, 478–502.

Davila, J., Hammen, C., Burge, D., Paley, B., & Daley, S.E. (1995). Poor interpersonal problem-solving as a mechanism of stress generation in depression among adolescent women. *Journal of Abnormal Psychology*, **104**, 592–600.

Downey, G., & Coyne, J.C. (1990). Children of depressed parents: an integrative review. *Psychological Bulletin*, **108**, 50–76.

Durbin, C.E., Klein, D.N., Hayden, E.P., Buckley, M.E., & Moerk, K.C. (2005). Temperamental emotionality in preschoolers and parental mood disorders. *Journal of Abnormal Psychology*, **114**, 28–37.

Eisenberg, N., Fabes, R.A., Guthrie, I.K., & Reiser, M. (2000). Dispositional emotionality and regulation: their role in predicting quality of social functioning. *Journal of Personality and Social Psychology*, **78**, 136–157.

Else-Quest, N.M., Hyde, J.S., Goldsmith, H.H., & Van Hulle, C.A. (2006). Gender differences in temperament: a meta-analysis. *Psychological Bulletin*, **132**, 33–72.

Fox, N.A., Henderson, H.A., Marshall, P.J., Nichols, K.E., & Ghera, M.M. (2005). Behavioral inhibition: linking biology and behavior within a developmental framework. *Annual Review of Psychiatry*, **56**, 235–262.

Fox, N.A., Nichols, K.E., Henderson, H.A. *et al.* (2005). Evidence for a gene-environment interaction in predicting behavioral inhibition in middle childhood. *Psychological Science*, **16**, 921–926.

Fredrickson, B.L. (2001). The role of positive emotions in positive psychology: the broaden-and-build theory of positive emotions. *American Psychologist*, **56**, 218–226.

Ge, X., Natsuaki, M.N., & Conger, R.D. (2006). Trajectories of depressive symptoms and stressful life events among male and female adolescents in divorced and non-divorced families. *Development and Psychopathology*, **18**, 253–273.

Gershuny, B.S., & Sher, K.J. (1998). The relation between personality and anxiety: findings from a 3-year prospective study. *Journal of Abnormal Psychology*, **107**, 252–262.

Gold, P.W., Goodwin, F.K., & Chrousos, G.P. (1988). Clinical and biochemical manifestations of depression: relations to the neurobiology of stress. *New England Journal of Medicine*, **319**, 348–353.

Goodyer, I.M., Herbert, J., Tamplin, A., & Altham, P.M.E. (2000). First episode major depression in adolescents: affective, cognitive and endocrine characteristics of risk status and predictors of onset. *British Journal of Psychiatry*, **176**, 142–149.

Goodwin, R.D., & Gotlib, I.H. (2004). Gender differences in depression: the role of personality factors. *Psychiatry Research*, **126**, 135–142.

Goodwin, R.D., Fergusson, D.M., & Horwood, J. (2004). Early anxious/withdrawn behaviors predict later internalizing disorders. *Journal of Child Psychology and Psychiatry and Allied Disciplines*, **45**, 874–883.

Hamburg, S. (1998). Inherited hypohedonia leads to learned helplessness: a conjecture updated. *Review of General Psychology*, **2**, 384–403.

Harris, T.O., Borsanyi, S., Messari, S. *et al.* (2000). Morning cortisol as a risk factor for subsequent major depressive disorder in adult women. *British Journal of Psychiatry*, **177**, 505–510.

Hayden, E.P., Klein, D.N., Durbin, C.E., & Olino, T.M. (2006). Low positive emotionality at age three predicts depressotypic cognitions in seven-year old children. *Development and Psychopathology*, **18**, 409–423.

Hirschfeld, R.M.A., Klerman, G.L., Lavori, P. *et al.* (1989). Premorbid personality assessments of first onset of major depression. *Archives of General Psychiatry*, **46**, 345–350.

Hirshfeld-Becker, D.R., Biederman, J., Henin, A. *et al.* (2006). Laboratory-observed behavioral disinhibition in the young offspring of parents with bipolar disorder: a high-risk pilot study. *American Journal of Psychiatry*, **163**, 265–271.

Holahan, C.J., Moos, R.H., Holahan, C.K., Brennan, P.L., & Schutte, K.K. (2005). Stress generation, avoidance coping, and depressive symptoms: a 10-year model. *Journal of Consulting and Clinical Psychology*, **73**, 658–666.

Jaffee, S.R., Moffitt, T.E., Caspi, A. *et al.* (2002). Differences in early childhood risk factors for juvenile-onset and adult-onset depression. *Archives of General Psychiatry*, **58**, 215–222.

Kardum, I., & Krapić, N. (2001). Personality traits, stressful life events, and coping styles in early adolescence. *Personality and Individual Differences*, **30**, 503–515.

Kasen, S., Cohen, P., Brook, J.S., & Hartmark, C. (1996). A multiple-risk interaction model: effects of temperament and divorce on psychiatric disorders in children. *Journal of Abnormal Child Psychology*, **24**, 121–150.

Katainen, S., Räikkönen, K., & Keltikangas-Järvinen, L. (1999). Adolescent temperament, perceived social support, and depressive tendencies as predictors of depressive tendencies in young adulthood. *European Journal of Personality*, **13**, 183–207.

Kendler, K.S., Neale, M.C., Kessler, R.C., Heath, A.C., & Eaves, L.J. (1993). A longitudinal twin study of personality and major depression in women. *Archives of General Psychiatry*, **50**, 853–862.

Khan, A.A., Jacobson, K.C., Gardner, C.O., Prescott, C.A., & Kendler, K.S. (2005). Personality and comorbidity of common psychiatric disorders. *British Journal of Psychiatry*, **186**, 190–196.

Klein, D.N., Durbin, C.E., Shankman, S.A., & Santiago, N.J. (2002). Depression and personality. In I.H. Gotlib & C.L. Hammen (Eds.), *Handbook of Depression and its Treatment* (pp. 115–140). New York: Guilford Press.

Klein, D.N., Lewinsohn, P.M., Rohde, P., Seeley, J.R., & Olino, T.M. (2005). Psychopathology in the adolescent and young adult offspring of a community sample of mothers and fathers with major depression. *Psychological Medicine*, **35**, 353–365.

Klein, M.H., Wonderlich, S., & Shea, M.T. (1993). Models of the relationships between personality and depression: toward a framework for theory and research. In M.H. Klein, D.J. Kupfer, & M.T. Shea (Eds.), *Personality and Depression: A Current View* (pp. 1–54). New York: Guilford Press.

Kochanska, G. (1991). Patterns of inhibition to the unfamiliar in children of normal and affectively ill mothers. *Child Development*, **62**, 250–263.

Krueger, R.F. (1999). Personality traits in late adolescence predict mental disorders in early adulthood: a prospective-epidemiological study. *Journal of Personality, 67*, 39–65.

Lahey, B.B. (2004). Commentary: role of temperament in developmental models of psychopathology. *Journal of Child and Adolescent Clinical Psychology, 33*, 88–93.

Lemery, K.S., Essex, M.J., & Smider, N.A. (2002). Revealing the relation between temperament and behavior problem symptoms by eliminating measurement confounding: expert ratings and factor analyses. *Child Development, 73*, 867–882.

Lengua, L.J., & Long, A.C. (2002). The role of emotionality and self-regulation in the appraisal-coping process: tests of direct and moderating effects. *Applied Developmental Psychology, 23*, 471–493.

Lengua, L.J., West, S.G., & Sandler, I.N. (1998). Temperament as a predictor of symptomatology in children: addressing contamination of measures. *Child Development, 69*, 164–181.

Lengua, L.J., Wolchik, S.A., Sandler, I.N., & West, S.G. (2000). The additive and interactive effects of parenting and temperament in predicting adjustment problems of children of divorce. *Journal of Clinical Child Psychology, 29*, 232–244.

Lewinsohn, P.M., Roberts, R.E., Seeley, J.R. *et al.* (1994). Adolescent psychopathology: II. Psychosocial risk factors for depression. *Journal of Abnormal Psychology, 103*, 302–315.

Lonigan, C.J., Phillips, B.M., & Hooe, E.S. (2003). Relations of positive and negative affectivity to anxiety and depression in children: evidence from a latent-variable longitudinal study. *Journal of Consulting and Clinical Psychology, 71*, 465–481.

Lonigan, C.J., Vasey, M.W., Phillips, B.M., & Hazen, R.A. (2004). Temperament, anxiety, and the processing of threat-relevant stimuli. *Journal of Child and Adolescent Clinical Psychology, 33*, 8–20.

Lynn, R., & Martin, T. (1997). Gender differences in extraversion, neuroticism, and psychoticism, in 37 nations. *Journal of Social Psychology, 137*, 369–373.

Martin, M. (1985). Neuroticism as a predisposition toward depression: a cognitive mechanism. *Personality and Individual Differences, 6*, 353–365.

McGuffin, P., Rijsdijk, F., Andrews, M. *et al.* (2003). The heritability of bipolar affective disorder and the genetic relationship to unipolar depression. *Archives of General Psychiatry, 60*, 497–502.

Meehl, P.E. (1975). Hedonic capacity: some conjectures. *Bulletin of the Menniger Clinic, 39*, 295–307.

Merikangas, K.R., Swendsen, J.D., Preisig, M.A., & Chazan, R.Z. (1998). Psychopathology and temperament in parents and offspring: results of a family study. *Journal of Affective Disorders, 51*, 63–74.

Mufson, L., Nomura, Y., & Warner, V. (2002). The relationship between parental diagnosis, offspring temperament, and offspring psychopathology: a longitudinal analysis. *Journal of Affective Disorders, 71*, 61–69.

Muris, P., Meesters, C., & Spinder, M. (2003). Relationships between child- and parent-reported behavioural inhibition and symptoms of anxiety and depression in normal adolescents. *Personality and Individual Differences, 34*, 759–771.

Muris, P., Roelofs, J., Rassin, E., Franken, I., & Mayer, B. (2005). Mediating effects of rumination and worry on the links between neuroticism, anxiety, and depression. *Personality and Individual Differences, 39*, 1105–1111.

Nelson, E.E., Leibenluft, E., McClure, E.B., & Pine, D.S. (2004). The social re-orientation of adolescence: a neuroscience perspective on the process and its relation to psychopathology. *Psychological Medicine*, **35**, 163–174.

Newman, D.L., Caspi, A., Moffitt, T.E., & Silva, P.A. (1997). Antecedents of adult interpersonal functioning: effects of individual differences in age 3 temperament. *Developmental Psychology*, **33**, 206–217.

Nolan, S.A., Roberts, J.E., & Gotlib, I.H. (1998). Neuroticism and ruminative response style as predictors of change in depressive symptomatology. *Cognitive Therapy and Research*, **22**, 445–455.

Nolen-Hoeksema, S. (2002). Gender differences in depression. In I.H. Gotlib & C.L. Hammen (Eds.), *Handbook of Depression and its Treatment* (pp. 492–509). New York: Guilford Press.

Ormel, J., Oldehinkel, A.J., & Vollebergh, W. (2004). Vulnerability before, during and after a major depressive episode: a 3-wave population-based study. *Archives of General Psychiatry*, **61**, 990–996.

Ouimette, P.C., Klein, D.N., Clark, D.C., & Margolis, E.T. (1992). Personality traits in the offspring of parents with unipolar affective disorder: an exploratory study. *Journal of Personality Disorders*, **6**, 91–98.

Ramklint, M., & Ekselius, L. (2003). Personality traits and personality disorders in early onset versus late onset major depression. *Journal of Affective Disorders*, **75**, 35–42.

Reinhertz, H.Z., Giaconia, R.M., Pakiz, B. *et al.* (1993). Psychosocial risks for major depression in late adolescence: a longitudinal community study. *Journal of the American Academy of Child and Adolescent Psychiatry*, **32**, 1155–1163.

Reinhertz, H.Z., Giaconia, R.M., Hauf, A.M.C., Wasserman, M.S., & Paradis, A.D. (2000). General and specific childhood risk factors for depression and drug disorders by early adulthood. *Journal of the American Academy of Child and Adolescent Psychiatry*, **39**, 223–231.

Rice, F., Harold, G.T., & Tharper, A. (2003). Negative life events as an account of age-related differences in the genetic aetiology of depression in childhood and adolescence. *Journal of Child Psychology and Psychiatry and Allied Disciplines*, **44**, 977–987.

Roberts, S.B., & Kendler, K.S. (1999). Neuroticism and self-esteem as indices of the vulnerability to major depression in women. *Psychological Medicine*, **29**, 1101–1109.

Rorsman, B., Grasbeck, A., Hagnell, O., Isberg, P.E., & Otterbeck, L. (1993). Premorbid personality traits and psychometric background factors in depression: the Lundby Study 1957–1972. *Neuropsychobiology*, **27**, 72–79.

Rosenbaum, J.F., Biederman, J., Hirshfeld-Becker, D.R. *et al.* (2000). A controlled study of behavioral inhibition in children of parents with panic disorder and depression. *American Journal of Psychiatry*, **157**, 2002–2010.

Rothbart, M.K., & Bates, J.E. (2006). Temperament in children's development. In W. Damon, R. Lerner, & N. Eisenberg (Eds.), *Handbook of Child Psychology, Sixth Edition: Social, Emotional, and Personality Development* (Vol. 3, pp. 99–166). New York: Wiley.

Rubin, K.H., Burgess, K.B., & Hastings, P.D. (2002). Stability and social-behavioral consequences of toddlers' inhibited temperament and parenting behaviors. *Child Development*, **73**, 483–495.

Ruiz-Caballero, J.A., & Bermúdez, J. (2001). Neuroticism, mood, and retrieval of negative personal memories. *Journal of General Psychology*, 122, 29–35.

Rusting, C.L. (1999). Interactive effects of personality and mood on emotion-congruent memory and judgment. *Journal of Personality and Social Psychology*, 77, 1073–1086.

Shankman, S.A., Tenke, C.E., Bruder, G.E. *et al.* (2005). Low positive emotionality as a risk marker for depression in young children: association with EEG asymmetry. *Development and Psychopathology*, 17, 85–98.

Shea, M.T., Leon, A.C., Mueller, T.I. *et al.* (1996). Does major depression result in lasting personality change? *American Journal of Psychiatry*, 153, 1404–1410.

Silberg, J., & Rutter, M. (2002). Nature-nurture interplay in the risks associated with parental depression. In S.H. Goodman & I.H. Gotlib (Eds.), *Children of Depressed Parents: Mechanisms of Risk and Implications for Treatment* (pp. 13–36). Washington, DC: American Psychological Association.

Silberg, J.L., Pickles, A., Rutter, M. *et al.* (1999). The influence of genetic factors and life stress on depression among adolescent girls. *Archives of General Psychiatry*, 56, 225–232.

Silberg, J., Rutter, M., & Eaves, L. (2001). Genetic and environmental influences on the temporal association between earlier anxiety and later depression in girls. *Biological Psychiatry*, 49, 1040–1049.

Steinberg, L. (2005). Cognitive and affective development in adolescence. *Trends in Cognitive Science*, 9, 69–74.

Steinberg, L., & Morris, A.S. (2001). Adolescent development. *Annual Review of Psychology*, 52, 83–110.

Tugade, M.M., & Fredrickson, B.L. (2004). Resilient individuals use positive emotions to bounce back from negative emotional experiences. *Journal of Personality and Social Psychology*, 86, 320–333.

van Os, J., Jones, P., Lewis, G., Wadsworth, M., & Murray, R. (1997). Developmental precursors of affective illness in a general population birth cohort. *Archives of General Psychiatry*, 54, 625–631.

Walker, E., & Bollini, A.M. (2002). Pubertal neurodevelopment and the emergence of psychotic symptoms. *Schizophrenia Research*, 54, 17–23.

Weissman, M.M., Warner, V., Wickramaratne, P., Moreau, D., & Olfson, M. (1997). Offspring of depressed parents: 10 years later. *Archives of General Psychiatry*, 54, 932–940.

Youngstrom, E., Izard, C., & Ackerman, B. (1999). Dysphoria-related bias in maternal ratings of children. *Journal of Consulting and Clinical Psychology*, 67, 905–916.

14

Familial processes related to affective development

Erin C. Hunter, Danielle M. Hessler, and Lynn Fainsilber Katz

The family is widely acknowledged to play a significant role in the affective development of children prior to the adolescent period (Denham *et al.*, 1992; Eisenberg *et al.*, 1998; Gottman *et al.*, 1997). Research from early and middle childhood indicates that children's affective development is influenced not only by the parent–child relationship, but also by relationships with siblings (Brown & Dunn, 1992; Denham *et al.*, 1992). Throughout the child's life, these family interactions shape children's understanding of emotions, expression of emotion, and their ability to regulate their emotions. Though relatively little is known about family influences on normative affective development in adolescence, research suggests that the family continues to be an important factor in the emotional lives of adolescents despite an expanding social world (Bronstein *et al.*, 1996; Katz & Hunter, 2007; Kobak & Sceery, 1988; Sheeber *et al.*, 2000).

The current chapter examines both theory and research related to family processes involved in children's affective development. The influences of different family members and subsystems will be explored, although the primary focus of the chapter will be on the parent–child relationship. Through teaching children how to self-soothe (Cole & Kaslow, 1988; Eisenberg *et al.*, 1996; Gottman *et al.*, 1997; Lewis & Ramsey, 1999; Thompson, 1994), coaching children in how to recognize and cope with emotion (Gottman *et al.*, 1997), reinforcing children's emotional displays (Sheeber *et al.*, 2000), or modeling how to express and regulate affect, parents play a significant role in children's developing knowledge about emotion. As there are few studies of family emotion socialization with normative adolescent populations, research on younger children will first be reviewed to provide an understanding of emotion socialization processes before turning to a discussion of the adolescent

Adolescent Emotional Development and the Emergence of Depressive Disorders, ed. Nicholas B. Allen and Lisa B. Sheeber. Published by Cambridge University Press. © Cambridge University Press 2009.

period. Finally, directions for future research are presented, including the investigation of how culture and specific family socialization behaviors, i.e. emotional expression, coaching, and contingent reactions, shape adolescent affective development.

What do we mean by "affective development?"

Among the core set of emotion skills children develop are: (1) the understanding of emotion in self and others; (2) the ability to regulate emotion; and (3) the ability to express emotions to others (Halberstadt *et al.*, 2001; Mayer & Salovey, 1997; Saarni, 1999). There has been some debate in the literature regarding specific definitions of these emotional abilities (e.g. Campos *et al.*, 2004; Cole *et al.*, 2004), but there is a general consensus regarding the basic constructs underlying these terms. Emotional awareness or understanding refers to children's ability to recognize their own and others' emotions as well as to understand the causes and social contexts of emotional experiences (Halberstadt *et al.*, 2001). Emotion regulation is the modification of the intensity, quality or duration of an emotional experience in the service of accomplishing one's goals (Thompson, 1994). Expression of emotion refers to children's ability to effectively convey or inhibit their emotional experiences in a socially and culturally appropriate manner (Halberstadt *et al.*, 2001).

Conceptual frameworks for understanding emotion socialization

Emotion theorists have described affective development as an inherently interpersonal process, indicating that it is within the context of social interactions that children learn to interpret, express, and manage their emotions (Campos *et al.*, 1983; Gottman & Fainsilber Katz, 1989; Saarni, 1990; Thompson, 1994). Particularly early in life, when the majority of social interactions occur with family members, children's emotional development is likely most strongly impacted by family processes. According to family systems theory (Minuchin, 1974), children's emotional development is influenced by the interactions and relationships between family members as an organized whole, as well as by that of distinct subsystems (e.g. parental, marital, and sibling).

The majority of theories regarding emotion socialization in families have focused on the role of parents. Three fundamental parental socialization behaviors have emerged in the literature: (1) parent emotion expression, (2) parent coaching of children's emotions, and (3) parent contingent reactions to children's emotions (Eisenberg *et al.*, 1998; Halberstadt, 1991). Parents' expressions of emotion highlight the emotional importance of certain events, model ways of expressing and managing emotions, and communicate acceptance of or discomfort with particular emotions (Barrett & Campos, 1991; Denham, 1989). Parental coaching of emotion, which involves labeling of emotions as well as discussion of children's emotional experiences, fosters children's ability to communicate about their emotional experiences (Denham, 1998). Parents' contingent responding to children's emotions reinforce or punish children's emotion-related behaviors, and thereby influence not only children's expressiveness but also the likelihood that they will seek support in coping with their emotions (Denham, 1998).

The concept of parental "meta-emotion philosophy" (PMEP), proposed by Gottman *et al.* (1996), encapsulates aspects of all three parental socialization behaviors described above (emotion expression, emotion coaching, and contingent reactions to children's emotions). It refers to an organized set of reactions, thoughts, and feelings parents have regarding their own and their child's experience and expression of emotion. It includes awareness, acceptance, and regulation of their own and their children's emotional experiences, as well as the degree of emotion coaching they display. Gottman *et al.* (1997) proposed that PMEP would have broad implications for the emotional well-being of children, including their ability to regulate emotional states, at both physiological and behavioral levels.

Less attention has been given to the role of siblings in children's emotional development. However, siblings are frequently a child's initial peer group, and are likely to influence the expression and management of children's emotional behaviors (Minuchin & Fishman, 1981). Research exploring the role of family processes on the emotional development of younger children is presented in the following section. As any discussion of family processes involved in children's emotional development necessitates inclusion of the reciprocal effects of the child on the family, a section on the role of child characteristics is also presented.

Emotion socialization findings in childhood

Emotion socialization by parents and siblings has been associated with several different aspects of young children's affective development, including their understanding, regulation, and expression of emotion.

The role of parents

Emotion understanding
Parents who provide explanations of emotions or show positive responses to their children's emotions have been found to have children with greater emotion understanding than do parents who do not provide explanations

or who show negative responses to their children's emotions (Denham *et al.*, 1997; Garner, 1999). Parental discussion of emotions has also been associated with children's understanding of emotions (e.g. Denham *et al.*, 1992, 1994; Martin & Green, 2005). Both the total number of emotion words used in parent–child interactions and the number of times parents provide explanations for children's emotional experiences are related to aspects of children's emotion understanding, including emotion labeling and affective perspective taking (Brown & Dunn, 1996; Dunn *et al.*, 1991). The level of importance mothers place on socializing their children's use of emotion language has also been associated with higher levels of later emotion understanding (Dunsmore & Karn, 2004).

Evidence regarding the associations between family members' expressions of positive and negative emotions and children's emotion understanding is mixed. Some studies have linked the expression of positive emotions in the home to higher levels of children's emotion understanding, while other studies have not (see Halberstadt & Eaton, 2002, for a review). Similarly, mixed findings have emerged with regard to the expression of negative emotions. While some studies have found the expression of negative emotions to be associated with deficits in children's understanding of emotions (Denham *et al.*, 1994; Dunn & Brown, 1994), others have noted a positive association (Denham & Grout, 1992). It has been suggested that a curvilinear relationship may exist, in which well-modulated expressions of negative emotions provide children with opportunities to learn about the experience and expression of emotion, while high or dysregulated levels of negative affect are distressing and interfere with children's processing of emotional information (Halberstadt *et al.*, 1999).

Behavioral indices of emotional regulation

Parental behaviors that are supportive or accepting of children's emotional experiences have been associated with better behavioral emotion regulation in children, whereas dismissing or rejecting parental socialization strategies have been associated with poor behavioral regulation. Mothers who use more frequent or sophisticated language about emotions or who are more accepting of their children's negative emotions were found to have children who were better able to regulate their emotions (Denham *et al.*, 1992; Ramsden & Hubbard, 2002). On the other hand, children whose mothers responded to negative affect with minimizing or punitive reactions were more likely to use avoidant strategies of coping with negative affect and less likely to use constructive behavioral regulation strategies (Eisenberg *et al.*, 1992, 1996). For instance, in a disappointment task with toddlers, the emotionally dismissing strategies of granting children's wishes and questioning children's emotions were associated with poorer self-regulation, while parental acceptance of children's disappointment and soothing behaviors were associated with better emotion regulation (Spinrad *et al.*, 2004). Similar results were found in a sample of African–American preschoolers, where high levels of maternal supportive behavior in reaction to children's negative emotions were associated with less avoidance on the part of girls, while negative reactions were associated with more aggression, less cognitive distraction, and less support seeking in boys (Smith & Walden, 1998).

Physiological indices of emotion regulation

Vagal tone, or respiratory sinus arrythmia (RSA), measures the parasympathetic influences on the heart that occur via the vagus nerve. Parasympathetic activation functions to decrease heart rate and restore calm in the body. Because the vagus nerve acts as a brake – slowing down one's heart rate – vagal tone has been conceptualized as an index of the child's ability to self-soothe when upset (Porges, 1995). Both baseline vagal tone and the ability to effectively suppress vagal tone under challenging circumstances have been associated with better emotion regulation abilities in children (Porges, 1995). Gottman *et al.* (1997) reported that parent socialization behaviors affect children's physiological regulation abilities. They found that parental meta-emotion philosophy related to children's physiological regulatory abilities at age 5, which in turn predicted behavioral emotion regulation at age 8. Specifically, children whose parents engaged in higher levels of emotion coaching and who utilized scaffolding/praising approaches demonstrated higher levels of emotion regulation as indicated by both higher basal vagal tone and greater ability to suppress vagal tone when engaging in tasks that demand impulse control and mental effort.

Emotional expression

Both parents' situation-specific and general level of expressivity have been related to children's expressivity, although whether the association is driven by parenting processes or genetic inheritance (or some interaction between these) still requires clarification. Parents who express more positive emotion have children who express more positive than negative emotion (Denham & Grout, 1992; Garner *et al.*, 1997; Halberstadt & Eaton, 2002). Parental expression of negative emotion has been positively correlated with both greater negative emotion expression (Denham, 1989; Denham *et al.*, 1997) and lower levels of positive affective expression in children (Garner *et al.*, 1997). However, under some circumstances low-intensity parental expression of negative affect may be associated with appropriate levels of positive and negative emotion expression in children (Denham & Grout, 1992). Maternal acceptance and encouragement of children's emotional expression has also been associated with lower levels of observed and reported anger expression by children during conflictual situations (Zahn-Waxler *et al.*, 1996).

The role of siblings

Siblings may play a unique role in socializing children's affective development given the amount of time spent together and the high level of both negative and positive affect expressed between siblings (Brown & Dunn, 1992). As early as preschool, children talk about emotions more with their siblings and peers than with their parents (Brown et al., 1996). Positive interactions with an older sibling and siblings' positive responsiveness to children's emotions have been associated with higher levels of children's emotion understanding (Brown & Dunn, 1996; Sawyer et al., 2002). Additionally, while it cannot be known whether the positive sibling relationship leads to increased opportunities for children to learn about emotions or rather that younger siblings with heightened emotion understanding are able to have better relationships with their siblings, friendly interactions and older sibling affection have been found to predict better affective perspective taking, a measure of emotion understanding (Dunn et al., 1991). It is less clear what role, if any, siblings play in socializing other aspects of children's emotional competence. One study examining children's emotion expression failed to find any associations between sibling relationship or behavior and children's spontaneous expression of emotion at school (Sawyer et al., 2002).

The influence of child characteristics on the family

Finally, it is important to consider bidirectional effects in family emotion socialization. Although the nature of the correlational results makes it difficult to discern the direction of the effects, it is likely that children's characteristics, such as their temperament, behavior, and gender, influence parental responding to their children's emotions. Mothers who perceive their children to be well regulated have been found to be more supportive of their children's emotions than mothers who perceive their children to be high in negative emotionality (Eisenberg & Fabes, 1994), suggesting that parents may have difficulty being supportive of children's negative emotions when children's emotions are intense. On the other hand, another study found that mothers were more likely to put additional effort into regulating their children's emotions when their child had a more difficult and emotionally reactive temperament, suggesting that these more difficult children may be pulling for more emotional support on the part of their parents in order to manage their emotions (Casey & Fuller, 1994). Children may also possess individual characteristics that result in the same parental socialization strategies or family emotional climate having a different impact on each particular child's affective development. For example, Denham et al. (1997) found that children who were more open and who positively reinforced their parents' emotions showed better emotional adjustment, suggesting that some children may be more open to benefiting from family emotion socialization.

Gender has also been found to influence family emotion socialization processes. Parents have been reported to utilize different socialization practices with sons than with daughters. Early studies reported that parents encouraged higher levels of emotional control in boys than girls (Block, 1979), specifically around the expression of sadness and fear (Birnbaum & Croll, 1984). Conversely, parents were more accepting of anger expression in sons than daughters (Birnbaum & Croll, 1984). Though societal expectations of gender roles have loosened over the past few decades, more recent studies have also found evidence of gender differences in family socialization practices. Mothers have been found to be more emotionally expressive of positive emotions (Garner *et al.*, 1997), and to talk more about feelings (Dunn *et al.*, 1991; Kuebli & Fivush, 1992) with daughters than with sons. However, maternal discussion of emotion appears to have a larger impact on their son's emotion understanding than their daughter's (Martin & Green, 2005). Parent emotional expressivity, on the other hand, has been found to have more influence on the emotion regulation abilities of girls than boys (Denham *et al.*, 1997). It is important to note, however, that many studies have failed to find gender differences in parent emotion socialization practices or its effects on children's affective development (e.g. Garner & Spears, 2000; Martin & Green, 2005).

Emotion socialization in adolescence: empirical evidence

Developmental changes during the adolescent period

Because adolescence is a period of heightened emotionality compared to middle childhood (Larson & Lampman-Petraitis, 1989; Larson *et al.*, 1990), increased demands are placed on adolescents' abilities to understand, express, and regulate their emotional experiences (Rosenblum & Lewis, 2003). Changes in relationship dynamics within the family also occur during adolescence. Peers begin to have increasing influence on the socialization of adolescent behavior (Buhrmester & Furman, 1987; Furman & Buhrmester, 1992), and adolescents appear to emotionally distance themselves from parents (Papini *et al.*, 1990; Steinberg, 1988). Compared to early and middle childhood, parents and adolescents display increased negativity towards one another (Montemayor *et al.*, 1993). Additionally, adolescents are less likely to openly express or disclose emotions with their mothers than children in middle childhood, which may be related to adolescents' perceptions that their mothers are not accepting of some of their emotional expressions, particularly expressions of anger (Zeman & Shipman, 1997). Likewise, early adolescents prefer emotional disclosure with their friends over disclosure to any adult, including their parents (Saarni, 1988). However, despite changes in the parent–child relationship, parental support has been found to better predict adolescent emotional adjustment than peer support (Helsen *et al.*, 2000).

Family influences on adolescent affective development

Research regarding family influences on adolescent emotional development is sparse relative to that focused on early and middle childhood. Additionally, the existing literature on emotion socialization in adolescence lacks the specificity seen in research with younger children; adolescent studies have typically reported relations with general emotional adjustment (e.g. externalizing, internalizing behaviors) instead of specific aspects of emotional competence such as emotion understanding, expressivity, or regulation abilities.

There is an extensive literature linking family processes to a wide range of psychological disorders in adolescence, including affective disorders (Barrera & Garrison-Jones, 1992; Cuffe *et al.*, 2005; Sheeber & Sorensen, 1998). Additionally, there is considerable evidence for the mediating role of family-based variables, such as parenting and parent–adolescent relationships, on the relation between stressors and psychological symptoms (see Grant *et al.*, 2005, for a review). However, fewer studies have focused on family emotion socialization processes in normative populations.

The majority of research on normative family emotion socialization has focused on the impact of family cohesion or connectedness on adolescents' emotional expression and regulation. Adolescents with secure attachments have been found to be less anxious, more emotionally regulated in peer interactions, more verbally expressive about emotions, and better able to match their facial emotion expressions with self-ratings of sadness and anger than adolescents with insecure attachments (Kobak & Sceery, 1988, Zimmermann, 1999; Zimmerman *et al.*, 2001). Securely attached adolescents have also been found to express less dysfunctional anger, show higher levels of engagement in discussions of disagreements, demonstrate less avoidance of discussions regarding problems, and have more adaptive interactions with their mothers (Kobak *et al.*, 1993). Family cohesiveness has been associated with increased sympathy and sadness in response to a compassion-evoking film clip in older adolescents (Eisenberg *et al.*, 1991). In a sample of Taiwanese adolescents and their families, parental support buffered adolescents from heightened anxiety reactions to a stressor (Yang & Yeh, 2006).

Parental expression and acceptance of emotion has also been linked to adolescent emotional functioning. Adolescents and their parents have been found to have similar emotional styles, both in terms of global emotional patterns and immediate emotional reactions (Larson & Richards, 1994). Growing up in an emotionally expressive and accepting home has been found to decrease adherence to stereotypical gender norms of emotional expression in adolescence, which in turn relates to higher levels of social and emotional adjustment (Bronstein *et al.*, 1996). Evidence also suggests that non-hostile emotion expression in the family buffers young adolescents against emotional problems (Bronstein *et al.*, 1993). Increased interparental hostility, on the other hand, has been related to increased hostility and less constructive problem-solving strategies in parent–child interactions (Schulz *et al.*, 2005). Maternal acceptance and expression of her own emotion has been associated with lower levels of depressive symptoms, higher self-esteem, and fewer externalizing problems in young adolescents (Katz & Hunter, 2007). Additionally, evidence suggests that maternal responding to adolescent emotional behavior affects adolescent emotion regulation abilities (Sheeber *et al.*, 2000). Parental warmth and positive expressivity has also been linked to better emotion regulation abilities and decreased externalizing problems (Eisenberg *et al.*, 2005).

Parental acceptance has emerged as a key factor in adolescents' perception of the parental–adolescent relationship (Forehand & Nousiainen, 1993), thus level of parent acceptance of emotion may affect the likelihood that the adolescent will turn to the parent for emotional support and advice. This could be important for adolescent emotional adjustment, as higher levels of maternal emotion coaching have been linked to less aversive and dysphoric behavior during mother–adolescent interactions (Katz & Hunter, 2007), while difficulty engaging in emotional discussion with parents has been related to increased emotional problems in adolescents (Ackard *et al.*, 2006).

The influence of the adolescent on the family

As previously outlined in the section on younger children, it is important to consider bidirectional effects in family emotion socialization. Adolescents' intra-individual characteristics, including their temperament, behavior, and gender, are likely to elicit different types of interactions with family members. Adolescents with resilient temperaments reported receiving more support from family members than did non-resilient adolescents (van Aken & Dubas, 2004). Additionally, adolescents' ability to regulate their emotional expressions has been found to influence parent–adolescent relationships. During parent–adolescent interactions, when adolescents were able to regulate their emotional expressions, their parents were less likely to display hostility and more likely to be positively engaged (Schulz *et al.*, 2005).

As with younger children, there is evidence that gender affects the ways in which families socialize adolescents to express and experience emotion (Shearer *et al.*, 2005). In shaping the expressions of anger and sadness, evidence suggests that parents utilize different socialization practices with boys and girls, with increased discouragement of expressions of sadness in boys and increased discouragement of expressions of anger in girls (Brody & Hall, 2000).

Studies have also found that overall, boys tend to avoid emotional expression and expect more belittling and less understanding in response to their emotional expressions than do girls (Zeman & Shipman, 1997). Adolescent girls tend to engage in more self-disclosure of emotional experiences than boys (Papini *et al.*, 1990), while adolescent boys appear to engage in more emotional distancing from their families than adolescent girls (Seiffge-Krenke, 1999), which is likely to result in more opportunities for families to respond to the emotional experiences of adolescent girls than adolescent boys.

Limitations and future directions

There is currently a dearth of information on the role of family socialization processes in normative adolescent affective development. Research with younger children has established the influential role the family plays in the development of children's emotion understanding, expression, and regulation (Brown & Dunn, 1996; Denham *et al.*, 1992; Denham & Grout, 1992). However, few studies have explored family influences on these dimensions of emotional competence in adolescence. Given both the developmental changes in the child, and differences inherent in the parenting of an adolescent versus a younger child, it is likely that familial socialization processes affecting emotional competence may differ during the adolescent period.

During adolescence, children become more independent from parents, are more likely to turn to friends for emotional support, and more frequently utilize self-coping strategies (Cole & Kaslow, 1988; Gross & Munoz, 1995). Yet family members remain important in the emotional lives of adolescents. As children mature into adolescence, it is likely that they require different types of emotional support from their families. The role of parents may shift during adolescence from that of a teacher, directly monitoring and correcting their child's behavior, to that of a consultant, operating as a resource to whom the adolescent can turn when faced with new or difficult situations. Evidence provides initial support for this role shift, with parental acceptance emerging as a key factor in both the quality of the parent–adolescent relationship and adolescent emotion regulation (Forehand & Nousiainen, 1993; Katz & Hunter, 2007).

Further research is warranted to better elucidate the influence of the parent–adolescent relationship on adolescent emotional competence, including the effects of parent socialization behaviors (e.g. emotion expression, coaching, and contingent responding) on adolescent emotional competence. It has been suggested that the impact of parent behaviors may differ as a function of the intensity of the behavior. For example, moderate levels of parent emotion expression may be beneficial for children while low and high levels of expression may negatively impact children's emotional competence

(Halberstadt *et al.*, 1999). The same principle, "everything is good in moderation," may also ring true for other aspects of parent socialization behaviors. Child emotional outcomes may depend on the intensity, frequency, and duration of exposure to parental socialization behaviors, with optimal child outcomes corresponding to moderate levels of parental socialization efforts. On the other hand, a single exposure to a parent behavior may have either a strong positive impact, such as having one open and intimate discussion regarding emotions with their child, or a strong negative impact, such as one incidence of parental rejection when the child is particularly vulnerable. Eisenberg and colleagues (1998) have suggested that the association between children's emotional competence and parental expression of negative emotion may be dependent upon many factors including the intensity of the parent's emotion, the type of negative emotion displayed, and whether or not the negative emotion is directed at the child. These factors should be further explored in future research to determine circumstances when negative parental emotional expression can be beneficial or detrimental to children's affective development.

There is also a need for further research investigating the differential effects of individual family members on adolescent emotional competence. To date, the majority of research on parental socialization behaviors has focused on mothers. However, recent research suggests fathers may make important contributions to children's emotional competence (Carlson, 2006; D'Angelo *et al.*, 1995; McDowell & Parke, 2000). Moreover, research with younger children highlights the impact of siblings on children's affective development (Brown & Dunn, 1996; Sawyer *et al.*, 2002; Dunn *et al.*, 1991). Some initial work has looked at the impact of siblings on adolescent emotional outcomes, though the majority of this research has focused on clinical symptoms (Branje *et al.*, 2004; Conger *et al.*, 1997; East & Khoo, 2005). The role of both fathers and siblings in adolescent affective development warrants further investigation, as well as possible interactions between the socialization behaviors of different family members.

Additional specificity in the aspects of adolescent emotional competence influenced by the family is also required. Much of the extant literature focuses on general adolescent adjustment problems (e.g. externalizing, internalizing behaviors) rather than how family processes relate to more specific aspects of emotional competence such as their emotional understanding, expressivity, or regulation abilities. The work relating to effects of family influences on emotional development in younger children needs to be extended into adolescent populations so that a picture can begin to form regarding the ways in which families shape the developing emotional abilities of adolescents. In particular, increased specificity is needed in describing the influence of particular family processes on the development of distinct components of adolescent emotional competence, including emotional understanding, expression, and regulation (both behavioral and physiological).

Currently, it is unclear to what extent relations between family socialization processes and children's emotional competence are driven by individual characteristics of the child. Temperament and gender have both been found to impact the way in which parents respond to their children's emotional experiences (Casey & Fuller, 1994; Dunn *et al.*, 1991; Eisenberg & Fabes, 1994; Martin & Green, 2005). However, the findings are often contradictory. For example, mothers' perceptions of their children as having a difficult temperament have been found to elicit both less support (Eisenberg & Fabes, 1994), and more support (Casey & Fuller, 1994). The effects of individual characteristics of children on parent behaviors may depend on interactions between characteristics of both the children and parents. The pairing of a temperamentally difficult parent and child may lead to less emotional support for the child. More research addressing the moderating role of child characteristics is necessary to better understand intra-individual child effects on the influence of family emotion socialization.

Additionally, cultural influences on family emotion socialization should be considered. The majority of research to date has primarily relied on White, middle-class populations. Research suggests that culture plays an important role in both the emotion socialization strategies utilised by parents, as well as the effect these strategies have on children's affective development. For example, parent expression of positive emotions has been associated with greater emotion regulation abilities in children in the USA, but not for children in Indonesia (Eisenberg *et al.*, 2001). Furthermore, in contrast to research conducted in the USA, emotion-dismissing behaviors in Nepalese parents were associated with low levels of child negative emotional expression (Cole & Tamang, 1998). These initial findings are intriguing and future cross-cultural research is needed to better understand the complexities of adaptive family emotion socialization strategies and children's affective development.

It is clear that we are just beginning to understand the ways in which family processes shape adolescent affective development. However, much work remains to be done to allow for increased understanding of the emotional lives of adolescents and their families. Better understanding of family processes relating to adolescent affective development will provide insight into how families can best interact with their adolescents to foster emotional competence and build lasting positive family relationships.

REFERENCES

Ackard, D., Neumark-Sztainer, D., Story, M., & Perry, C. (2006). Parent–child connectedness and behavioral and emotional health among adolescents. *American Journal of Preventive Medicine*, **30**, 59–66.

Barrera, M., & Garrison-Jones, C. (1992). Family and peer social support as specific correlates of adolescent depressive symptoms. *Journal of Abnormal Child Psychology*, **20**, 1–16.

Barrett, K.C., & Campos, J.J. (1991). A diacritical function approach to emotions and coping. In E.M. Cummings, A.L. Greene, & K.H. Karraker (Eds.), *Life-span Developmental Psychology: Perspectives on Stress and Coping* (pp. 21–41). Hillsdale, NJ: Lawrence Erlbaum.

Birnbaum, D.W., & Croll, W.L. (1984). The etiology of children's stereotypes about sex differences in emotionality, *Sex Roles*, **10**, 677–691.

Block, J.H. (1979). Another look at sex differentiation in the socialization behaviors of mothers and fathers. In J. Sherman & F.L. Denmark (Eds.), *Psychology of Women: Future of Research* (pp. 29–87). New York: Psychological Dimensions.

Branje, S.J.T., van Lieshout, C.F.M., van Aken, M.A.G., & Haselager, G.J.T. (2004). Perceived support in sibling relationships and adolescent adjustment. *Journal of Child Psychology and Psychiatry*, **45**, 1385–1396.

Brody, L.R., & Hall, J.A. (2000). Gender, emotion, and expression. In M. Lewis & J. Haviland-Jones (Eds.), *Handbook of Emotions* (2nd edn, pp. 338–349). New York: Guilford Press.

Bronstein, P., Fitzgerald, M., Briones, M., Pieniadz, J., & D'Ari, A. (1993). Family emotional expressiveness as a predictor of early adolescent social and psychological adjustment. *Journal of Early Adolescence*, **13**, 448–471.

Bronstein, P., Briones, M., Brooks, T., & Cowan, B. (1996). Gender and family factors as predictors of late adolescent emotional expressiveness and adjustment: a longitudinal study. *Sex Roles*, **34**, 739–765.

Brown, J.R., & Dunn, J. (1992). Talk to your mother or your sibling? Developmental changes in early family conversations about feelings. *Child Development*, **63**, 336–349.

Brown, J.R., & Dunn, J. (1996). Continuities in emotion understanding from 3–6 years. *Child Development*, **67**, 789–802.

Brown, J.R., Donelan-McCall, N., & Dunn, J. (1996). Why talk about mental states? The significance of children's conversations with friends, siblings, and mothers. *Child Development*, **67**, 836–849.

Buhrmester, D., & Furman, W. (1987). The development of companionship and intimacy. *Child Development*, **58**, 1101–1113.

Campos, J.J., Barrett, K.C., Lamb, M.E., Goldsmith, H.H., & Stenberg, C. (1983). Socioemotional development. In P. Mussen (Series Ed.), J.J. Campos, & M.H. Haith (Vol. Eds.), *Handbook of Child Psychology: Vol. 2. Infancy and Developmental Psychobiology* (pp. 783–915). New York: John Wiley.

Campos, J.J., Frankel, C.B., & Camras, L. (2004). On the nature of emotion regulation. *Child Development*, **75**, 377–394.

Carlson, M.J. (2006). Family structure, father involvement and adolescent behavioral outcomes. *Journal of Marriage and Family*, **68**, 137–154.

Casey, R.J., & Fuller, L.L. (1994). Maternal regulation of children's emotions. *Journal of Nonverbal Behavior*, **18**, 57–89.

Cole, P.M., & Kaslow, N.J. (1988). Interactional and cognitive strategies for affect regulation: Developmental perspective on childhood depression. In L.B. Alloy (Ed.), *Cognitive Processes in Depression* (pp. 310–343). New York: Guilford Press.

Cole, P.M., & Tamang, B.L. (1998). Nepali children's ideas about emotional displays in hypothetical challenges. *Developmental Psychology*, **34**, 640–646.

Cole, P.M., Martin, S.E., & Dennis, T.A. (2004). Emotion regulation as a scientific construct: methodological challenges and directions for child development research. *Child Development*, **75**, 317–333.

Conger, K.J., Conger, R.D., & Scaramella, L.V. (1997). Parents, siblings, psychological control, and adolescent adjustment. *Journal of Adolescent Research*, **12**, 113–138.

Cuffe, S.P., McKeown, R.E., Addy, C.L., & Garrison, C.Z. (2005). Family and psychological risk factors in a longitudinal epidemiological study of adolescents. *Journal of the American Academy of Child and Adolescent Psychiatry*, **44**, 121–129.

D'Angelo, L.L., Weinberger, D.A., & Feldman, S.S. (1995). Like father, like son? Predicting male adolescents' adjustment from parents' distress and self-restraint. *Developmental Psychology*, **31**, 883–896.

Denham, S.A. (1989). Maternal affect and toddlers' social-emotional competence. *American Journal of Orthopsychiatry*, **59**, 368–376.

Denham, S.A. (1998). *Emotional Development in Young Children*. New York: Guilford Press.

Denham, S.A., & Grout, L. (1992). Mothers' emotional expressiveness and coping: relations with preschoolers' social-emotional competence. *Genetic, Social, and General Psychology Monographs*, **118**, 73–101.

Denham, S.A., Cook, M., & Zoller, D. (1992). Baby looks very sad: implication of conversations about feelings between mother and preschooler. *British Journal of Developmental Psychology*, **10**, 301–315.

Denham, S.A., Zoller, D., & Couchoud, E.A. (1994). Socialization of preschoolers' emotion understanding. *Developmental Psychology*, **30**, 928–936.

Denham, S.A., Mitchell-Copeland, J., Strandberg, K., Auerbach, S., & Blair, K. (1997). Parental contributions to preschoolers' emotional competence: direct and indirect effects. *Motivation and Emotion*, **21**, 65–86.

Dunn, J., & Brown, J. (1994). Affect expression in the family, children's understanding of emotions and their interactions with others. *Merrill-Palmer Quarterly*, **40**, 120–137.

Dunn, J., Brown, J., & Beardsall, L. (1991). Family talk about feeling states and children's later understanding of others' emotions. *Developmental Psychology*, **27**, 448–455.

Dunn, J., Brown, J., Slomkowski, C., Tesla, C., & Youngblade, L. (1991). Young children's understanding of other people's feelings and beliefs: individual differences and their antecedents. *Child Development*, **62**, 1352–1366.

Dunsmore, J.C., & Karn, M.A. (2004). The influence of peer relationships and maternal socialization on kindergartner's developing emotion knowledge. *Early Education and Development*, **15**, 39–56.

East, P.L., & Khoo, S.T. (2005). Longitudinal pathways linking family factors and sibling relationship qualities to adolescent substance use and sexual risk behaviors. *Journal of Family Psychology*, **19**, 571–580.

Eisenberg, N., & Fabes, R.A. (1994). Mothers' reactions to children's negative emotions: relations to children's temperament and anger behavior. *Merrill-Palmer Quarterly*, **40**, 138–156.

Eisenberg, N., Fabes, R.A., Schaller, M. *et al.* (1991). Personality and socialization correlates of vicarious emotional responding. *Journal of Personality and Social Psychology,* **61,** 459–470.

Eisenberg, N., Fabes, R.A., Carlo, G., & Karbon, M. (1992). Emotional responsivity to others: behavioral correlates and socialization antecedents. *New Directions for Child Development,* **55,** 57–73.

Eisenberg, N., Fabes, R.A., & Murphy, B.C. (1996). Parents' reactions to children's negative emotions: relations to children's social competence and comforting behavior. *Child Development,* **67,** 2227–2247.

Eisenberg, N., Cumberland, A., & Spinrad, T. (1998). Parental socialization of emotion. *Psychological Inquiry,* **9,** 241–273.

Eisenberg, N., Liew, J., & Pidada, N. (2001). The relations of regulation and negative emotionality to Indonesian children's social functioning. *Child Development,* **72,** 1747–1763.

Eisenberg, N., Zhou, Q., Spinrad, T.L., Valiente, C., Fabes, R.A., & Liew, J. (2005). Relations among positive parenting, children's effortful control, and externalizing problems: a three-wave longitudinal study. *Child Development,* **76,** 1055–1071.

Forehand, R., & Nousiainen, S. (1993). Maternal and paternal parenting: Critical dimensions in adolescent functioning. *Journal of Family Psychology,* **7,** 213–221.

Furman, W., & Buhrmester, D. (1992). Age and sex differences in perceptions of networks of personal relationships. *Child Development,* **63,** 103–115.

Garner, P.W. (1999). Continuity in emotion knowledge from preschool to middle-childhood and relation to emotion socialization. *Motivation and Emotion,* **23,** 247–266.

Garner, P.W., & Spears, F.M. (2000). Emotion regulation in low-income preschoolers. *Social Development,* **9,** 246–264.

Garner, P.W., Robertson, S., & Smith, G. (1997). Preschool children's emotional expressions with peers: the roles of gender and emotion socialization. *Sex Roles,* **36,** 675–691.

Gottman, J.M., & Fainsilber Katz, L. (1989). Effects of marital discord on young children's peer interaction and health. *Developmental Psychology,* **25,** 373–381.

Gottman, J.M., Katz, L.F., & Hooven, C. (1996). Parental meta-emotion structure and the emotional life of families: theoretical models and preliminary analyses. *Journal of Family Psychology,* **10,** 243–268.

Gottman, J.M., Katz, L.F., & Hooven, C. (1997). *Meta-emotion: How Families Communicate Emotionally.* Mahwah, NJ: Lawrence Erlbaum Associates.

Grant, K.E., Compas, B.E., Thurm, A.E. *et al.* (2005). Stressors and child and adolescent psychopathology: evidence of moderating and mediating effects. *Clinical Psychology Review,* **26,** 257–283.

Gross, J.J., & Munoz, R.E. (1995). Emotion regulation and mental health. *Clinical Psychology: Science and Practice,* **2,** 151–164.

Halberstadt, A.G. (1991). Towards an ecology of expressiveness: family expressiveness in particular and a model in general. In R.S. Feldman & B. Rime (Eds.), *Fundamentals in Nonverbal Behavior* (pp. 106–160). Cambridge, UK: Cambridge University Press.

Halberstadt, A.G., & Eaton, K.L. (2002). A meta-analysis of family expressiveness and children's emotion expressiveness and understanding. *Marriage and Family Review,* **34,** 35–62.

Halberstadt, A.G., Crisp, V.W., & Eaton, K.L. (1999). Family expressiveness: a retrospective and new directions for research. In P. Philippot, R.S. Feldman, & E.J. Coats (Eds.), *The Social Context of Nonverbal Behavior* (pp. 109–155). New York: Cambridge University Press.

Halberstadt, A.G., Denham, S.A., & Dunsmore, J.C. (2001). Affective social competence. *Social Development*, **10**, 79–119.

Helsen, M., Vollebergh, W., & Meeus, W. (2000). Social support from parents and friends and emotional problems in adolescence. *Journal of Youth and Adolescence*, **29**, 319–335.

Katz, L.F., & Hunter, E.C. (2007). Maternal meta-emotion philosophy and adolescent depressive symptomatology. *Social Development*, **16**(2), 343–360.

Kobak, R., & Sceery, A. (1988). Attachment in late adolescence: working models, affect regulation, and representation of self and others. *Child Development*, **59**, 135–146.

Kobak, R.R., Cole, H.E., Ferenz-Gillies, R., Fleming, W.S., & Gamble, W. (1993). Attachment and emotion regulation during mother-teen problem solving: a control theory analysis. *Child Development*, **64**, 231–245.

Kuebli, J., & Fivush, R. (1992). Gender differences in parent-child conversations about past emotions. *Sex Roles*, **27**, 683–698.

Larson, R., & Lampman-Petraitis, C. (1989). Daily emotional stress as reported by children and adolescents. *Child Development*, **60**, 1250–1260.

Larson, R.W., & Richards, M.H. (1994). Family emotions: do young adolescents and their parents experience the same states? *Journal of Research on Adolescence*, **4**, 567–583.

Larson, R.W., Raffaelli, M., Richards, M.H., Ham, M., & Jewell, L. (1990). Ecology of depression in late childhood and early adolescence: a profile of daily states and activities. *Journal of Abnormal Psychology*, **99**, 92–102.

Lewis, M., & Ramsey, D.S. (1999). Effect of maternal soothing on infant stress reactivity. *Child Development*, **70**(1), 11–20.

Martin, R.M., & Green, J.A. (2005). The use of emotion explanations by mothers: relation to preschoolers' gender and understanding of emotions. *Social Development*, **14**, 229–249.

Mayer, J.D., & Salovey, P. (1997). What is emotional intelligence? In P. Salovey & D. Sluyter (Eds.), *Emotional Development and Emotional Intelligence: Implications for Educators* (pp. 3–31). New York: Basic Books.

McDowell, D.J., & Parke, R.D. (2000). Differential knowledge of display rules for positive and negative emotions: influences from parents, influences on peers. *Social Development*, **9**, 415–432.

Minuchin, S. (1974). *Families and Family Therapy*. Cambridge, MA: Harvard University Press.

Minuchin, S., & Fishman, H.C. (1981). *Family Therapy Techniques*. Cambridge, MA: Harvard University Press.

Montemayor, R., Eberly, M., & Flannery, D.J. (1993). Effects of pubertal status and conversation topic on parent and adolescent affective expression. *Journal of Early Adolescence*, **13**, 431–447.

Papini, D.R., Farmer, F.F., Clark, S.M., Micka, J.C., & Barnett, J.K. (1990). Early adolescent age and gender differences in patterns of emotional disclosure to parents and friends. *Adolescence*, **15**, 959–1001.

Porges, S. W. (1995). Orienting in a defensive world: mammalian modifications of our evolutionary heritage: a Polyvagal theory. *Psychophysiology*, **32**, 301–318.

Ramsden, S. R., & Hubbard, J. A. (2002). Family expressiveness and parental emotion coaching: their role in children's emotion regulation and aggression. *Journal of Abnormal Child Psychology*, **30**, 657–667.

Rosenblum, G., & Lewis, M. (2003). Emotional development in adolescence. In G. Adams & M. Berzonsky (Eds.), *Blackwell Handbook on Adolescence* (pp. 269–289). Malden, MA: Blackwell Publishers.

Saarni, C. (1988). Children's understanding of the interpersonal consequences of dissemblance of nonverbal emotional-expressive behaviour. *Journal of Nonverbal Behavior*, **12**, 275–294.

Saarni, C. (1990). Emotional competence: how emotions and relationships become integrated. In R. A. Thompson (Ed.), *Socioemotional Development. Nebraska Symposium on Motivation* (pp. 115–182). Lincoln, NE: University of Nebraska Press.

Saarni, C. (1998). Issues of cultural meaningfulness in emotional development. *Developmental Psychology*, **34**, 647–652.

Saarni, C. (1999). *The Development of Emotional Competence.* New York: Guilford Press.

Sawyer, K. S., Denham, S., DeMulder, E. *et al.* (2002). The contribution of older siblings' reactions to emotions to preschoolers' emotional and social competence. *Marriage and Family Review*, **34**, 183–212.

Schulz, M. S., Waldinger, R. J., Hauser, S. T., & Allen, J. P. (2005). Adolescents' behavior in the presence of interparental hostility: developmental and emotion regulatory influences. *Development and Psychopathology*, **17**, 489–507.

Seiffge-Krenke, I. (1999). Families with daughters, families with sons: different challenges for family relationships and marital satisfaction? *Journal of Youth and Adolescence*, **28**, 325–342.

Shearer, C. L., Crouter, A. C., & McHale, S. M. (2005). Mothers' and fathers' perceptions of relationship change in parent-child relationships during adolescence. *Journal of Adolescent Research*, **20**, 662–684.

Sheeber, L., & Sorenson, E. (1998). Family relationships of depressed adolescents: a multimethod assessment. *Journal of Clinical Child Psychology*, **27**, 268–277.

Sheeber, L., Allen, N., Davis, B., & Sorensen, E. (2000). Regulation of negative affect during mother-child problem-solving interactions: adolescent depressive status and family processes. *Journal of Abnormal Child Psychology*, **28**, 467–479.

Smith, M., & Walden, T. (1998). Developmental trends in emotion understanding among a diverse sample of African-American preschool children. *Journal of Applied Developmental Psychology*, **19**, 177–197.

Spinrad, T., Stifter, C., Donelan-McCall, N., & Turner, L. (2004). Mothers' regulation strategies in response to toddlers' affect: links to later emotion self-regulation. *Social Development*, **13**, 40–55.

Steinberg, L. (1988). Reciprocal relations between parent-child distance and pubertal maturation. *Developmental Psychology*, **24**, 122–128.

Thompson, R. A. (1994). Emotion regulation: a theme in search of definition. *Monographs of the Society for Research in Child Development*, **59**(2–3), 25–52.

van Aken, M., & Dubas, J. S. (2004). Social cognition in adolescence: its developmental significance. *European Journal of Developmental Psychology*, **1**, 331–348.

Yang, Y., & Yeh, K. (2006). Differentiating the effects of enacted parental support on adolescent adjustment in Taiwan: moderating role of relationship intimacy. *Asian Journal of Social Psychology*, **9**, 161–166.

Zahn-Waxler, C., Friedman, R.J., Cole, P.M., Mizuta, I., & Hiruma, N. (1996). Japanese and United States preschool children's responses to conflict and distress. *Child Development*, **67**, 2462–2477.

Zeman, J., & Shipman, K. (1997). Social-contextual influences on expectancies for managing anger and sadness: the transition from middle childhood to adolescence. *Developmental Psychology*, **33**, 917–924.

Zimmermann, P. (1999). Structure and functioning of internal working models of attachment and their role for emotion regulation. *Attachment and Human Development*, **1**, 55–71.

Zimmermann, P., Maier, M.A., Winter, M., & Grossmann, K.E. (2001). Attachment and adolescents' emotion regulation during a joint problem-solving task with a friend. *International Journal of Behavioral Development*, **25**, 331–343.

15

Adolescent mood disorders and familial processes

Martha C. Tompson, James W. McKowen,
and Joan Rosenbaum Asarnow

Rates of depressive disorders increase markedly during adolescence. Epidemiological data indicate that prior to adolescence 1–3% of children suffer from major depressive disorder, and rates of dysthymic and minor depressive disorders are somewhat higher (Birmaher *et al.*, 1996; Fleming & Offord, 1990; McCracken, 1992). Prevalence of these disorders is markedly increased in pediatric settings and among youth referred for psychiatric treatment (McCracken, 1992). Roughly 20% of our nation's youth can be expected to have suffered from depressive episodes by age 18 (Lewinsohn *et al.*, 1993), highlighting the significance of this public health problem. Increasing attention has been paid to the problem of bipolar disorders in youth in recent years; current studies underscore the complexity of this diagnosis in adolescents; and debates continue about the validity of "narrow-spectrum" versus "broad-spectrum" diagnostic approaches (Carlson & Meyer, 2006). Available epidemiologic data suggest that fewer than 1% of adolescents experience bipolar disorders, which present most frequently as bipolar II disorder and cyclothymia (Seeley and Lewinsohn, see Chapter 3, this volume). The present chapter focuses on the family context in which youth mood disorders develop and are maintained. Our goals are threefold. First, we describe some contextual issues that impact our understanding of family processes in youth mood disorder. Second, we briefly review the literature on family processes in youth with depression and bipolar disorders and youth at risk due to parental mood disorder. Third, and finally, we relate these findings to a broader model of family processes in youth mood disorders and outline significant limitations in the existing literature.

Adolescent Emotional Development and the Emergence of Depressive Disorders, ed. Nicholas B. Allen and Lisa B. Sheeber. Published by Cambridge University Press. © Cambridge University Press 2009.

The context of youth depression

During adolescence youth face the challenge of moving from childhood to adulthood. A number of developmental shifts and tasks are characteristic of the adolescent years, including solidifying personal identity (Harter, 1999), becoming physically and sexually mature, increasing intimate relationships outside the family, and developing educational and occupational skills necessary for work and financial independence (Burt, 2002). These tasks of adolescence are negotiated upon the shifting ground of the developing self and evolving environment. One developmental shift is increased cognitive capacity. The adolescent is developing a greater ability to take others' perspectives, to use abstractions and higher order constructs in understanding the world, and to engage in increasingly complex reasoning both in intellectual and social matters (Kesek, Zelazo, and Lewis, see Chapter 8, this volume). A second developmental shift is from family as the primary unit of socialization to increased associations with peers, romantic partners, and the larger social world (Furman, McDunn, and Young, see Chapter 16, this volume). Despite this shift, families remain a vital source of support, and family relations are more powerfully associated with adolescent depressive symptoms than are peer relations (Barrera & Garrison-Jones, 1992; Gore et al., 1993; McFarlane et al., 1994).

Family relationships established at earlier time points can support the adolescent in negotiating the tasks of development or can contribute to the development of maladaptation. In the optimal scenario earlier attachment processes provide a secure base from which the adolescent can continue the development of emotion regulation strategies and solidify his or her identity. Conversely, negative parent–child relations may contribute to the development of either cognitive vulnerabilities, such as negative self-concept, or to significant deficits in the capacity for appropriate self-regulation. In the face of the inevitable stressors of adolescence, these vulnerabilities or deficits may "set the stage" for the manifestation of depressive symptoms or disorder.

The task of parenting adolescents involves balancing the sometimes competing goals of nurturing their growth while protecting them from the many dangers of this period. Despite the general good health of the adolescent period, adolescents are at increasing risk for motor vehicle accidents, homicide, and suicide (Irwin et al., 2002). The tripling of the death rate from the ages of 10–14 years (21.1/100 000) to 15–19 years (69.8/100 000) underscores the impact of these risks (Grunbaum et al., 2002). Most deaths during adolescence are due to preventable causes, including risky driving, substance use/abuse, and unsafe sexual practices (Irwin et al., 2002). Thus, parents must give the youth space to grow and yet provide protection, warmth, and guidance in navigating the dangers of this period.

In recent years the protection afforded to adolescents has been compromised by additional societal factors. First, increases in the numbers of single parents and working mothers has resulted in parents often experiencing competing demands and having fewer resources available for monitoring and spending time with their children (Irwin *et al.*, 2002). Second, support systems may be more taxed and provide fewer resources. For example, increasingly larger high-school class sizes may lead to decreases in both teacher–student interaction and monitoring of student behavior by school personnel (Irwin *et al.*, 2002). Overall, decreased family and societal resources may be available during a developmental period when rates of depression and high-risk behaviors increase.

In discussing family psychosocial factors and processes, one must determine the appropriate unit for analysis. Parental divorce (Aseltine, 1996; Siegel & Griffin, 1984) and associated family structures (Cuffe *et al.*, 2005), parental marital conflict (Jekielek, 1998), and parental psychopathology (for review see Goodman & Gotlib, 2002) all show associations with youth depression. These family risk variables bring with them a host of sequelae that provide numerous potential pathways for the development of youth depression. The present chapter focuses on the parent–child relationship and youth depression.

Review of data on family factors

In investigating the association between family processes and depression in youth two primary strategies have been undertaken – "bottom-up studies," in which the family environment is measured in depressed youth, and "top-down studies," in which the impact of parental depression on youth outcome is examined. We first examine the studies of youth with depression and then those studies of youth with depressed parents.

Depressed youth

In an early study of case records of severely depressed youth during their early childhood through pre-adolescent years, Poznanski & Zrull (1970) noted the association between depression and long-standing negative family relationships, including rejection, marital discord, physical punishment, and neglect. More recent literature with larger samples and more explicit diagnostic criteria suggests that families of depressed children report high levels of stress and negative life events (for review, see Hammen, 1997, 2002), low family cohesion (Cole & McPherson, 1993), high levels of coercion, control (Dadds *et al.*, 1992; Hops *et al.*, 1990), and conflict (Kashani *et al.*, 1988; Racusin & Kaslow, 1991) and low rates of positive reinforcement (Cole & Rehm, 1986). The direction of effects is not entirely clear. Recent research examining depressive symptoms in youth suggest that family difficulties may antedate and increase risk for symptom exacerbation (Sheeber *et al.*, 1997; Stice *et al.*, 2004). However, depressive symptoms may also contribute to parent–child conflict (Rudolph & Hammen, 1999).

The increased negativity and conflict in parent–child relationships are evident in studies of both pre-adolescents and adolescents. Diagnosed depressed pre-adolescent youth report higher levels of verbally aggressive conflicts with their mothers than do non-diagnosed youth, and conflict is significantly correlated with the severity of depression (Kashani *et al.*, 1988). Compared with the parents of anxious youth, parents of depressed pre- and early-adolescent youth paint a picture of excessive control over life choices and self-expression (Amanat & Butler, 1984).

High levels of Expressed Emotion (EE), defined as critical and/or emotionally overinvolved attitudes on the part of family members toward the child, may be a particularly important construct to investigate. High family EE predicts poorer outcome in a variety of psychiatric disorders in adults (for reviews, see Butzlaff & Hooley, 1998; Hooley & Gotlib, 2000; Miklowitz *et al.*, 1996), particularly among individuals with mood disorders (Butzlaff & Hooley, 1998). Two studies have examined parental EE as a predictor of the course of youth depression, and one has examined its association with course among adolescents with bipolar disorder. First, among pre- and early-adolescent youth hospitalized for major depression and/or dysthymia, high parental EE predicted increased risk of relapse and non-recovery in the year following hospital discharge (Asarnow *et al.*, 1993). Second, among adolescents referred for outpatient depression treatment, low parental EE was associated with higher social functioning and, among those without comorbid ADHD, lower persistence of depression at one-year follow-up (McCleary & Sanford, 2002). Finally, in an open trial of a family-based intervention for bipolar disorder, youth with high EE parents had higher symptom ratings (both mania and depression) across 3-, 6-, 9-, 12-, 18-, and 24-month follow-up points compared to youth with low EE parents (Miklowitz *et al.*, 2006). Overall, these early data suggest that parental EE may be associated with a more negative course among youth with mood disorders.

There is a growing literature using direct observation of youth and their parents discussing a topic of disagreement in the laboratory. As a whole, this literature suggests that families with a depressed child interact differently than families without a depressed child (Kaslow *et al.*, 1994). First, interactions between depressed youth and their parents are more negative and conflictual. Depressed pre and early-adolescents demonstrate depressed affect (Dadds *et al.*, 1992; Sanders *et al.*, 1992) and may be more guilt-inducing and blaming (Hamilton *et al.*, 1997) during interaction tasks. In turn, mothers of depressed youth may be more negative, and this negativity may increase with increases in child's depressive behavior (Dadds *et al.*, 1992); however, findings of parental negativity are not always evident (Hamilton *et al.*, 1997).

Second, parents of depressed youth provide less positive feedback than parents of non-depressed youth (Cole & Rehm, 1986). Third, limited available studies have examined the possibility that patterns of interaction within families of depressed youth may reinforce depressive behavior. For example, Sheeber and colleagues (Sheeber *et al.*, 1998) found that, compared with non-depressed peers, mothers of depressed adolescents increased facilitative behavior (happy/caring affect and approving/affirming statements) and fathers of depressed adolescents decreased aggressive behavior in response to adolescent depressive behavior during problem-solving discussions. However, using similar methods, Slesnick & Waldron (1997) found that depressive content on the part of non-depressed youth had a *greater* impact on suppressing parental aversive content than did depressive content on the part of depressed youth. Thus, support for the model in which depressive behavior is reinforced in ongoing family transactions is mixed, and further research is needed to clarify whether, and under what circumstances, depression may develop and be maintained within family interactions.

Careful attention needs to be paid to the possible role of gender in moderating the relationship between family interactions and youth depression. In a recent prospective study, Davis and colleagues (2000) examined family interaction patterns and their relationship to youth's depressive symptoms one year later. They found that girls who took on a peacemaking and caretaking role within their parents' relationship were at increased risk for depressive outcomes. Specifically, those girls who increased their facilitative behavior toward their mother following their father's depressive behavior toward the mother and those who suppressed anger toward their mother when the mother directed depressive behavior toward the father demonstrated significant increases in depressive symptoms from baseline to the one-year follow-up point. In contrast, boys who respond to mother's depressive behavior in an angry fashion seem to have a limited repertoire of coping skills for dealing with negative family transactions, and this limited repertoire may increase depression risk. Specifically those boys who are more likely to demonstrate aggressive behavior toward the mother after she directed depressive behavior toward the father showed significant increases in depression from baseline to the one-year follow-up. These findings underscore the importance of including gender as a variable when examining the association between depression and family roles and interactional behavior.

In addition to high conflict and negativity, low family cohesion, closeness and social support are associated with depression in youth. These findings appear in studies of both pre-adolescents and adolescents, and in studies using both cross-sectional and longitudinal designs. Among adolescents, depressive symptoms are inversely correlated cross-sectionally with perceptions of family cohesion (Friedich *et al.*, 1982) and social support and caring from family (Avison & McAlpine, 1992; Windle, 1992). However, some data suggest that these associations are primarily evident among girls rather than boys (Avison & McAlpine, 1992; Windle, 1992). These family relationship impairments appear to represent a relatively stable risk factor for depression (Hops *et al.*, 1990), to add to previous depressive symptoms in predicting current depressive symptoms (Garrison *et al.*, 1990), and, when persistent, may be associated with new onsets of depression over time (McFarlane *et al.*, 1994). Although mother–child relationships are the focus of most studies, father–child relationships may be equally important (Cole & McPherson, 1993), and there is a need for more research to examine their role. The degree to which low family cohesion and support may be specific to depression is not clear. Some studies have shown links between family cohesion and suicidality specifically (Asarnow *et al.*, 1987; Kandel *et al.*, 1991) and others to severity of psychopathology more generally (Barber & Buehler, 1996; Carbonell *et al.*, 1998; Prange, Greenbaum, & Silver, 1992).

Few data exist on family functioning among youth with bipolar disorders. Examining older adolescents' reports of family functioning, Robertson *et al.* (2001) compared adolescents with bipolar disorder to adolescents with major depressive disorder and adolescents with no psychiatric disorder. All mood-disordered individuals were stabilized on medications. Although adolescents with bipolar disorders reported significantly more minor hassles than adolescents in the other two groups, there were no other differences between groups. These findings underscore the need to examine the role of mood disorder type and phase in understanding the role of family factors.

Children of depressed parents

Studies estimate that children of depressed parents are 2–5 times more likely to develop any psychological disorder (Cummings & Davies, 1992) and three times more likely to develop depression than are children whose parents are not depressed (Downey & Coyne, 1990). Given the high rates of depression among women and the availability of mothers in research, most of the research on parental depression in families has focused on maternal depression (Hammen *et al.*, 1987) and underscores its strong association with child functioning across development. Infants with depressed mothers demonstrate higher levels of insecure attachment than do infants of non-depressed mothers (Cohn *et al.*, 1986; Field *et al.*, 2002; Larsen & O'Hara, 2002). Among young children, maternal depression and bipolar disorder are associated with increased behavior problems over time (Radke-Yarrow *et al.*, 1992). Five longitudinal studies in particular have included pre-adolescent and adolescent children of depressed parents, followed them to examine the stability of symptoms and functional outcomes, and used structured diagnostic assessments (Beardslee *et al.*, 1993; Billings & Moos, 1986; Hammen *et al.*, 1990; Lee & Gotlib, 1991; Wickramaratne & Weissman, 1998). These find that compared with children of non-depressed parents, those with depressed parents often show elevated levels of psychological symptoms (Lee & Gotlib, 1991), frequently experience academic difficulties (Weissman *et al.*, 1988), and have higher rates of diagnosis, recurrence, and chronicity of depression. Even remitted parental depression may be associated with poorer functioning (Billings & Moos, 1986) and more internalizing symptoms than no history of parental depression (Lee & Gotlib, 1991). Overall, findings from these studies underscore the risk conferred by parental depression and suggest that these difficulties do not necessarily subside with parental recovery from depression. However, the majority of methodologically sophisticated studies of parental depression have focused on hospital- and clinic-based populations that may not be representative of the larger population of depressed persons (Downey & Coyne, 1990; Goodman & Gotlib, 1999). Although some large studies of depression in community samples have been conducted or are underway (e.g. Hammen *et al.*, 2004), additional studies of parental depression ascertained in community samples are needed.

Parental bipolar disorder has been less thoroughly examined than parental unipolar depression as a risk factor for the development of psychopathology in youth. However, a review of high-risk studies examining children of bipolar parents noted high rates of psychopathology, particularly mood disorders (DelBello & Geller, 2001).

Although genetic and biological risk mechanisms may contribute to the association between parental and youth mood disorder, psychosocial factors in families may also be operative (Goodman & Gotlib, 2002). Parental depression and bipolar disorder are associated with a host of additional life stressors which may impact children's well-being, including divorce (Harlow *et al.*, 2002), marital conflict (Coyne *et al.*, 2002; Hoover & Fitzgerald, 1981; Whisman, 2001) and spousal psychopathology (Fendrich *et al.*, 1990; Merikangas & Spiker, 1982). Thus, parental depression may be an index of broader genetic and environmental risk. Work by Rudolph, Hammen and colleagues (Hammen, 1997; Rudolph *et al.*, 2000) supports the notion that the relationship between maternal depression and youth depression may be mediated by life stress and negative family relationships. Overall, this work underscores the need to understand the complex web of risk factors often accompanying parental depression.

The literature examining child and parent self-reports suggests that parental depression, whether measured diagnostically or dimensionally, is associated with more negative reports of family relationships. Depressed mothers report less cohesive and satisfying family relationships and higher family stress than do non-depressed mothers in families of both pre-adolescent (Henderson *et al.*, 2003; Stein *et al.*, 2000) and adolescent youth (Shiner & Marmorstein, 1998), and more symptomatic mothers report poorer family functioning (Kinsman & Wildman, 2001). More recent studies have attempted to evaluate the psychosocial pathways by which maternal depression may impact youth depression. Hammen and colleagues (2004) indicate that maternal depression may exert direct effects on parenting quality, including warmth, hostility, acceptance, and psychological control. In turn, the relationship between parenting quality and youth depression is partially mediated by youth social competence and youth interpersonal stress. As well, longitudinal research suggests that increased family adversity, experienced in families where mothers have high depressive symptoms, may also increase depressive symptoms in youth; thus far support for this hypothesis has emerged for adolescent girls but not for boys (Fergusson et al., 1995).

The data on parental bipolar disorder are more limited and equivocal. One small study found that youth with a bipolar parent reported lower cohesion and lower expressiveness than did youth with parents without psychiatric disorder (Romero et al., 2005), and another study reported lower cohesion and higher conflict than did the normative sample (Chang et al., 2001).

Expressed Emotion has only rarely been examined as a risk factor for either depression diagnosis or outcome among youth with depressed parents – only three studies appear in the literature. There are no studies of EE among parents with bipolar disorder. First, McCleary & Sanford (2002), in their study of depressed youth, found no association between parental mood disorder, either current or past, and parental EE status. Second, in a large cross-sectional study of at-risk children, Schwartz and colleagues (1990) found that although maternal EE and depression were associated, they made independent contributions to children's risk for depression, conduct disorder, and substance abuse. Third, examining mothers' expressed attitudes about their pre-adolescent children, Goodman and colleagues (1994) found that overall mothers with a history of depression used significantly more affectively charged negative descriptions and critical/hostile comments, and described more overinvolvement. Further, use of these statements was negatively associated with youths' ratings of global self-worth and self-perceptions of competence. Results of these limited studies of EE among depressed parents suggest that parental EE may increase the risk of youth mood disorder through decreases in youth self-esteem.

Observational studies suggest depressed parents are frequently less attentive to their children's emotional needs, and more critical, controlling, and negative in their communication patterns (Kaslow et al., 1994) than non-depressed parents. Studies conducted with infants, toddlers, preschoolers, school-aged youth, and adolescents converge. Depressed mothers have more negative interactions with their infants (Field et al., 2002; Zahn-Waxler et al., 1984); interactions with infants are, on average, characterized by less responsivity and poorer ability to sustain interactions (Cox et al., 1987). With their toddler and preschool-aged offspring, mothers with dysphoric symptoms show less joint attention (Goldsmith & Rogoff, 1997), and these children may be at a slightly increased risk for insecure attachment generally (van Ijzendoorn *et al.*, 1999) and more strongly increased risk for disorganized attachment specifically (Lyons-Ruth *et al.*, 2002). Among 8–16-year-old children, current parental mood is a significant predictor of negative remarks (Gordon *et al.*, 1989) during parent–child interactions; depressed mothers demonstrate greater proportions of negative, critical statements and overall negative communication than non-depressed mothers (Conrad & Hammen, 1989; Hamilton *et al.*, 1993). These negative behaviors – criticism, guilt-induction, and intrusiveness – are associated with more reciprocal child criticism (Hamilton *et al.*, 1993). Children of depressed mothers are more self-critical, and children's perceptions of maternal behaviors, as well as actual negative maternal behaviors toward the child, may be associated with a depressogenic attributional style (Jaenicke *et al.*, 1987). Furthermore, maternal criticism in an interaction task was significantly correlated with children's self-blame and self-criticisms. These findings underscore both the bidirectional negativity that can be associated with maternal depression and the risk to the developing child's sense of self. Further study is needed to clearly establish if maternal communication and interaction patterns predict child-onset depressions and/or depression vulnerability.

Among adolescents, several studies examining parent–child interaction suggest that consideration needs to be given to gender – both of the depressed parent and of the target child – in understanding the impact of parental depression. First, Jacob & Johnson (1997) found that while overall families with a depressed parent are less positive and congenial than families without a depressed parent, these differences were particularly pronounced when mothers, as opposed to fathers, were depressed. Furthermore, families with a daughter were more negative than families with a son. Second, Tarullo and colleagues (1994) found that mothers with depression were significantly less engaged with daughters than with sons. Third, Hops and colleagues (Hops *et al.*, 1990) found that older children showed increased dysphoric affect in families with a depressed mother, and adolescent girls showed the highest rates of happy affect when in normal families but the lowest rates of happy affect in depressed families. Overall, the studies of family interaction, both in youth with and without depressed parents suggest that adolescent girls may be more at risk for the occurrence of negative family transactions and more susceptible to the effect of these transactions in fueling depression; however, others have failed to find gender-specific effects.

Convergence of findings

At the same time as youth with depressed parents exhibit high rates of depressive disorders, parents of depressed youth are also likely to suffer from depression, relative to parents of controls with no mental illness (Klein *et al.*, 2001; Kovacs *et al.*, 1997; Mitchell *et al.*, 1989; Puig-Antich *et al.*, 1989; Todd *et al.*, 1993; Wickramaratne *et al.*, 2000; Williamson *et al.*, 1995), and in some instances when compared with parents of youth with other forms of psychiatric disorder (Harrington *et al.*, 1993; Klein *et al.*, 2001; Kovacs *et al.*, 1997). Indeed, Puig-Antich and colleagues (1985) found that one-half to two-thirds of parents of depressed children have diagnosable depression. Evidence of this convergence has led Coyne *et al.* (1994) to conclude "the apparent specificity of the association between depression in parents and depression in children, together with the high rates of depression in the parents of depressed children and in the children of depressed parents, suggest that these ostensibly separate literatures are based on the same families" (p. 45). Indeed, to date findings on family processes among depressed youth and youth with depressed parents yield similar conclusions.

Overall, studies of family relationships among depressed youth and youth with depressed parents support a bidirectional model. Negative parent–child relationships may be a risk factor for depression (McFarlane *et al.*, 1994; Schwartz *et al.*, 1990) and for the maintenance of symptoms in already depressed youth (Asarnow *et al.*, 1993; McCleary & Sanford, 2002). The family environment plays a particularly crucial role in providing children both feedback on their own characteristics and information about what they can anticipate from others in relationships. Depressed children and children at risk due to parental depression are likely to be exposed to criticism and other negative expressed emotions (Asarnow *et al.*, 1994, 2001; Goodman *et al.*, 1994). High levels of parental criticism and low levels of parental positive feedback and support could lead to internalization of a more negative self-concept, reduced sense of mastery, low expectations of social support, and subsequently, greater depression (Goodman *et al.*, 1994; Hammen *et al.*, 2004). Over time, these interactions form a family climate in which children are increasingly likely to internalize negative conceptions of relationships and, more generally, negative cognitions and expectations (Jaenicke *et al.*, 1987). This compromised self-concept and the propensity to generate negative cognitions represent vulnerability factors proximal to the youth, and may increase risk for the development of depressive symptoms, particularly in the face of the many stressors of the adolescent period. The adolescent in a distressed family environment may have more difficulty navigating the complicated developmental tasks of the adolescent period and developing a positive and effective sense of self.

With the onset of depression, youth may have increasingly negative, less effective interactions with family members. While depressive behavior may decrease parental negativity by reducing parental demands during specific interactions (Slesnick & Waldron, 1997), in the long term it can erode relationships and increase negativity. Youth with depression often present with irritable, as well as dysphoric, mood and may be negative and guilt inducing in their interactions with their parents (Hamilton *et al.*, 1993, 1997). This may increase the likelihood that parents will respond in kind and develop negative attitudes and interactional patterns. In turn, parental negativity and criticism increase the risk that the depression will linger, further fueling negative parent–child relationships. Thus, a negative interactional cycle may ensue, with negative moods and behavior worsening family interactional processes and dysfunctional interactional processes worsening mood and behavior.

Gender differences in the association between family relationships and depression are apparent in a number of studies. Girls may be more sensitive to the negative impact of conflictual and unsupportive family relationships due to the intensity of the mother–daughter relationship in particular (Youniss & Ketterlinus, 1987) and to societal demands that increasingly focus on their role in maintaining harmonious interpersonal relationships, particularly with family (Davies & Windle, 1997). Although boys may be less likely to develop depression in the face of negative family relationships, these difficult family environments may increase risk for the manifestation of other forms of psychopathology, including conduct and substance abuse problems (Hartung & Widiger, 1998). However, not all studies indicate significant gender differences (Sheeber *et al.*, 1997), and further work in this area is needed.

The current literature has a number of limitations. First, much of it has focused on depressive symptoms in youth. While important, it is not clearly understood how continuous symptom measures may relate to diagnoses. Future studies need to include both symptom measures and assessment of "caseness." Second, although the number of longitudinal investigations has increased, many of these prospective studies involve relatively short follow-up periods limiting our ability to examine the interrelations between family factors, youth self-concept, and depressive symptoms over time. Third, and relatedly, the direction of effects still needs clarification. Although family factors may impact risk of youth depression, youth depression, as well as parent depression, may also negatively impact family relationships. Fourth, many studies rely primarily on youth self-reports, thus providing a measure of youth perceptions of family relationships. Recent attempts to assess family processes using multiple methods and informants will improve our understanding of the relationship between youth depression and family processes. Fifth, the interaction between family factors and genetic vulnerability has yet to be clarified, and further investigations using more complex bio-psycho-social models are sorely needed. Sixth, few data exist to facilitate understanding of the association between family processes and bipolar disorders in youth. Seventh, it is not known whether and to what extent ethnic and cultural differences, as well as the effects of socioeconomic status may exert an impact. Studies need to be conducted that include large enough samples of ethnic minority youth to examine ethnic and cultural variables. Finally, the majority of youth with depressive disorders present with comorbid disorders and/or histories of other forms of mental health disorders. These comorbid disorders are also likely to influence and be influenced by family factors, and few studies have been large enough to adequately disentangle depression effects and effects of other specific forms of comorbid psychopathology.

Clinically, an enhanced understanding of family factors and their association with youth depression may lead to more effective intervention and prevention strategies. There is a general consensus that effective treatment of youth living in families requires some intervention and guidance for parents. The literature reviewed here suggests that this is particularly important in the treatment of depressed youth, as well as in depression prevention efforts. Most successful intervention trials for depressed children and adolescents have included some family component and a small number of studies suggest the promise of family treatments or other treatments augmented by family treatment for youth depression. However, the literature supporting efficacy of family-focused interventions is quite limited and some studies in adolescents raise questions regarding the benefits of a family-focused approach (for review, see Asarnow et al., 2005). The research reviewed above highlights the fact that youth depression is often associated with family stress and that depression in youth and parents often co-occur. As this literature becomes further developed, it may lead to more specific and individually tailored intervention strategies that are rooted in evaluation of the family environment and child and parent vulnerabilities and strengths. More comprehensive developmental models which incorporate biological factors and other individual, family, and social factors are needed. Research aimed at untangling the complex processes through which family factors influence child and adolescent depression, as well as development, will also enhance our understanding of normal development and risk.

REFERENCES

Amanat, E., & Butler, C. (1984). Oppressive behaviors in the families of depressed children. *Family Therapy*, **11**(1), 65–77.

Asarnow, J.R., Carlson, G.A., & Guthrie, D. (1987). Coping strategies, self-perceptions, hopelessness, and perceived family environments in depressed and suicidal children. *Journal of Consulting and Clinical Psychology*, **55**(3), 361–366.

Asarnow, J.R., Goldstein, M.J., Tompson, M.C., & Guthrie, D. (1993). One-year outcomes of depressive disorders in child psychiatric in-patients: evaluation of the prognostic power of a brief measure of expressed emotion. *Journal of Child Psychology and Psychiatry*, **34**(2), 129–137.

Asarnow, J.R., Tompson, M.C., & Hamilton, E.B. (1994). Family expressed emotion, childhood-onset depression, and childhood-onset schizophrenia spectrum disorders: is expressed emotion a nonspecific correlate of child psychopathology or a specific risk factor for depression? *Journal of Abnormal Child Psychology*, **22**(2), 129–146.

Asarnow, J.R., Tompson, M.C., & Woo, S. (2001). Is expressed emotion a specific risk factor for depression or a nonspecific correlate of psychopathology? *Journal of Abnormal Child Psychology*, **29**(6), 573–583.

Asarnow, J.R., Tompson, M.C., & Berk, M.S. (2005). Adolescent depression: family-focused treatment strategies. In W.M. Pinsof & J. Lebow (Eds.), *Family Psychology: The Art of the Science* (pp. 425–450). New York: Oxford University Press.

Aseltine, R.H.J. (1996). Pathways linking parental divorce with adolescent depression. *Journal of Health and Social Behavior*, **37**(2), 133–148.

Avison, W.R., & McAlpine, D.D. (1992). Gender differences in symptoms of depression among adolescents. *Journal of Health Social Behavior*, **33**(2), 77–96.

Barber, B.K., & Buehler, C. (1996). Family cohesion and enmeshment: different constructs, different effects. *Journal of Marriage and the Family*, **58**, 433–441.

Barrera, M., Jr., & Garrison-Jones, C. (1992). Family and peer social support as specific correlates of adolescent depressive symptoms. *Journal of Abnormal Child Psychology*, **20**(1), 1–16.

Beardslee, W.R., Keller, M.B., Lavori, P.W., Staley, J., & Sacks, N. (1993). The impact of parental affective disorder on depression in offspring: a longitudinal follow-up in a nonreferred sample. *Journal of the American Academy of Child and Adolescent Psychiatry*, **32**(4), 723–730.

Billings, A.G., & Moos, R.H. (1986). Children of parents with unipolar depression: a controlled 1-year follow-up. *Journal of Abnormal Child Psychology*, **14**(1), 149–166.

Birmaher, B., Ryan, N.D., Williamson, D.E. *et al.* (1996). Childhood and adolescent depression: a review of the past 10 years. Part I. *Journal of the American Academy of Child and Adolescent Psychiatry*, **35**(11), 1427–1439.

Burt, M.R. (2002). Reasons to invest in adolescents. *Journal of Adolescent Health*, **31**(6 Suppl.), 136–152.

Butzlaff, R.L., & Hooley, J.M. (1998). Expressed emotion and psychiatric relapse: a meta-analysis. *Archives of General Psychiatry*, **55**(6), 547–552.

Carbonell, D.M., Reinherz, H.Z., & Giaconia, R.M. (1998). Risk and resilience in late adolescents. *Child and Adolescent Social Work Journal*, **15**, 251–272.

Carlson, G.A., & Meyer, S.E. (2006). Phenomenology and diagnosis of bipolar disorder in children, adolescents, and adults: complexities and developmental issues. *Development and Psychopathology*, **18**(4), 939–970.

Chang, K.D., Blasey, C., Ketter, T.A., & Steiner, H. (2001). Family environment of children and adolescents with bipolar parents. *Bipolar Disorder*, **3**(2), 73–78.

Cohn, J.F., Matias, R., Tronick, E.Z., Connell, D., & Lyons-Ruth, K. (1986). Face-to-face interactions of depressed mothers and their infants. *New Directions for Child Development*, **34**, 31–45.

Cole, D.A., & Rehm, L.P. (1986). Family interaction patterns and childhood depression. *Journal of Abnormal Child Psychology*, **14**(2), 297–314.

Cole, D.A., & McPherson, A.E. (1993). Relation of family subsystems to adolescent depression: implementing a new family assessment strategy. *Journal of Family Psychology*, **7**(1), 119–133.

Conrad, M., & Hammen, C. (1989). Role of maternal depression in perceptions of child maladjustment. *Journal of Consulting and Clinical Psychology*, **57**(5), 663–667.

Cox, A.D., Puckering, C., Pound, A., & Mills, M. (1987). The impact of maternal depression in young children. *Journal of Child Psychology and Psychiatry*, **28**(6), 917–928.

Coyne, J.C., Schwoeri, L., & Downey, G. (1994). Depression, the marital relationship, and parenting: an interpersonal view. In G.P. Sholevar & L. Schwoeri (Eds.), *The Transmission of Depression in Families and Children: Assessment and Intervention*. Northvale, NJ: J. Aronson.

Coyne, J.C., Thompson, R., & Palmer, S.C. (2002). Marital quality, coping with conflict, marital complaints, and affection in couples with a depressed wife. *Journal of Family Psychology*, **16**(1), 26–37.

Cuffe, S.P., McKeown, R.E., Addy, C.L., & Garrison, C.Z. (2005). Family and psychosocial risk factors in a longitudinal epidemiological study of adolescents. *Journal of the American Academy of Child and Adolescent Psychiatry*, **44**(2), 121–129.

Cummings, M.E., & Davies, P.T. (1992). Parental depression, family functioning, and child adjustment: risk factors, processes, and pathways. In D. Cicchetti & S.L. Toth (Eds.), *Developmental Perspectives on Depression* (pp. 283–322). Rochester, NY: University of Rochester Press.

Dadds, M.R., Sanders, M.R., Morrison, M., & Rebgetz, M. (1992). Childhood depression and conduct disorder: II. An analysis of family interaction patterns in the home. *Journal of Abnormal Psychology*, **101**(3), 505–513.

Davies, P.T., & Windle, M. (1997). Gender-specific pathways between maternal depressive symptoms, family discord, and adolescent adjustment. *Developmental Psychology*, **33**(4), 657–668.

Davis, B., Sheeber, L., Hops, H., & Tildesley, E. (2000). Adolescent responses to depressive parental behaviors in problem-solving interactions: implications for depressive symptoms. *Journal of Abnormal Child Psychology*, **28**(5), 451–465.

DelBello, M.P., & Geller, B. (2001). Review of studies of child and adolescent offspring of bipolar parents. *Bipolar Disorder*, **3**(6), 325–334.

Downey, G., & Coyne, J.C. (1990). Children of depressed parents: an integrative review. *Psychology Bulletin*, **108**(1), 50–76.

Fendrich, M., Weissman, M.M., Warner, V., & Mufson, L. (1990). Two-year recall of lifetime diagnoses in offspring at high and low risk for major depression. The stability of offspring reports. *Archives of General Psychiatry*, **47**(12), 1121–1127.

Fergusson, D.M., Horwood, L.J., & Lynskey, M.T. (1995). Maternal depressive symptoms and depressive symptoms in adolescents. *Journal of Child Psychology and Psychiatry*, **36**(7), 1161–1178.

Field, T., Hernandez-Reif, M., & Feijo, L. (2002). Breastfeeding in depressed mother-infant dyads. *Early Child Development and Care*, **172**(6), 539–545.

Fleming, J.E., & Offord, D.R. (1990). Epidemiology of childhood depressive disorders: a critical review. *Journal of American Academy of Child and Adolescent Psychiatry*, **29**(4), 571–580.

Freidrich, W., Reams, R., & Jacobs, J. (1982). Depression and suicidal ideation in early adolescents. *Journal of Youth and Adolescence*, **11**(5), 403–407.

Garrison, C.Z., Jackson, K.L., & Marsteller, F. (1990). A longitudinal study of depressive symptomatology in young adolescents. *Journal of the American Academy of Child and Adolescent Psychiatry*, **29**(4), 581–585.

Goldsmith, D.F., & Rogoff, B. (1997). Mothers' and toddlers' coordinated joint focus of attention: variations with maternal dysphoric symptoms. *Developmental Psychology*, **33**(1), 113–119.

Goodman, S.H., & Gotlib, I.H. (1999). Risk for psychopathology in the children of depressed mothers: a developmental model for understanding mechanisms of transmission. *Psychology Review*, **106**(3), 458–490.

Goodman, S.H., & Gotlib, I.H. (2002). *Children of Depressed Parents: Mechanisms of Risk and Implications for Treatment*. Washington, DC: American Psychological Association.

Goodman, S.H., Adamson, L.B., Riniti, J., & Cole, S. (1994). Mothers' expressed attitudes: associations with maternal depression and children's self-esteem and psychopathology. *Journal of the American Academy of Child and Adolescent Psychiatry*, **33**(9), 1265–1274.

Gordon, D., Burge, D., Hammen, C. et al. (1989). Observations of interactions of depressed women with their children. *American Journal of Psychiatry*, **146**(1), 50–55.

Gore, S., Aseltine, R.H., & Colten, M.E. (1993). Gender, social-relational involvement, and depression. *Journal of Research on Adolescence*, **3**(2), 101–125.,

Grunbaum, J.A., Kann, L., Kinchen, S.L. et al. (2002). Youth risk behavior surveillance. *Morbidity and Mortality Weekly Report*, **51**, 1–64.

Hamilton, E.B., Jones, M., & Hammen, C. (1993). Maternal interaction style in affective disordered, physically ill, and normal women. *Family Process*, **32**(3), 329–340.

Hamilton, E.B., Asarnow, J.R., & Tompson, M.C. (1997). Social, academic, and behavioral competence of depressed children: relationship to diagnostic status and family interaction style. *Journal of Youth and Adolescence*, **26**(1), 77–87.

Hammen, C. (1997). Children of depressed parents: the stress context. In S.A. Wolchik & I.N. Sandler (Eds.), *Handbook of Children's Coping: Linking Theory and Intervention* (pp. 131–157). New York: Plenum Press.

Hammen, C. (2002). Context of stress in families of children with depressed parents. In S.H. Goodman & I.H. Gotlib (Eds.), *Children of Depressed Parents: Mechanisms of Risk and Implications for Treatment* (pp. 175–199). Washington, DC: American Psychological Association.

Hammen, C., Gordon, D., Burge, D. et al. (1987). Maternal affective disorders, illness, and stress: risk for children's psychopathology. *American Journal of Psychiatry*, **144**(6), 736–741.

Hammen, C., Burge, D., Burney, E., & Adrian, C. (1990). Longitudinal study of diagnoses in children of women with unipolar and bipolar affective disorder. *Archives of General Psychiatry*, **47**(12), 1112–1117.

Hammen, C., Shih, J.H., & Brennan, P.A. (2004). Intergenerational transmission of depression: test of an interpersonal stress model in a community sample. *Journal of Consulting and Clinical Psychology*, **72**(3), 511–522.

Harlow, B.L., Cohen, L.S., Otto, M.W. et al. (2002). Demographic, family, and occupational characteristics associated with major depression: the Harvard study of moods and cycles. *Acta Psychiatria Scandanavica*, **105**(3), 209–217.

Harrington, R.C., Fudge, H., Rutter, M.L. et al. (1993). Child and adult depression: a test of continuities with data from a family study. *British Journal of Psychiatry*, **162**, 627–633.

Harter, S. (1999). *The Construction of the Self: A Developmental Perspective*. New York, NY: Guilford Press.

Hartung, C.M., & Widiger, T.A. (1998). Gender differences in the diagnosis of mental disorders: conclusions and controversies of the DSM-IV. *Psychology Bulletin,* **123**(3), 260–278.

Henderson, A.D., Sayger, T.V., & Horne, A.M. (2003). Mothers and sons: a look at the relationship between child behavior problems, marital satisfaction, maternal depression, and family cohesion. *Family Journal: Counseling and Therapy for Couples and Families,* **11**(1), 33–34.

Hooley, J.M., & Gotlib, I.H. (2000). A diathesis-stress conceptualization of expressed emotion and clinical outcome. *Applied and Preventive Psychology,* **9**(3), 135–151.

Hoover, C.F., & Fitzgerald, R.G. (1981). Marital conflict of manic-depressive patients. *Archives of General Psychiatry,* **38**(1), 65–67.

Hops, H., Tildesley, E., Lichtenstein, E., Ary, D., & Sherman, L. (1990). Parent-adolescent problem-solving interactions and drug use. *American Journal of Drug and Alcohol Abuse,* **16**(3–4), 239–258.

Irwin, C.E., Jr., Burg, S.J., & Uhler Cart, C. (2002). America's adolescents: where have we been, where are we going? *Journal of Adolescent Health,* **31**(6 Suppl.), 91–121.

Jacob, T., & Johnson, S. (1997). Parenting influences on the development of alcohol abuse and dependence. *Alcohol Health Research World,* **21**(3), 204–209.

Jaenicke, C., Hammen, C., Zupan, B. et al. (1987). Cognitive vulnerability in children at risk for depression. *Journal of Abnormal Child Psychology,* **15**(4), 559–572.

Jekielek, S.M. (1998). Parental conflict, marital disruption and children's emotional well-being. *Social Forces,* **76**(3), 905–936.

Kandel, D.B., Raveis, V.H., & Davies, M. (1991). Suicidal ideation in adolescence: depression, substance use, and other risk factors. *Journal of Youth and Adolescence Special Issue: The Emergence of Depressive Symptoms during Adolescence,* **20**(2), 289–309.

Kashani, J.H., Burbach, D.J., & Rosenberg, T.K. (1988). Perception of family conflict resolution and depressive symptomatology in adolescents. *Journal of the American Academy of Child and Adolescent Psychiatry,* **27**(1), 42–48.

Kaslow, N.J., Deering, C.G., & Racusin, G.R. (1994). Depressed children and their families. *Clinical Psychology Review,* **14**(1), 39–59.

Kinsman, A.M., & Wildman, B.G. (2001). Mother and child perceptions of child functioning: relationship to maternal distress. *Family Process,* **40**(2), 163–172.

Klein, D.N., Lewinsohn, P.M., Seeley, J.R., & Rohde, P. (2001). A family study of major depressive disorder in a community sample of adolescents. *Archives of General Psychiatry,* **58**(1), 13–20.

Kovacs, M., Devlin, B., Pollock, M., Richards, C., & Mukerji, P. (1997). A controlled family history study of childhood-onset depressive disorder. *Archives of General Psychiatry,* **54**(7), 613–623.

Larsen, K.E., & O'Hara, M.W. (2002). The effects of postpartum depression on close relationships. In J.H. Harvey & A. Wenzel (Eds.), *A Clinician's Guide to Maintaining and Enhancing Close Relationships* (pp. 157–176). Mahwah, NJ: Lawrence Erlbaum Associates.

Lee, C.M., & Gotlib, I.H. (1991). Adjustment of children of depressed mothers: a 10-month follow-up. *Journal of Abnormal Psychology,* **100**(4), 473–477.

Lewinsohn, P.M., Rohde, P., Seeley, J.R., & Fischer, S.A. (1993). Age-cohort changes in the lifetime occurrence of depression and other mental disorders. *Journal of Abnormal Psychology,* **102**(1), 110–120.

Lyons-Ruth, K., Lyubchik, A., & Wolfe, R. (2002). Parental depression and child attachment: hostile and helpless profiles of parent and child behavior among families at risk. In S.H. Goodman & I.H. Gotlib (Eds.), *Children of Depressed Parents: Mechanisms of Risk and Implications for Treatment* (pp. 89–120). Washington, DC: American Psychological Association.

McCleary, L., & Sanford, M. (2002). Parental expressed emotion in depressed adolescents: prediction of clinical course and relationship to comorbid disorders and social functioning. *Journal of Child Psychology and Psychiatry,* **43**(5), 587–595.

McCracken, J.T. (1992). The epidemiology of child and adolescent mood disorders. *Child and Adolescent Psychiatric Clinics of North America,* **1**(1), 53–71.

McFarlane, A.H., Bellissimo, A., & Norman, G.R. (1994). Adolescent depression in a school-based community sample: preliminary findings on contributing social factors. *Journal of Youth and Adolescence,* **23**(6), 601–620.

Merikangas, K.R., & Spiker, D.G. (1982). Assortative mating among in-patients with primary affective disorder. *Psychology Medicine,* **12**(4), 753–764.

Miklowitz, D.J., Frank, E., & George, E.L. (1996). New psychosocial treatments for the outpatient management of bipolar disorder. *Psychopharmacology Bulletin,* **32**(4), 613–621.

Miklowitz, D.J., Biuckians, A., & Richards, J.A. (2006). Early-onset bipolar disorder: a family treatment perspective. *Development and Psychopathology,* **18**(4), 1247–1265.

Mitchell, J., McCauley, E., Burke, P., Calderon, R., & Schloredt, K. (1989). Psychopathology in parents of depressed children and adolescents. *Journal of the American Academy of Child and Adolescent Psychiatry,* **28**(3), 352–357.

Poznanski, E., & Zrull, J.P. (1970). Childhood depression. Clinical characteristics of overtly depressed children. *Archives of General Psychiatry,* **23**(1), 8–15.

Prange, M.E., Greenbaum, P.E., & Silver, S.E. (1992). Family functioning and psychopathology among adolescents with severe emotional disturbances. *Journal of Abnormal Child Psychology,* **20**(1), 83–102.

Puig-Antich, J., Lukens, E., Davies, M. *et al.* (1985). Psychosocial functioning in prepubertal major depressive disorders: I. Interpersonal relationships during the depressive episode. *Archives of General Psychiatry,* **42**(5), 500–507.

Puig-Antich, J., Goetz, D., Davies, M. *et al.* (1989). A controlled family history study of prepubertal major depressive disorder. *Archives of General Psychiatry,* **46**(5), 406–418.

Racusin, G.R., & Kaslow, N.J. (1991). Assessment and treatment of childhood depression. In P.A. Keller & L.G. Ritt (Eds.), *Innovations in Clinical Practice: A Source Book: Vol. 10* (pp. 223–243). Sarasota, FL: Professional Resource Exchange.

Radke-Yarrow, M., Nottelmann, E., Martinez, P., Fox, M.B., & Belmont, B. (1992). Young children of affectively ill parents: a longitudinal study of psychosocial development. *Journal of the American Academy of Child and Adolescent Psychiatry,* **31**, 68–77.

Robertson, H.A., Kutcher, S.P., Bird, D., & Grasswick, L. (2001). Impact of early onset bipolar disorder on family functioning: adolescents' perceptions of family dynamics, communication, and problems. *Journal of Affective Disorders,* **66**(1), 25–37.

Romero, S., Delbello, M.P., Soutullo, C.A., Stanford, K., & Strakowski, S.M. (2005). Family environment in families with versus families without parental bipolar disorder: a preliminary comparison study. *Bipolar Disorders*, **7**(6), 617–622.

Rudolph, K.D., & Hammen, C. (1999). Age and gender as determinants of stress exposure, generation, and reactions in youngsters: a transactional perspective. *Child Development*, **70**(3), 660–677.

Rudolph, K.D., Hammen, C., Burge, D. *et al.* (2000). Toward an interpersonal life-stress model of depression: the developmental context of stress generation. *Developmental Psychopathology*, **12**(2), 215–234.

Sanders, M.R., Dadds, M.R., Johnston, B.M., & Cash, R. (1992). Childhood depression and conduct disorder: I. Behavioral, affective, and cognitive aspects of family problem-solving interactions. *Journal of Abnormal Psychology*, **101**(3), 495–504.

Schwartz, C.E., Dorer, D.J., Beardslee, W.R., Lavori, P.W., & Keller, M.B. (1990). Maternal expressed emotion and parental affective disorder: risk for childhood depressive disorder, substance abuse, or conduct disorder. *Journal of Psychiatry Research*, **24**(3), 231–250.

Sheeber, L., & Sorensen, E. (1998). Family relationships of depressed adolescents: a multimethod assessment. *Journal of Clinical Child Psychology*, **27**(3), 268–277.

Sheeber, L., Hops, H., Andrews, J., Alpert, T., & Davis, B. (1998). Interactional processes in families with depressed and non-depressed adolescents: reinforcement of depressive behavior. *Behaviour Research and Therapy*, **36**(4), 417–427.

Sheeber, L.B., Hops, H., Alpert, A., Davis, B., & Andrews, J.A. (1997). Family support and conflict: prospective relations to adolescent depression. *Journal of Abnormal Child Psychology*, **25**, 333–344.

Shiner, R.L., & Marmorstein, N.R. (1998). Family environments of adolescents with lifetime depression: associations with maternal depression history. *Journal of the American Academy of Child and Adolescent Psychiatry*, **37**(11), 1152–1160.

Siegel, L.J., & Griffin, N.J. (1984). Correlates of depressive symptoms in adolescents. *Journal of Youth and Adolescence*, **13**(6), 475–498.

Slesnick, N., & Waldron, H.B. (1997). Interpersonal problem-solving interactions of depressed adolescents and their parents. *Journal of Family Psychology*, **11**(2), 234–245.

Stein, D., Williamson, D.E., Birmaher, B. *et al.* (2000). Parent-child bonding and family functioning in depressed children and children at high risk and low risk for future depression. *Journal of the American Academy of Child and Adolescent Psychiatry*, **39**(11), 1387–1395.

Stice, E., Ragan, J., & Randall, P. (2004). Prospective relations between social support and depression: differential direction of effects for parent and peer support? *Journal of Abnormal Psychology*, **113**(1), 155–159.

Tarullo, L.B., DeMulder, E.K., Martinez, P.E., & Radke-Yarrow, M. (1994). Dialogues with preadolescents and adolescents: mother–child interaction patterns in affectively ill and well dyads. *Journal of Abnormal Child Psychology*, **22**(1), 33–51.

Todd, R.D., Neuman, R., Geller, B., Fox, L.W., & Hickok, J. (1993). Genetic studies of affective disorders: should we be starting with childhood onset probands? *Journal of the American Academy of Child and Adolescent Psychiatry*, **32**(6), 1164–1171.

van Ijzendoorn, M.H., Schuengel, C., & Bakermans-Kranenburg, M.J. (1999). Disorganized attachment in early childhood: meta-analysis of precursors, concomitants, and sequelae. *Development and Psychopathology*, **11**(2), 225–249.

Weissman, M.M., Warner, V., & Wickramaratne, P. (1988). Early-onset major depression in parents and their children. *Journal of Affective Disorders*, **15**(3), 269–277.

Whisman, M.A. (2001). Marital adjustment and outcome following treatments for depression. *Journal of Consulting and Clinical Psychology*, **69**(1), 125–129.

Wickramaratne, P.J., & Weissman, M.M. (1998). Onset of psychopathology in offspring by developmental phase and parental depression. *Journal of the American Academy of Child and Adolescent Psychiatry*, **37**(9), 933–942.

Wickramaratne, P.J., Greenwald, S., & Weissman, M.M. (2000). Psychiatric disorders in the relatives of probands with prepubertal-onset or adolescent-onset major depression. *Journal of the American Academy of Child and Adolescent Psychiatry*, **39**(11), 1396–1405.

Williamson, D.E., Birmaher, B., Anderson, B.P., al-Shabbout, M., & Ryan, N.D. (1995). Stressful life events in depressed adolescents: the role of dependent events during the depressive episode. *Journal of the American Academy of Child and Adolescent Psychiatry*, **34**(5), 591–598.

Windle, M. (1992). Temperament and social support in adolescence: interrelations with depressive symptoms and delinquent behaviors. *Journal of Youth and Adolescence*, **21**(1), 1–21.

Youniss, J., & Ketterlinus, R.D. (1987). Communication and connectedness in mother- and father-adolescent relationships. *Journal of Youth and Adolescence*, **16**(3), 265–280.

Zahn-Waxler, C., Cummings, E.M., & Iannotti, R. (1984). Young offspring of depressed parents: a population at risk for affective problems. *New Directions for Child Development*, **26**, 81–105.

16

The role of peer and romantic relationships in adolescent affective development

Wyndol Furman, Christine McDunn, and Brennan J. Young

Before and after I was involved with Colin Sugarman, I heard a thousand times that a boy, or a man, can't make you happy, that you have to be happy on your own before you can be happy with another person. All I can say is, I wish it were true
(Sittenfeld, 2005, p. 419).

These sentiments of Lee, the protagonist in Curtis Sittenfeld's (2005) coming of age novel *Prep*, are not atypical of adolescent girls or boys. Boyfriends, girlfriends, friends, and other peers are central to the social and affective lives of adolescents. They are primary triggers and recipients of adolescents' affect. In this chapter we explore the normative links between adolescent peer relationships and affective experiences. Our chapter complements the one by La Greca, Davila, and Siegel (see Chapter 17, this volume) which focuses on the links between these processes and the emergence of depressive disorders. We begin with a discussion of general peer relations, and then consider sociometric status, peer groups, friendships, and romantic relationships in particular. We describe the nature of these relationships in adolescence, developmental changes within them, and their potential implications for affective development. Finally, we describe the limitations of our current knowledge and implications for subsequent research.

Consistent with Scherer (1984), we use the term *affect* to refer to valenced states in general, including emotions, emotional episodes, moods, dispositional states (e.g. hating), and traits (e.g. agreeableness). The existing literature on peer and romantic relationships typically does not differentiate among these facets of affect. Although much of the research has focused on depressed affect, we include research on other negative affects and positive affects when available. We also briefly discuss the small literature on the role of adolescent peers in the development of affect-regulation skills.

Adolescent Emotional Development and the Emergence of Depressive Disorders, ed. Nicholas B. Allen and Lisa B. Sheeber. Published by Cambridge University Press. © Cambridge University Press 2009.

Peer relationships

Early adolescence marks a shift in the importance of peer relationships. Interaction with family members decreases substantially; ninth graders spend time with family members half as often as fifth graders do (Larson & Richards, 1991). Similarly, ratings of support from mothers, fathers, and siblings decrease during adolescence, and the frequency of negative interactions with parents increases. In contrast, ratings of support from friends and romantic partners increase. In elementary school, parents are perceived as the most supportive; in junior high, friends and parents are comparable; in high school friends are the most supportive, followed by mothers and romantic partners (Furman & Buhrmester, 1992).

The changes in these patterns of interactions also are reflected in affective experiences. Overall, affective states become more negative in junior high than in late elementary school (Larson & Lampman-Petraitis, 1989). However, affective states with friends or peers are relatively more positive than those with family members, and they become increasingly more positive from elementary school to high school (Larson & Richards, 1991).

Although interactions with peers are generally characterized by positive affect, peers are also a frequent source of negative affect. In fact, negative affect generated by peer interactions increases from pre-adolescence to adolescence, and for girls such negative affect occurs more often with peers than family members in adolescence (Larson & Asmussen, 1991).

Peer relationships have several distinct features that may account for the affective experiences that are associated with them. Relationships with peers are relatively egalitarian in nature, whereas in relationships with adults, an imbalance exists in the distribution of power and knowledge. Peer relationships are also voluntary in nature, and can be initiated or terminated at the choice of either person. In contrast, most familial relationships are not voluntary, at least not until adulthood.

As a consequence of these features, peer relationships entail much more give and take than other relationships. They appear to provide opportunities for enhancing positive affective experiences, yet also opportunities for affect getting out of control (Larson, 1983). Peer interactions also provide chances for growth and self-knowledge as youth confront and master the strong affects of adolescence (Douvan & Adelson, 1966). Because of their similar developmental status, adolescent peers may also be in a better position than parents to understand the intensity and intricacies of each other's affective life.

The processes of establishing and maintaining peer relationships have significant implications for adolescent affective development. Adolescents need to learn how to be sensitive toward others' wishes and needs and be willing to negotiate areas of conflict in order to maintain a relationship that is mutually satisfactory.

Although peer relations are central in adolescence, spending a moderate amount of time alone is normative. In fact, the amount of time young adolescents spend alone increases 50% between fifth and seventh grade (Larson & Richards, 1991). Some time alone is associated with healthy psychosocial adjustment, but when excessive, it is associated with negative mood states and poor adjustment (Larson & Csikszentmihalyi, 1978). Approximately 10% of children and early adolescents report feeling very lonely (Kupersmidt *et al.*, 1999). Lonely adolescents are more depressed, report poorer quality relationships, and are less emotionally sensitive than their peers (Ernst & Cacioppo, 1999).

Sociometric status

Up to this point, we have described experiences with peers as if they were relatively uniform. Adolescents' social status in the broad network of peers, however, substantially influences their experiences, including their affective experiences. Measures of sociometric status typically identify five social groups: (a) popular – those who are liked by many and disliked by few, (b) neglected – those who are neither liked nor disliked, (c) controversial – those who are both widely liked and widely disliked by others, (d) rejected – those who are liked by few and disliked by many, and (e) average (Coie *et al.*, 1982).

Sociometric status has been associated with distinct behavioral profiles. Popular children, for example, skillfully initiate and maintain social interactions and demonstrate good understanding of social situations (Asher *et al.*, 1984). They respond to their peers with cooperation and sensitivity (Rubin *et al.*, 2006). As a result, popular children are often admired by their peers and are considered fun to hang out with, kind and trustworthy (Lease *et al.*, 2002; Rubin *et al.*, 2006). Thus, they elicit positive interactions, which may contribute to their confidence in affectively regulating themselves and having peers there to support them.

Neglected children tend to be ignored by their peers. These children are rarely named as friends but are not actively disliked (Bierman, 2004). Some investigators have found that neglected children are not very distinguishable from others (see Rubin *et al.*, 2006), but others have found them to be withdrawn, socially isolated, and struggling with social anxiety (Inderbitzen *et al.*, 1997). When coping with a stressful event, neglected adolescents are more likely to receive instrumental support from their peers than emotional support (Munsch & Kinchen, 1995), possibly reflecting a lack of depth and closeness in their peer relationships.

Controversial children are aggressive and disruptive and thus are prone to alienate their peers (Coie & Dodge, 1988). Nevertheless, these children have some redeeming qualities in the eyes of their peers. Controversial children show more pro-social behaviors than rejected children and show similar levels of cooperation, leadership, helpfulness, and social sensitivity as average and popular children (Coie & Dodge, 1988). Controversial children also have less social anxiety than rejected and neglected children (Inderbitzen *et al.*, 1997).

The majority of sociometric research has focused upon children who are rejected by their peers. Unlike the status of neglected children which tends to be transient (Bierman, 2004), peer rejection tends to persist throughout childhood and adolescence (Bukowski & Newcomb, 1984) and often results in negative psychosocial outcomes (see Bierman, 2004; Parker & Asher, 1987).

Peer rejection may occur as the result of several interpersonal difficulties. The most commonly identified characteristic of rejected children is aggression, including unregulated anger, frustration, disruptiveness, verbal acts, and physical aggression (Rubin *et al.*, 2006). Socially withdrawn behavior can also elicit peer rejection. Those who are sullen and reticent to engage peers are often rejected (Deater-Deckard, 2001). Social withdrawal becomes an increasingly common source of rejection during middle childhood and adolescence (Ladd, 1999).

Finally, although a distinct construct, peer victimization is consistently related to peer rejection (Deater-Deckard, 2001). Children who are socially withdrawn and peer-rejected become easy targets of physical and relational/social aggression (Rubin *et al.*, 2006). In turn, victimization has been shown to predict increases in internalizing symptoms such as depression and social anxiety (Hodges & Perry, 1999; La Greca & Harrison, 2005). Similarly, children who are aggressive and peer-rejected are often themselves victims of aggression. The disruptive and irritating behavior of aggressive-rejected children can provoke retaliatory behavior from peers (Rubin *et al.*, 2006).

Perceived popularity

Recently, researchers have recognized the importance of distinguishing between sociometric popularity and perceived popularity in adolescence. Whereas sociometric popularity represents how well-liked an adolescent is among peers, perceived popularity serves as an index of social reputation and salience (Cillessen & Mayeux, 2004). Sociometric popularity is assessed by nominations of who adolescents actually like, whereas perceived popularity is assessed by having them identify the popular students in their grade. Perceived popularity is only moderately associated with being well-liked by peers, especially in adolescence (LaFontana & Cillessen, 1999). It is, however, associated with being attractive, athletic, having desirable possessions, and being accepted by others who are perceived as popular (Rose *et al.*, 2004). Moreover, the connection between sociometric status and aggression becomes more complex in adolescence. Overt and relational aggression are negatively related to sociometric status and perceived popularity among elementary school children (Cillessen & Mayeux, 2004; Rose *et al.*, 2004). Relational aggression continues to be negatively related to sociometric popularity in middle school, but it is *positively* related to perceived popularity. For those adolescents who are perceived to be popular, indirect and relational aggression may be a means to obtain – and to maintain – their status. These individuals are socially sophisticated and dominant, often arriving at their position at the expense of lower status peers (Farmer *et al.*, 2003). Nevertheless, they are not necessarily well-liked (Parkhurst & Hopmeyer, 1998). As yet, little is known about the affective experiences of children with perceived popularity, but the links with relational aggression suggest a different picture will emerge from that of sociometric popularity.

Peer groups

Cliques

Cliques also become more common and more established in early adolescence (Gavin & Furman, 1989). Approximately half of adolescents are members of a clique, although a significant number are not connected to any specific clique or are liaisons between cliques. Cliques are relatively stable over the course of a given school year, and members tend to be homogenous both in terms of demographic characteristics and personal attributes (Ennett & Bauman, 1996).

These small groups of friends provide regular social interactions, which are primarily positive in nature (Gavin & Furman, 1989). Such positive interactions peak during early and middle adolescence, when group membership is most valued (Gavin & Furman, 1989). Small group interactions may contribute to the development of affect regulation as friends interpret experiences and influence behaviors by discussing their own ideas concerning how to act, feel, and express affect (Simon *et al.*, 1992). Group expectations concerning social norms may be communicated and clarified through the use of humor or gossip about others. In effect, affective socialization becomes a negotiated process as adolescents discuss alternative ways of handling situations.

Antagonistic interactions within cliques also occur and, in fact, peak in early and middle adolescence; group conformity is emphasized the most during this time (Gavin & Furman, 1989). Moreover, a clear status hierarchy exists within cliques; those with higher status determine membership and find ways to tease and control the lower status members, thus reinforcing their place in the hierarchy (Eder, 1985).

Antagonistic interactions with peers who are not part of the clique are equally commonplace and increase from pre-adolescence through late adolescence. Although boys engage in more negative interactions with those outside of their cliques, girls are more troubled by such interactions (Gavin & Furman, 1989).

Interestingly, we know relatively little about the effects of clique membership or clique dynamics on affective or psycho-social adjustment, as most investigators have either examined the role of dyadic friendships or peer-group status. The descriptive information on cliques, however, suggests that these social groups are a major context for affective experiences and potentially contribute to adjustment problems, such as depression.

Mixed-gender groups

Another significant change in early adolescence is the formation of mixed-gender groups. During childhood, most children interact primarily with friends and peers of the same gender (Maccoby, 1990). A distinct shift in peer relations occurs during early adolescence as interest in, and interactions with, other-gender peers increase. Initially, early adolescents spend time thinking about members of the other gender, and it is not until later that they actually begin to spend much time with them (Richards *et al.*, 1998). Typically, these interactions begin when same-gender friend groups start to "hang out" with groups of other-gender peers (Connolly *et al.*, 2004). As adolescents get older, partying on weekend nights with several other-gender peers or a romantic partner is increasingly associated with positive affect, whereas being alone on the weekend nights is associated with loneliness (Larson & Richards, 1998).

Through the course of childhood, girls and boys develop somewhat different ways of structuring relationships and expressing and regulating affect (Maccoby, 1990). The different styles of boys and girls can clash, and the two genders must find ways to accommodate each other. Such accommodations may be particularly difficult for girls, who have been used to facilitative reactions to their partners and may feel less powerful in their interactions with boys. Girls' cooperative style is likely to lead to demoralizing experiences with boys, which may contribute to the marked increase in depression in girls in early adolescence. Additionally, girls are taught to value relationships more than boys (Block, 1983). The imbalance in relationship importance between genders may result in girls having a relatively greater preoccupation with relationships, particularly romantic ones, and perhaps becoming more vulnerable to negative experiences that occur within relationships (Gilligan, 1996).

Crowds

A final developmental change associated with adolescence is the emergence of crowds. Crowds are reputation-based labels given to individuals with similar perceived stereotypical behaviors, attitudes, and personality (Brown, 1990; Brown *et al.*, 1994). Although different crowds may exist, some types are found in most American high schools: "populars," "jocks," "brains," "druggies," and "loners" (Brown, 1999). One's crowd label affects how peers expect an adolescent to behave, and influences overall status among peers. Although crowd membership is based on reputation and not interactions per se, they do channel adolescents' interactions, and friends are often in the same crowd (Brown *et al.*, 1994). Crowds also provide a means of bolstering one's identity, as the attributes and members of one's own crowd are looked at favorably and other crowds may be denigrated. Crowd membership is also associated with affective experiences; those in high-status crowds are less depressed, anxious, and lonely and display decreases in these internalizing symptoms over time (La Greca & Harrison, 2005; Prinstein & La Greca, 2002).

Friendships

Friendships are defined as voluntary dyadic relationships in which both members have positive affective feelings toward the other. Most are with peers of the same sex, although other-sex friendships become increasingly salient in adolescence as well.

Friendships first emerge much earlier in life, but undergo significant developmental changes during pre-adolescence with the emergence of chumships (Sullivan, 1953). A chumship is a collaborative relationship, in which each person adjusts his or her behavior in order to meet the needs of the other so as to attain satisfying and shared outcomes. Such relationships are based on extensive self-disclosure and consensual validation of personal worth. The need for such intimate exchange is thought to be motivated by the desire to experience love and avoid loneliness (Buhrmester & Furman, 1986). During pre-adolescence the focus of chumships or friendships often centers on shared activities, with a child's best friend typically being the person with whom he or she spends the most time. Consistent activity with the same person indirectly promotes interpersonal sensitivity and provides validation of each individual's self-worth (Sullivan, 1953).

A primary component of chumships and adolescent friendships is intimate self-disclosure. Theoretically, pre-adolescents begin to express thoughts and affect within their friendships as they recognize and value the intimacy, trust, mutual support, and loyalty that can be found within these close relationships (Youniss & Volpe, 1978). Such affective expressions increase further in adolescence. Intimate disclosures are associated with feeling less lonely (Franzoi & Davis, 1985). Moreover, supportive interactions with friends are associated with lower feelings of social anxiety (La Greca & Harrison, 2005).

Adolescents may actively recruit or engage their friends to boost arousal or to cheer them up. Sometimes friends repeatedly discuss the problems they are experiencing (Rose, 2002). Such co-rumination often entails mutually encouraging each other to discuss problems, speculating about problems, and focusing on the negative feelings of problems. Co-rumination increases from childhood to adolescence with girls being more likely to co-ruminate with their friends than boys. Although co-rumination is associated with closeness in adolescent friendships, it is also associated with internalizing symptoms. As such, co-rumination may provide an account for why adolescent girls have closer friendships than boys (Furman & Buhrmester, 1992), yet more internalizing symptoms as well.

Approximately one-third of adolescent boys report that their friendships are characterized by an absence of support (Youniss & Smollar, 1985). The consequences of such relationships have not received much attention to date.

Conflict is common in adolescent friendships and is not, by itself, related to relationship quality (Laursen, 1993, 1995). Important, however, is the manner in which conflict is resolved (Perry *et al.*, 1992). Unbridled affective expression, power assertion, and third-party mediation result in disengagement and poorer quality friendships (Shulman & Laursen, 2002).

Though disagreements still occur, open conflict among late adolescents becomes less common (Collins & Steinberg, 2006). This decrease may be due to increased awareness of the negative impact conflict may have on relationships and to increased skill in conflict resolution. In healthy, late adolescent relationships, conflict resolution often involves compromise and presents an opportunity for adolescents to adjust their expectancies within a particular relationship (Collins & Steinberg, 2006). Such resolution often leads to increased intimacy and understanding.

Although friendships do end because of conflicts or friendship violations, they more typically end less dramatically due to diverging interests or friends moving away. In any case, the dissolution of friendships is frequently associated with depression, loneliness, physiological dysregulation, guilt, and anger (Laursen *et al.*, 1996; Parker & Seal, 1996).

Romantic relationships

Of course, one of the most noteworthy features of adolescence is the emergence of romantic relationships. Surprisingly, relatively little research had been done on this topic until recently (see Brown *et al.*, 1999), and most of the work to date has focused on heterosexual relationships. In this section, we principally describe heterosexual relationships, but discuss gay and lesbian relationships when research is available.

As noted in the prior section, interest in and interactions with other-gender peers increases during early adolescence. Initially, adolescents simply spend time thinking about the other gender and then increasingly interact with them. These interactions first occur in mixed-gender groups (Connolly *et al.*, 2004); then dating begins, often in the company of other peers. Today such dating is much less formal or planned than in the past, but it still has the feature of romantic or sexual interest. Finally, adolescents begin to form dyadic romantic relationships, especially as they reach middle adolescence. These relationships also increase in their typical length over the course of adolescence (Carver *et al.*, 2003) and become more intense and central over time, as interdependence and closeness between romantic partners increases with age (Furman & Buhrmester, 1992; Laursen & Williams, 1997).

We know less about the developmental course of romantic experiences for gay and lesbian youth. On average, self-labeling as a sexual minority occurs at an average age of 16 for boys and 17½ for girls (Savin-Williams & Diamond, 2000). In the past, few sexual minority youth had romantic relationships with same-gender peers during adolescence because of the limited opportunities to do so (Sears, 1991), but the opportunities appear to be increasing in some locations, especially with the increase in internet dating. Importantly, sexual attraction, sexual behavior, and sexual identity are not as closely related to one another as traditionally thought (Savin-Williams, 2006). Many gay and lesbian youth report that they had dated and had sexual experiences with other-gender peers during adolescence (Russell & Consolacion, 2003). Lesbians particularly report a high degree of fluidity in their sexual behavior and identity (Diamond, 2000). Experiences with the other sex may help clarify sexual orientation for gay, lesbian, and bisexual youths and can provide a cover for their sexual identity (Diamond *et al.*, 1999). Conversely, some youth who identify as heterosexual may be attracted to or engage in sexual behavior with same sex peers.

For both homosexual and heterosexual youth, romantic experiences can be highly rewarding. Adolescents commonly report that romantic partners provide support, companionship, and intimacy (Feiring, 1996; Hand & Furman, in press), and they become increasingly supportive over the course of adolescence. By middle adolescence, the degree of support is comparable to relationships with mothers and second only to friends (Furman & Buhrmester, 1992). In late adolescence, romantic relationships are the most supportive relationship for boys and are among the most supportive relationships for girls. Members of the other gender are also the most common source of strong positive affect for heterosexual adolescents (Wilson-Shockley, 1985 cited in Larson *et al.*, 1999), and presumably same-gender peers are the most common source of strong positive affect for sexual minorities. Such positive affect can have beneficial effects on thinking and judgment, but can also cloud judgments, such as decision-making about sexual behavior (Larson *et al.*, 1999).

At the same time, other-gender peers are also the most common source of strong negative affect for heterosexual adolescents (Wilson-Shockley, 1985 cited in Larson *et al.*, 1999), although we do not yet know who is the most common source of strong negative emotions for sexual minorities. Adolescents also have more negative interactions with romantic partners than with close friends (Kuttler & La Greca, 2004), and the frequency of such negative interactions is linked to social anxiety (La Greca & Harrison, 2005). Disappointments in such relationships can be associated with negative affect (Larson & Asmussen, 1991); for example, a lack of intimacy is associated with a cognitive vulnerability to depression in girls (Williams *et al.*, 2001).

In effect, romantic experiences are a primary source of both positive and negative experiences, and as such are an emotional cauldron for adolescents. Not surprisingly, adolescents experience more frequent mood swings than adults, and such mood swings are associated with having a romantic partner, thinking about romantic relationships, and thinking about their appearance (Larson *et al.*, 1980). Because romantic experiences are both central and new in adolescents' social worlds, they provide a series of challenging experiences that are affectively-laden.

For example, there is the issue of finding a romantic partner. Most adolescents would like to be romantically interested in someone and have someone interested in them. Unreciprocated love is thought to be a significant source of negative affect (Larson & Asmussen, 1991; Seiffge-Krenke, 1995). A lack of interest may be particularly disappointing to early adolescent girls, many of whom expect to be in love all the time (Simon *et al.*, 1992). Certainly, romantic relationships are a key topic of conversation among most adolescents (Eder, 1993; Thompson, 1994). Not having a romantic interest makes it more difficult to participate in the ongoing peer exchanges and could be detrimental to their status in the group, especially in early and middle adolescence (Brown, 1999). If they rarely or never have a romantic interest, their peers may make negative attributions about why they do not, and they themselves may be affectively troubled by not having such an interest.

Interestingly, we know relatively little about the experiences and adjustment of non-daters except by comparison to the experiences and adjustment of daters, and that picture is mixed. As noted previously, romantic relationships are a source of both positive and negative affect and interactions. Moreover, romantic experiences are associated with facets of social competence (Furman *et al.*, 2007; Neeman *et al.*, 1995) and are thought to contribute to psychosocial development and adjustment (see Furman & Shaffer, 2003). At the same time, romantic involvement, especially in early adolescence, is associated with poor academic performance, externalizing and internalizing symptoms, and substance use (see Furman *et al.*, 2007; Neeman *et al.*, 1995). Non-normative behavior seems more associated with adverse outcomes. For example, relatively early romantic involvement with boys by girls is associated with depressive symptoms, but platonic involvement with boys is not (Compian *et al.*, 2004).

As yet, only limited information is available concerning the extent to which these findings regarding adjustment and romantic experiences reflect the effects of romantic experiences per se or differences in those who are and are not romantically involved at different ages. The mixture of positive and negative correlates can be understood, however, by recognizing that the emergence of romantic experiences is a developmental task undertaken in the peer social world. Accordingly, romantic experiences would be expected to be associated with social competence, but also associated with the risky behaviors that occur in peer contexts.

Of course, not only is the presence or absence of romantic involvement important, but the identity of the romantic partner also has significant affective consequences. Adolescent romantic relationships tend to be closely supervised by mixed-gender groups, especially in early adolescence (Brown, 1999). Dating a particularly popular person could improve one's status in the peer network (Brown, 1999). Conversely, disapproval of a new partner by peers may also lead to a decrease in one's status and potentially negative affective consequences. Additionally, girls' early dating partners are frequently older boys, who may be more likely to exploit young adolescents, which often leads to adverse affective consequences (Pawlby et al., 1997).

Sexual minorities face particular challenges. They have relatively fewer role models than heterosexual youth to emulate and fewer partners with whom to develop relationships. Moreover, they are frequently teased, harassed, or ostracized by heterosexual peers because of their sexual preferences. Sexual minority adolescent males have fewer friends, and sexual minority adolescents tend to lose more friends (Diamond, 2004). Sometimes they develop passionate same-gender friendships – intense yet avowedly non-sexual relationships – which may serve purposes similar to romantic relationships of heterosexual youth (Diamond et al., 1999). Sexual minorities report higher levels of negative affect than heterosexual youth (Diamond, 2004). These differences in affect are mediated by greater fears of not finding a desired type of romantic relationship, perceived lack of control in romantic relationships, the loss of friends, and greater fears of losing friends.

Romantic relationships also entail some severe risks. More than 25% of adolescents are victims of dating violence or aggression (see Wolfe & Feiring, 2000) and estimates of sexual victimization range from 14–43% of girls and 0.3–36% for boys (Hickman et al., 2004). Dating violence is associated with anxiety, depression, suicidal ideation, and posttraumatic stress symptoms (Callahan et al., 2003; Holt & Espelage, 2005; Howard & Wang, 2003).

Finally, one common romantic experience that elicits strong, negative affect is a romantic breakup (Larson et al., 1999). Although adolescent romantic relationships begin and end frequently, making such breakups a normative experience, not all adolescents are able to effectively cope with this type of loss. In fact, romantic dissolution is one of the strongest predictors of adolescent depression and suicide attempts (Monroe et al., 1999). As yet, we know relatively little about why some adolescent breakups have major effects and other ones do not. However, the literature on adult romantic dissolution suggests that factors such as gender, the quality and investment in the relationship, and the manner in which a break-up occurs may be influential (Frazier & Cook, 1993; Simpson, 1987). In any case, as these descriptions indicate, romantic experiences are associated with significant affective experiences from the beginning stages of initiation through the end of a relationship.

Peer and romantic relationships, affect, and affect regulation

It seems safe to say that peer and romantic relationships are related to affective experiences and affect regulation. However, the specific nature of these links and the theoretical models accounting for these relationships are yet to be delineated. In effect, much of the literature consists of demonstrations that some facet of peer relations is associated with some aspect of affective experience. Such work has all the intrinsic limitations of correlational research, including several ones particularly relevant to this topic.

First, although we have talked about sociometric status, crowds, friendships, and romantic relationships in separate sections, they are intrinsically related. For example, popular children are more likely to have friends (Franzoi et al., 1994), be part of a high-status crowd (La Greca et al., 2001), and enter romantic relationships (Franzoi et al., 1994). Conversely, rejected children are more likely to be friendless (Zettergren, 2005) or victimized (Deater-Deckard, 2001). Moreover, experiences in one type of relationship affect the other relationships. For example, 52% of girls and 32% of boys report having felt excluded by a friend because of the friend's romantic involvement (Roth & Parker, 2001). Finally, one aspect of peer relations may moderate the impact of another aspect of peer relations. For example, having friends buffers a child from the negative effects of being victimized (Hodges et al., 1997). Similarly, the negative aspects of early romantic involvement may be limited to those adolescents who are not well accepted by their peers (Brendgen et al., 2002). In a similar vein, it is often not clear if the links are specific to a particular aspect of adjustment or maladjustment, such as depression, or if the links may be more general. Moreover, research with adolescents has focused more on affective experiences than affect regulation. Happily, more recent studies have begun to examine the role of multiple facets of peer relations or multiple aspects of affective experiences or adjustment simultaneously (La Greca & Harrison, 2005). As yet, however, relatively little work exists on affect regulation (vs. affective experiences).

Second, the organization of this chapter would seem to suggest that peer relations affect experiences, but such inferences cannot be drawn from correlational and cross-sectional studies. In fact, relatively few studies have examined such links longitudinally, but existing work suggests the links may be reciprocal in nature (Vernberg, 1990). Longitudinal examinations will also help determine the effects of relationship experiences at different developmental periods. For example, most studies have examined contemporary peer experiences, but peer relations prior to adolescence may be at least as important, especially as many facets of peer relations are at least moderately stable (see Rubin *et al.*, 2006).

Third, research needs to directly examine the processes that may lead to depression or have other affective consequences and not just examine the affective experiences associated with individual differences in early adolescents' peer relations. For example, research has shown that adolescents who are romantically involved are more likely to be depressed (Joyner & Udry, 2000). Yet, more detailed analyses suggest that it is romantic breakups that account for the association of depression with romantic involvement; similarly, having friendships may reduce feelings of loneliness, but specific processes in friendship such as co-rumination may contribute to the emergence or maintenance of depressive symptoms (Rose, 2002).

In a related vein, existing work has primarily examined the links between affective experiences and relatively stable, general characteristics of a person, such as sociometric status or quality of relationships. Larson and colleagues are among the few investigators to examine links between adolescents' moods in different interactional contexts using electronic pagers (Larson & Richards, 1991). It is important to complement existing work with molecular work examining such links in ongoing interactions. For example, it would be important to examine how adolescents react to specific acts of disclosure or rejection.

In sum, the particular pathways between relationships and affective experiences are not well delineated yet, but the salience of peer and romantic relationships in adolescence suggests that they are likely to be implicated in the emergence of affective disorders, such as depression. It is hoped that this chapter can stimulate further work leading to a greater understanding of these pathways and the roles that peer and romantic relationships play.

REFERENCES

Asher, S. R., Hymel, S., & Renshaw, P. D. (1984). Loneliness in children. *Child Development*, **55**, 1456–1464.

Bierman, K. L. (2004). *Peer Rejection*. New York, NY: Guilford Press.

Block, J. H. (1983). Differential premises arising from differential socialization of the sexes: some conjectures. *Child Development*, **54**, 1335–1354.

Brendgen, M., Vitaro, F., Doyle, A. B., Markiewicz, D., & Bukowski, W. M. (2002). Same-sex peer relations and romantic relationships during early adolescence: interactive links to emotional, behavioral, and academic adjustment. *Merrill-Palmer Quarterly*, **48**, 77–103.

Brown, B.B. (1990). Peer groups and peer cultures. In S.S. Feldman & G.R. Elliot (Eds.), *At the Threshold: The Developing Adolescent* (pp. 171–196). Cambridge, MA: Harvard University.

Brown, B.B. (1999). "You're going out with who?": Peer group influences on adolescent romantic relationships. In W. Furman, B.B. Brown, & C. Feiring (Eds.), *The Development of Romantic Relationships in Adolescence* (pp. 291–329). Cambridge, UK: Cambridge University Press.

Brown, B.B., Mory, M.S., & Kinney, D. (1994). Casting adolescent crowds in a relational perspective: caricature, channel, and context. In R. Montemayor, G.R. Adams, & G.P. Gullota (Eds.), *Advances in Adolescent Development, Volume 6: Relationships During Adolescence* (pp. 123–167). Thousand Oaks, CA: Sage.

Brown, B.B., Feiring, C., & Furman, W. (1999). Missing the love boat: why researchers have shied away from adolescent romance. In W. Furman, B.B. Brown, & C. Feiring (Eds.), *The Development of Romantic Relationships in Adolescence* (pp. 1–18). New York, NY: Cambridge University Press.

Buhrmester, D., & Furman, W. (1986). The changing functions of friends in childhood. A neo-Sullivan perspective. In V.J. Derlega & B.A. Winstead (Eds.), *Friendship and Social Interaction* (pp. 41–62). New York, NY: Springer-Verlag.

Bukowski, W.M., & Newcomb, A.F. (1984). A longitudinal study of the utility of social preference and social impact sociometric classification schemes. *Developmental Psychology*, **20**, 941–952.

Callahan, M.R., Tolman, R.M., & Saunders, D.G. (2003). Adolescent dating violence victimization and psychological well-being. *Journal of Adolescent Research*, **18**, 664–681.

Carver, K., Joyner, K., & Udry, J.R. (2003). National estimates of adolescent romantic relationships. In P. Florsheim (Ed.), *Adolescent Romantic Relationships and Sexual Behavior: Theory, Research, and Practical Implications* (pp. 291–329). New York, NY: Cambridge University Press.

Cillessen, A.H., & Mayeux, L. (2004). From censure to reinforcement: developmental changes in the association between aggression and social status. *Child Development*, **75**(1), 147–163.

Coie, J.D., & Dodge, K.A. (1988). Multiple sources of data on social behavior and social status. *Child Development*, **59**, 815–829.

Coie, J.D., Dodge, K.A., & Coppotelli, H. (1982). Dimensions and types of social status: a cross-age perspective. *Developmental Psychology*, **18**, 557–570.

Collins, A., & Steinberg, L. (2006). Adolescent development in interpersonal context. In N. Eisenberg (Ed.) & W. Damon (Series Ed.), *Handbook of Child Psychology: Vol. 3. Social, Emotional, and Personality Development* (6th edn, pp. 1003–1067). Hoboken, NJ: Wiley.

Compian, L., Gowen, L.K., & Hayward, C. (2004). Peripubertal girls' romantic and platonic involvement with boys: associations with body image and depression symptoms. *Journal of Research on Adolescence*, **14**, 23–47.

Connolly, J., Craig, W., Goldberg, A., & Pepler, D. (2004). Mixed-gender groups, dating, and romantic relationships in early adolescence. *Journal of Research on Adolescence*, **14**, 185–207.

Deater-Deckard, K. (2001). Annotation: recent research examining the role of peer relationships in the development of psychopathology. *Journal of Child Psychology and Psychiatry*, **43**, 565–579.

Diamond, L.M. (2000). Sexual identity, attractions, and behavior among young sexual-minority women over a 2-year period. *Developmental Psychology*, **36**, 241–250.

Diamond, L.M. (2004). Sexual-minority and heterosexual youths' peer relationships: experiences, expectations, and implications for well-being. *Journal of Research in Adolescence*, **14**, 313–340.

Diamond, L.M., Savin-Williams, R.C., & Dubé, E.M. (1999). Sex, dating, passionate friendships, and romance: intimate peer relations among lesbian, gay, and bisexual adolescents. In W. Furman, B.B. Brown, & C. Feiring (Eds.), *The Development of Romantic Relationships in Adolescence* (pp. 175–210). Cambridge, UK: Cambridge University Press.

Douvan, E., & Adelson, J. (1966). *The Adolescent Experience.* New York, NY: Wiley.

Eder, D. (1985). The cycle of popularity: interpersonal relations among female adolescents. *Sociology of Education*, **5**, 154–165.

Eder, D. (1993). "Go get ya a French!": Romantic and sexual teasing among adolescent girls. In Deborah Tannen (Ed.), *Gender and Conversational Interaction* (pp. 17–31). New York, NY: Oxford University Press.

Ennett, S.T., & Bauman, K.E. (1996). Adolescent social networks: school, demographic and longitudinal considerations. *Journal of Adolescent Research*, **11**, 194–215.

Ernst, J.M., & Cacioppo, J.T. (1999). Lonely hearts: psychological perspectives on loneliness. *Applied and Preventive Psychology*, **8**, 1–22.

Farmer, T.W., Estell, D.B., Bishop, J.L., O'Neal, K.K., & Cairns, B.D. (2003). Rejected bullies or popular leaders? The social relations of aggressive subtypes of rural African American early adolescents. *Developmental Psychology*, **39**, 992–1004.

Feiring, C. (1996). Concepts of romance in 15-year-old adolescents. *Journal of Research on Adolescence*, **6**, 181–200.

Franzoi, S.L., & Davis, M.H. (1985). Adolescent self-disclosure and loneliness: private self-consciousness and parental influences. *Journal of Personality and Social Psychology*, **48**, 768–780.

Franzoi, S.L., Davis, M.H., & Vasquez-Suson, K.A. (1994). Two social worlds: social correlates and stability of adolescent status groups. *Journal of Personality and Social Psychology*, **67**, 462–473.

Frazier, P.A., & Cook, S.W. (1993). Correlates of distress following heterosexual relationship dissolution. *Journal of Social and Personal Relationships*, **10**, 55–67.

Furman, W., & Buhrmester, D. (1992). Age and sex differences in perceptions of networks of personal relationships. *Child Development*, **63**, 103–115.

Furman, W., & Shaffer, L. (2003). The role of romantic relationships in adolescent development. In P. Florsheim (Ed.), *Adolescent Romantic Relations and Sexual Behavior: Theory, Research, and Practical Implications* (pp. 3–22). Mahwah, NJ: Lawrence Erlbaum Associates.

Furman, W., Ho, M.H., & Low, S.M. (2007). The rocky road of adolescent romantic experience: dating and adjustment. In R. Engels, M. Kerr, & H. Stattin (Eds.), *Friends, Lovers and Groups: Key Relationships in Adolescence* (pp. 47–60). Chichester, UK: John Wiley.

Gavin, L., & Furman, W. (1989). Age difference in adolescents' perceptions of their peer groups. *Developmental Psychology*, **25**, 827–834.

Gilligan, C. (1996). The centrality of relationship in human development: a puzzle, some evidence, and a theory. In G. Noam & K. Fischer (Eds.), *Development and*

Vulnerability in Close Relationships (pp. 237–261). Hillsdale, NJ: Lawrence Erlbaum Associates.

Hand, C.S. & Furman, W. (in press). Rewards and costs in adolescent other-sex friendships: comparisons to same-sex friendships and romantic relationships. *Social Development*.

Hickman, L.J., Jaycox, L.H., & Aronoff, J. (2004). Dating violence among adolescents: prevalence, gender distribution, and prevention program effectiveness. *Trauma, Violence, and Abuse*, **5**, 123–142.

Hodges, E.V.E., & Perry, D.G. (1999). Personal and interpersonal antecedents and consequences of victimization by peers. *Journal of Personality and Social Psychology*, **76**, 677–685.

Hodges, E.V.E., Malone, M.J., & Perry, D.G. (1997). Individual risk and social risk as interacting determinants of victimization in the peer group. *Developmental Psychology*, **33**, 1032–1039.

Holt, M.K., & Espelage, D.L. (2005). Social support as a moderator between dating violence victimization and depression/anxiety among African American and Caucasian adolescents. *School Psychology Review*, **34**, 309–328.

Howard, D.E., & Wang, M.Q. (2003). Risk procedures of adolescent girls who were victims of dating violence. *Adolescence*, **38**, 1–14.

Inderbitzen, H.M., Walters, K.S., & Bukowski, A.L. (1997). The role of social anxiety in adolescent peer relations: differences among sociometric status groups and rejected subgroups. *Journal of Clinical Child Psychology*, **26**, 338–348.

Joyner, K., & Udry, R. (2000). You don't bring me anything but down: adolescent romance and depression. *Journal of Health and Social Behavior*, **41**, 369–391.

Kupersmidt, J.B., Sigda, K.B., Sedikides, C., & Voegler, M.E. (1999). Social self-discrepancy theory and loneliness during childhood and adolescence. In Rotenberg & Hymel (Eds.), *Loneliness in Children and Adolescents* (pp. 263–279). New York, NY: Cambridge University Press.

Kuttler, A.F., & La Greca, A.M. (2004). Linkages among adolescent girls' romantic relationships, best friendships, and peer networks. *Journal of Adolescence*, **27**, 395–414.

Ladd, G.W. (1999). Peer relationships and social competence during early and middle childhood. *Annual Review of Psychology*, **50**, 339–359.

La Greca, A.M., & Harrison, H.M. (2005). Adolescent peer relations, friendships, and romantic relationships: do they predict social anxiety and depression? *Journal of Clinical Child and Adolescent Psychology*, **34**, 49–61.

La Greca, A.M., Prinstein, M.J., & Fetter, M.D. (2001). Adolescent peer crowd affiliation: linkages with health-risk behaviors and close friendships. *Journal of Pediatric Psychology*, **26**, 131–143.

LaFontana, K.M., & Cillessen, A.H. (1999). Children's interpersonal perceptions as a function of sociometric and peer-perceived popularity. *Journal of Genetic Psychology*, **160**, 225–242.

Larson, R. (1983). Adolescents' daily experience with family and friends: contrasting opportunity systems. *Journal of Marriage and the Family*, **45**(4), 739–750.

Larson, R., & Lampman-Petraitis, C. (1989). Daily emotional states as reported by children and adolescents. *Child Development*, **60**, 1250–1260.

Larson, R., & Richards, M. (1991). Daily companionship in late childhood and early adolescence: changing developmental contexts. *Child Development*, **62**(2), 284–300.

Larson, R., Csikszentmihalyi, M., & Graef, R. (1980). Mood variability and the psycho-social adjustment of adolescents. *Journal of Youth and Adolescence*, 9(6), 469–490.

Larson, R.W., & Asmussen, L. (1991). Anger, worry, and hurt in early adolescence: an enlarging world of negative emotions. In M.E. Coltern & S. Gore (Eds.), *Adolescent Stress: Causes and Consequences* (pp. 21–41). New York: Aldine.

Larson, R.W., & Csikszentmilhalyi, M. (1978). Experiential correlates of time alone in adolescence. *Journal of Adolescence*, 46, 677–693.

Larson, R.W., & Richards, M. (1998). Waiting for the weekend: Friday and Saturday night as the emotional climax of the week. In A. Crouter & R. Larson (Eds.), *Temporal Rhythms in Adolescence: Clocks, Calendars, and the Coordination of Daily Life* (pp. 37–51). San Francisco, CA: Jossey-Bass.

Larson, R.W., Clore, G.L., & Wood, G.A. (1999). The emotions of romantic relation-ships: Do they wreck havoc on adolescents? In W. Furman, B.B. Brown, & C. Feiring (Eds.), *The Development of Romantic Relationships in Adolescence* (pp. 19–49). Cambridge, UK: Cambridge University Press.

Laursen, B. (1993). Conflict management among close peers. In B. Laursen (Ed.), *Close Friendships in Adolescence* (pp. 39–54). San Francisco, CA: Jossey-Bass.

Laursen, B. (1995). Conflict and social interaction in adolescent relationships. *Journal of Research on Adolescence*, 5, 55–70.

Laursen, B., & Williams, V. (1997). Perceptions of interdependence and closeness in family and peer relationships among adolescents with and without romantic partners. In S. Shulman & W.A. Collins (Eds.), *New Directions for Child and Adolescent Development, Vol. 9: Romantic Relationships in Adolescence* (pp. 3–20). San Francisco, CA: Jossey-Bass.

Laursen, B., Hartup, W., & Koplas, A. (1996). Towards understanding peer conflict. *Merrill–Palmer Quarterly*, 42, 76–102.

Lease, A.M., Musgrove, K.T., & Axelrod, J.L. (2002). Dimensions of social status in preadolescent peer groups: likability, perceived popularity, and social dominance. *Social Development*, 11, 508–533.

Maccoby, E.E. (1990). Gender and relationships: a developmental account. *American Psychologist*, 45, 513–520.

Monroe, S.M., Rohde, P., Seeley, J.R., & Lewinsohn, P.M. (1999). Life events and depression in adolescence: relationship loss as a prospective risk factor for first onset of major depressive disorder. *Journal of Abnormal Psychology*, 108, 606–614.

Munsch, J., & Kinchen, K.M. (1995). Adolescent sociometric status and social support. *Journal of Early Adolescence*, 15, 181–202.

Neeman, J., Hubbard, J., & Masten, A.S. (1995). The changing importance of romantic relationship involvement to competence from late childhood to late adolescence. *Development and Psychopathology*, 7, 727–750.

Parker, J.G., & Asher, S.R. (1987). Peer relations and later personal adjustment: are low-accepted children at risk? *Psychological Bulletin*, 102, 357–389.

Parker, J.G., & Seal, J. (1996). Forming, losing, renewing, and replacing friendships: applying temporal parameters to the assessment of children's friendship experiences. *Child Development*, 67, 2248–2268.

Parkhurst, J.T., & Hopmeyer, A. (1998). Sociometric popularity and peer-perceived popularity: two distinct dimensions of peer status. *Journal of Early Adolescence*, 18, 125–144.

Pawlby, S.J., Mills, A., & Quinton, D. (1997). Vulnerable adolescent girls: opposite-sex relationships. *Journal of Child Psychology and Psychiatry*, **38**, 909–920.

Perry, D.G., Perry, L.C., & Kennedy, E. (1992). Conflict and the development of antisocial behavior. In C.U. Shantz & W. Hartup (Eds.), *Conflict in Child and Adolescent Development* (pp. 301–329). New York, NY: Cambridge University Press.

Prinstein, M.J., & La Greca, A.M. (2002). Peer crowd affiliation and internalizing distress in adolescence: a longitudinal follow-back study. *Journal of Research on Adolescence*, **12**, 325–351.

Richards, M.H., Crowe, P.A., Larson, R., & Swarr, A. (1998). Developmental patterns and gender differences in the experience of peer companionship during adolescence. *Child Development*, **69**, 154–163.

Rose, A.J. (2002). Co-rumination in the friendships of girls and boys. *Child Development*, **73**, 1830–1843.

Rose, A.J., Swenson, L.P., & Waller, E.M. (2004). Overt and relational aggression and perceived popularity: developmental differences in concurrent and prospective relations. *Developmental Psychology*, **40**, 378–387.

Roth, M.A., & Parker, J.G. (2001). Affective and behavioral responses to friends who neglect their friends for dating partners: influences of gender, jealousy, and perspective. *Journal of Adolescence*, **24**, 281–296.

Rubin, K.H., Bukowski, W., & Parker, J.G. (2006). Peer interactions, relationships, and groups. In N. Eisenberg (Ed.) & W. Damon (Series Ed.), *Handbook of Child Psychology: Vol. 3. Social, Emotional, and Personality Development* (6th edn, pp. 571–645). New York, NY: Wiley.

Russell, S.T., & Consolacion, T.B. (2003). Adolescent romance and emotional health in the U.S.: beyond binaries. *Journal of Clinical Child and Adolescent Psychology*, **32**, 499–508.

Savin-Williams, R.C. (2006). Who's gay? Does it matter? *Current Directions in Psychological Science*, **15**, 40–44.

Savin-Williams, R.C., & Diamond, L.M. (2000). Sexual identity trajectories among sexual-minority youths: gender comparisons. *Archives of Sexual Behavior*, **29**, 607–627.

Scherer, K. (1984). On the nature and function of emotion: a component process approach. In K. Escherer & P.E. Ekman (Eds.), *Approaches to Emotion* (pp. 293–317). Hillsdale, NJ: Lawrence Erlbaum Associates.

Sears, J.T. (1991). *Growing up Gay in the South: Race, Gender, and Journeys of the Spirit*. New York, NY: Harrington Park Press.

Seiffge-Krenke, I. (1995). *Stress, Coping, and Relationships in Adolescence*. Hillsdale, NJ: Lawrence Erlbaum Associates.

Shulman, S., & Laursen, B. (2002). Adolescent perceptions of conflict in interdependent and disengaged friendships. *Journal of Research on Adolescence*, **12**, 353–372.

Simon, R.W., Eder, D., & Evans, C. (1992). The development of feeling norms underlying romantic love among adolescent females. *Social Psychological Quarterly*, **55**, 29–46.

Simpson, J.A. (1987). The dissolution of romantic relationships: factors involved in relationship stability and emotional distress. *Journal of Personality and Social Psychology*, **53**, 683–692.

Sittenfeld, C. (2005). *Prep*. New York: Random House.

Sullivan, H.S. (1953). *The Interpersonal Theory of Psychiatry*. New York, NY: W.W. Norton.

Thompson, S. (1994). Changing lives, changing genres: teenage girls' narratives about sex and romance, 1978–1986. In A.S. Rossi (Ed.), *Sexuality across the Life Course* (pp. 209–232). Chicago, IL: University of Chicago Press.

Vernberg, E.M. (1990). Psychological adjustment and experiences with peers during early adolescence: reciprocal, incidental, or unidirectional relationships? *Journal of Abnormal Child Psychology*, **18**, 187–198.

Williams, S., Connolly, J., & Segal, Z.V. (2001). Intimacy in relationships and cognitive vulnerability to depression in adolescent girls. *Cognitive Therapy and Research*, **25**, 477–496.

Wolfe, D.A., & Feiring, C. (2000). Dating violence through the lens of adolescent romantic relationships. *Child Maltreatment*, **5**, 360–363.

Youniss, J., & Smollar, J. (1985). *Adolescent Relations with Mothers, Fathers, and Friends*. Chicago, IL: University of Chicago Press.

Youniss, J., & Volpe, J. (1978). A relational analysis of children's friendships. In Damon, W. (Ed.), *Social Cognition* (pp. 1–22). San Francisco, CA: Jossey-Bass.

Zettergren, P. (2005). Childhood peer status as predictor of midadolescence peer situation and social adjustment. *Psychology in the Schools*, **42**, 745.

17

Peer relations, friendships, and romantic relationships: implications for the development and maintenance of depression in adolescents

Annette M. La Greca, Joanne Davila, and Rebecca Siegel

Adolescence is a critical period in development, marked by an expansion of peer networks, increased importance of close friendships, and the emergence of romantic relationships. As adolescents transition from middle school to high school, the size and diversity of their peer networks increase and peer crowd affiliation becomes important (La Greca & Prinstein, 1999). During adolescence, close friends surpass parents as the primary source of social support, and contribute to adolescents' self-concept and well-being (Furman & Buhrmester, 1992; Furman, McDunn, & Young, see Chapter 16, this volume). Moreover, dating relationships emerge and become increasingly important. By age 16, most adolescents have had a romantic relationship (Carver *et al.*, 2003). Such relationships may have mental health benefits, including the provision of social support, the enhancement of self-esteem, preparation for adult relationships, and the development of intimacy (Collins, 2003; Connolly & Goldberg, 1999).

Although peer relations, friendships, and romantic relationships may be beneficial to adolescents' social and emotional functioning, they also can represent significant stressors. Romantic relationships explain 25–34% of the strong emotions that high-school students experience, and about 42% of these strong emotions are negative feelings, such as anxiety, anger, jealousy, and depression (Larson *et al.*, 1999). The presence of a romantic relationship is associated with feelings of depression, especially among girls (Davila *et al.*, 2004).

This chapter reviews the literature on adolescents' peer relations, close friendships, and romantic relationships in order to understand their implications for the development and maintenance of depressive symptoms and disorders. The significance of peers is consistent with several theories of

Adolescent Emotional Development and the Emergence of Depressive Disorders, ed. Nicholas B. Allen and Lisa B. Sheeber. Published by Cambridge University Press. © Cambridge University Press 2009.

depression. Interpersonal theories (Coyne, 1976; Hammen, 1991) emphasize the role of interpersonal behaviors in the maintenance and exacerbation of depressive symptoms; attachment theory (Bowlby, 1969, 1973, 1980) and stress-diathesis frameworks (Lewinsohn *et al.*, 2001; Monroe & Simons, 1991) also address the importance of rejection experiences and interpersonal stress in the development and maintenance of depression. These frameworks are considered within the review that follows.

This chapter is organized into three main sections. The first reviews the role of the larger peer group, including adolescents' peer acceptance/rejection, peer crowd affiliations, and peer victimization; the second reviews literature on adolescents' close friendships; and the third reviews the role of romantic relationships. The chapter ends with a summary and suggestions for future research.

The larger peer group

The broadest level of social functioning we examine is adolescents' experiences with the larger peer group; that is, the large set of adolescents with whom an adolescent regularly interacts. The peer group is important for adolescent social and emotional development because youngsters derive a sense of *belonging and acceptance* from peers (La Greca & Prinstein, 1999). However, peers can also be a source of stress. Adolescents who are actively rejected, and those who are victimized by peers, display much higher rates of psychological difficulties and internalized distress than other adolescents (Hecht *et al.*, 1998; La Greca & Harrison, 2005; Prinstein *et al.*, 2001).

Although ample evidence links "interpersonal problems with peers" and depression, much less attention has been devoted to underlying mechanisms that account for this relationship. Problematic peer relations could be a marker for, a correlate of, or a causal pathway to psychopathology in youth (Coie, 1990). In our view, problematic peer relations actively contribute to depression in youth and, furthermore, such problematic relationships may also result from feelings of depression.

Acceptance and rejection

Peer relations have been evaluated along two distinct dimensions: acceptance and rejection. Acceptance refers to the degree to which an individual is actively liked by peers, whereas rejection reflects peers' active dislike (Newcomb *et al.*, 1993; Furman, McDunn, and Young, see Chapter 16, this volume).

There are several pathways by which youngsters may come to be rejected by peers (La Greca & Prinstein, 1999), although it is apparent that rejected youth are at risk for current and future psychological difficulties (Coie, 1990;

Parker & Asher, 1987). Community samples show that peer-rejected adolescents report more depressive symptoms than other adolescents. Specifically, rejected adolescents report lower self-esteem, lower perceived support, more self-perceived ineffectiveness, and greater anhedonia than do adolescents with average (Hecht *et al.*, 1998) or popular peer status (East *et al.*, 1987). Studies of neglected adolescents (low in acceptance but not rejection) have been mixed; some (Hecht *et al.*) have found levels of depressive symptoms comparable to that of rejected adolescents, while others have not (East *et al.*). Longitudinal studies also have linked childhood peer rejection to symptoms of internalized distress in adolescence, suggesting a causal role for peer rejection (Coie *et al.*, 1992; Kupersmidt & Patterson, 1991).

Prospective studies also indicate that symptoms of depression predict subsequent peer rejection. Vernberg (1990) followed early adolescents over a school year, finding that depressive symptoms early in the year predicted higher levels of peer rejection 6 months later. Similarly, Little & Garber (1995) found that symptoms of depression among early adolescents predicted an increase in peer rejection over a 3-month period.

Among clinical samples, depressed adolescents have been found to have interpersonal difficulties with peers, and depressed adolescents' social behaviors may contribute to problematic peer relations. For example, depressed adolescents are rejected more frequently by peers and are less popular than their non-depressed peers (Field *et al.*, 2001; Little & Garber, 1995). Moreover, laboratory studies examining adolescents' opinions of unfamiliar peers find that clinically depressed adolescents are rated more negatively than non-depressed adolescents (Connolly *et al.*, 1992).

Although evidence supports a bi-directional relationship between peer rejection and depressive affect, there may be important variables that moderate this relationship, including gender. For example, some studies have found a stronger relationship between peer rejection and depression for girls than for boys (Kupersmidt & Patterson, 1991; Lopez & DuBois, 2005). In addition, Connolly and colleagues (1992) found that depressed adolescent girls were viewed by peers as less skilled at making friends and less interested in getting to know others than were non-depressed girls, but the same was not true for boys. Similarly, Baker *et al.* (1996) found that dysphoric adolescent girls were viewed as more critical and were more often rejected by their non-depressed partners in a research setting than were non-dysphoric adolescent girls; boys were not examined in this study.

Other factors also may moderate the relationship between peer rejection and depression. Prinstein & Aikins (2004) found that peer rejection predicted symptoms of depression, but only in adolescent girls who placed high importance on their social status or who exhibited a depressogenic attributional style. In addition, Little & Garber (1995) found that depressive symptoms only predicted peer rejection for adolescents who had low levels of life stress, suggesting that peers may be more compassionate (and less rejecting) towards depressed adolescents who experience a significant stressor.

Others have posited that adolescents' self-perceptions may account for the relationship between peer rejection and adolescent depression. Specifically, Lopez & Dubois (2005) found that both peer victimization and perceived peer rejection contributed to depressive symptoms among adolescents, but only for girls whose self-esteem was influenced by these negative peer experiences. Kistner *et al.* (1999) found that peer-rated acceptance in childhood did not predict adolescents' dysphoria 7 years later, however, *perceived* peer acceptance in childhood did.

In summary, evidence supports a bi-directional association between peer rejection and depression. Adolescents who have a depressogenic attributional style, who value peer relations, and who are girls, may be more vulnerable to experiencing depression in reaction to peer rejection. Moreover, once depressed, the interpersonal behaviors of adolescents, especially girls, appear to perpetuate problems with peers.

Adolescent peer crowds

During adolescence, peer relationships expand substantially. Adolescents interact with a wide range of peers, in school and other settings, and may affiliate with a peer crowd.

Peer crowd affiliations represent the primary attitudes or behaviors by which an adolescent is known to peers (Brown, 1989). Peer crowds include a high-status, image-oriented crowd (Populars), an athletically oriented crowd (Jocks), an academically oriented crowd (Brains), a crowd that rebels against social norms (Alternatives or Non-conformists), a deviant, rule-breaking crowd (Burnouts or Druggies), and sometimes a crowd of misfits who keep to themselves (Loners). Adolescents cite acceptance, support, friendship development, and social interactions as benefits of peer crowd affiliation (Brown *et al.*, 1986).

Because peer crowd affiliation may be reputation based, crowd affiliations also reflect adolescents' acceptance within the larger peer system. Jocks and Populars represent high status crowds, whereas Burnouts and Alternatives typically reflect low status crowds (La Greca *et al.*, 2001). Although peer crowds are distinct from adolescents' smaller peer networks (or cliques) and close friendships (La Greca & Prinstein, 1999; Furman, McDunn, and Young, see Chapter 16, this volume), most adolescents have one or more close friends who affiliate with the same crowd (La Greca *et al.*, 2001).

A growing body of research has examined linkages between peer crowd affiliations and adolescents' distress, including symptoms of depression. Specifically, peer crowd affiliations, and especially affiliating with a high-status crowd, may confer some protection against feelings of depression.

Adolescents affiliating with high-status crowds report higher self-esteem, less loneliness (Brown & Lohr, 1987; Prinstein & La Greca, 2002), and lower levels of depressive symptoms (La Greca & Harrison, 2005) than other adolescents. Moreover, the "benefit" of affiliating with a high-status crowd appears to be *independent* of other indicators of social competence, as the linkage between peer crowd affiliation and low levels of depression remains even when the qualities of adolescents' friendships and romantic relationships are controlled (La Greca & Harrison, 2005).

It is not surprising that adolescents affiliating with high status crowds report fewer depressive symptoms. Such adolescents are regarded highly by their peers (La Greca *et al.*, 2001; Prinstein & La Greca, 2002), and may be connected to a large, social network that facilitates social interactions (Brown *et al.*, 1986).

In contrast, adolescents who affiliate with *low status* crowds report more depressive affect and lower self-esteem than others (Brown & Lohr, 1987; Prinstein & La Greca, 2002), although this is not always the case (La Greca & Harrison, 2005). Perhaps for some adolescents, the negative social status associated with certain peer crowds is offset by the positive aspects of "belonging" to a crowd. Even adolescents from low-status crowds report that support, friendship, and companionship were positive benefits of crowd affiliation (Brown *et al.*, 1986).

In summary, adolescents affiliating with high-status peer crowds report fewer depressive symptoms, and those affiliating with low-status crowds sometimes report more depressive symptoms, than other adolescents. Little is known about underlying mechanisms that account for these findings, although it is possible that the esteem, status, and regard that are associated with certain peer crowds might play a role. In addition, athletic abilities, sociability, or temperamental characteristics that facilitate adolescents' belonging to high-status crowds might be protective against depression. Further research is needed to understand the contribution of peer crowd affiliations to the development of depression.

Peer victimization/negative peer experiences

The third aspect of the peer system that has implications for adolescent depression is victimization and/or aversive experiences with peers, such as exclusion and aggression. Although related, peer victimization differs from peer rejection in that victimization focuses on negative experiences that are specifically directed toward an adolescent, whereas rejection reflects the prevailing attitudes of peers toward an adolescent (Lopez & DuBois, 2005). Although rejected adolescents experience peer victimization, more accepted adolescents can also be targets of victimization (Prinstein & Cillessen, 2003). Studies consistently link peer victimization with adolescents' reports of depression and anxiety (La Greca & Harrison, 2005; Prinstein *et al.*, 2005; Vernberg, 1990).

Initial research focused on *overt* peer victimization, such as physical violence and threats, finding that boys are often the aggressors and the victims (Nansel *et al.*, 2001). Recently, research has expanded to include *relational* victimization, such as friendship withdrawal and exclusion, and *reputational* victimization, such as rumor spreading (Prinstein *et al.*, 2001; Vernberg *et al.*, 1999). Among adolescents, relational victimization is more common than overt (La Greca & Harrison, 2005; Prinstein *et al.*, 2001).

In community studies, adolescents' reports of peer victimization have been associated with internal distress, including feelings of loneliness, social anxiety, and low self-worth (Graham & Juvonen, 1998). Both overt and relational victimization have been related to adolescents' reports of depression, loneliness, and low self-esteem (Prinstein *et al.*, 2001). Moreover, relational victimization has been strongly associated with adolescents' reports of social anxiety and depression, even when other aspects of adolescents' social status are controlled (La Greca & Harrison, 2005). Although these studies document a strong relationship between peer victimization and depressive symptoms, depressed adolescents are also *more likely to perceive* and overestimate rates of peer victimization relative to their peers' estimates (De Los Reyes & Prinstein, 2004).

The few available prospective studies suggest that aversive peer experiences and peer victimization lead to *increases* in depression over time. Vernberg (1990) evaluated early adolescents at two time points during the school year, finding that aversive peer experiences, evaluated in the context of less contact with friends and less closeness with a best friend, predicted increases in depressive affect over time. Vernberg also found reciprocal effects, in that initial levels of depressive symptoms predicted increases in aversive peer experiences. With older adolescents, Harrison (2006) found that peer victimization predicted *increases* in depressive symptoms over a 2-month period and this relationship was stronger for adolescents who were high in rejection sensitivity (the tendency to expect, perceive, and overreact to rejection; Ayduk *et al.*, 2001). Together these studies suggest that problematic peer relations contribute to depressive affect, which in turn contributes to more aversive peer experiences.

Critique and summary

Evidence clearly supports a relationship between problematic peer relations and adolescents' depressive symptoms. Peer rejection, peer victimization, and low peer status contribute to depressive affect, and this linkage may be stronger for girls and for adolescents who display certain cognitive vulnerabilities (rejection sensitivity, depressogenic attribution style). Evidence also indicates that depressed adolescents, especially girls, elicit more negative reactions from peers (more rejection, more victimization) than non-dysphoric youth. These findings are consistent with interpersonal theories of depression (Hammen, 1991) that highlight the role of interpersonal behaviors in the maintenance and exacerbation of depressive symptoms, and with stress-diathesis perspectives (Lewinsohn *et al.*, 2001) that emphasize rejection experiences and interpersonal stress in the development and maintenance of depression. Further research would benefit from theory-driven studies examining underlying mechanisms that could explain why some youth develop depressive symptoms in response to peer rejection/aversive experiences, while others do not. Also in need of investigation are the ways in which depressed adolescents' interpersonal behaviors and cognitive vulnerabilities contribute to peer problems.

Close friendships

Intimate friendships arise in early adolescence and become increasingly important over time. Through close friendships, adolescents learn how to express and regulate emotion and how to interpret and react to others' emotional expression (Newcomb & Bagwell, 1995). Secure friendships also help adolescents develop the social skills needed for intimate relationships later in life (Hartup, 1992; Furman, McDunn, and Young, see Chapter 16, this volume).

Although studies are scarce, it appears that simply having a close friendship may protect adolescents from feelings of depression. Bishop & Inderbitzen (1995) found that adolescents with at least one reciprocal close friend had higher self-esteem (an indicator of low depression) than those who had no close friends. Others have found that close friendships moderate the relationship between certain stressors, such as peer victimization, and feelings of depression. One study of third through seventh graders (Hodges *et al.*, 1997) found that, among victimized youth, having more close friends was related to lower levels of internalizing symptoms compared with youth who had fewer close friends; however, among the youth with low levels of peer victimization, the number of friends was unrelated to internalizing symptoms. This suggests that friends may both buffer the negative consequences of peer victimization and also protect adolescents from being victimized.

In contrast, however, La Greca & Harrison (2005) did not find that the positive qualities of adolescents' closest friendship moderated the relationship between peer victimization and depressive symptoms. The qualities of best friendships (support, disclosure) may potentially *reinforce* depressive feelings for adolescents who discuss and revisit problems or focus on negative feelings, a process referred to as co-rumination (Rose, 2002; Furman, McDunn, and Young, see Chapter 16, this volume).

Moreover, close friendships may also represent significant stressors. Friends who engage in more conflict and negative interactions than positive experiences report less social satisfaction than others (Parker & Asher, 1993). Conflictual friendships are also less stable, thus depriving some adolescents of the benefits of close, long-lasting friendships (Ladd, 1999).

In fact, negative interactions with close friends are associated with symptoms of depression. Adolescents who are involved in controlling friendships, which are characterized by peer pressure and social dominance, report low self-esteem and feelings of depression (Hussong, 2000). La Greca & Harrison (2005) found that negative interactions with a best friend (e.g. conflict, exclusion) predicted adolescents' depressive symptoms, even after controlling for other aspects of social functioning (e.g. rejection, peer victimization). It is not clear, however, whether negative interactions with friends contributed to or resulted from adolescents' feelings of depression.

Several investigators have examined clinically depressed adolescents, finding that their close friendships are impaired. Field and colleagues (2001) found that depressed adolescents reported fewer friends than non-depressed peers. Even after recovery, dysthymic adolescents reported less peer support than those without a history of mood disorders or than those with a history of major depressive disorder (Klein *et al.*, 1997).

Only one study has examined the peer relationships of youth with bipolar disorder, finding that children and adolescents with bipolar disorder had "few or no friends" significantly more frequently than youth with attention deficit hyperactivity disorder (ADHD) or normal controls (Geller *et al.*, 2000). The bipolar youth also had more impaired social skills than youth with ADHD and those with no psychiatric diagnosis. Research is needed to examine specific peer relationship problems in depressed adolescents.

The above findings indicate that the connections between close friendships and depressive symptoms are complex and may depend, in part, on the adolescents' attributes and the characteristics of the close friends. For example, having a close friend who exhibits symptoms of depression can increase depressive symptoms in adolescents, a phenomenon referred to as "contagion." Stevens & Prinstein (2005) found that, among 4th through 6th graders, a best friend's depressive affect predicted increases in youngsters' depressive affect 11 months later. In addition, a depressogenic attributional style reported by a reciprocal friend was longitudinally associated with youngsters' own problematic attributional style.

Other interpersonal behaviors, such as excessive reassurance-seeking, may be important. Prinstein and colleagues (2005) used a transactional, interpersonal framework for understanding gender differences in depression. Sociometric nominations and ratings of friendship quality were evaluated over three annual time points for a large cohort of adolescents, revealing that initial levels of reassurance-seeking and depressive symptoms predicted deteriorating friendship quality among girls and low friendship stability. Moreover, reassurance-seeking combined with poor peer experiences predicted increases in girls' depressive symptoms. As these and other findings indicate, the connections between adolescents' friendships and their depressive feelings are complex.

In terms of potential moderators, findings on gender differences in the relationship between close friendships and depressive symptoms have been mixed. Some studies found a stronger relationship between positive friendship qualities and fewer symptoms of depression in girls than in boys (Franzoi & Davis, 1985; Moran & Eckenrode, 1991), but others have not (Townsend *et al.*, 1988). Still others have found that positive friendship qualities increased positive affect in adolescent boys but not girls (Hussong, 2000).

In summary, although research is relatively limited, evidence suggests that having a close friend may protect adolescents from feelings of depression, that negative interactions in best friendships are associated with depressive symptoms, and that the close friendships of depressed adolescents are impaired. It is likely that there are bi-directional and transactional influences between friendship experiences and adolescents' depressive affect. Negative experiences with close friends could contribute to depressive affect; in turn, the interpersonal behaviors of depressed teens (e.g. excessive reassurance seeking) or their cognitive vulnerabilities (e.g. attributional style) might interfere with the development and maintenance of close friendships. Future research would benefit from studies that address the reciprocal influences of depression and friendship qualities, and that examine variables that moderate these linkages.

Romantic relationships

The association between adolescent romance and depression is of interest because depression is a prevalent problem whose rates increase during adolescence (particularly for girls) and because depression is associated with romantic dysfunction at later ages (Nolen-Hoeksema & Girgus, 1994; Whisman, 2001). We review existing literature on adolescent romance and depression, focusing on heterosexual youth, as studies of sexual minority youth are sparse.

There is limited but growing evidence that involvement in dating and romantic relationships during adolescence, particularly if frequent or steady, is associated with internalizing and depressive symptoms, and this is true among early and later adolescents and particularly among girls (Compian *et al.*, 2004; Davila *et al.*, 2004; Joyner & Udry, 2000; Quatman *et al.*, 2001). Even engaging in statistically normative romantic behaviors (e.g. flirting, kissing) is associated with depressive symptoms for early adolescent girls (Steinberg & Davila, 2008). In contrast, there is no evidence for an association between depressive symptoms and romantic involvement in adulthood.

In fact, romantic involvement is often associated with fewer symptoms (Umberson & Williams, 1999). So, why would romantic relationships be associated with greater depressive symptoms in adolescence?

One model emphasizes the importance of following the normative trajectory of romantic development (Welsh *et al.*, 2003), suggesting that adolescents who conform to developmentally appropriate norms will evidence better psychological adjustment compared with adolescents who engage in non-normative behavior. However, the mechanisms for this effect have not been examined. Perhaps youth who follow a non-normative trajectory, especially those who engage in later stage behaviors at an earlier phase, may not have the emotional or cognitive capacity to manage such experiences, particularly if stressful. Also, when young people engage in early dyadic dating they may reduce or lose social interaction with peers (Zimmer-Gembeck, 1999), resulting in a reduction or loss of support and socialization experiences. This may limit skills development and decrease chances of success in dating relationships. Brendgen *et al.* (2002) found that the association between romantic involvement and low self-esteem was strongest among early adolescents who reported low levels of acceptance by same-sex peers. Whether the same is true for depression has not been tested. Moreover, adolescents who are not receiving adequate support from family members or friends might seek out romantic relationships at an early age. These potential mechanisms need further evaluation.

Given that romantic involvement is associated with depression at all ages during adolescence (Davila *et al.*, 2004; Joyner & Udry, 2000) and with even normative experiences (Steinberg & Davila, 2008), normative trajectory models may not fully explain the association. One possibility is to explore characteristics of adolescents or their social worlds that may serve as moderators. For example, Davila *et al.* found that romantic involvement was associated more strongly with depressive symptoms among adolescents with a more preoccupied style of relating. People with a preoccupied style are needy yet fear rejection (Collins & Read, 1990). Consequently, they are often unhappy in relationships, feeling that they are not getting their needs met and worrying about rejection. So a relationship, regardless of its qualities, may always feel bad to the preoccupied person and thus result in dysphoria. In addition, Steinberg and Davila found that the association between depressive symptoms and normative romantic experiences was stronger for girls with emotionally unavailable parents, suggesting that when parents are not available to help youth regulate emotions and cope with stress (that romantic experiences may bring), young people will fail to develop such skills and be vulnerable to depression (see Doyle *et al.*, 2003). Therefore, romantic involvement at any point in adolescence may challenge young people's interpersonal, emotional, and cognitive resources or present adolescents with stressful circumstances, thereby increasing risk for depression particularly among adolescents with compromised personal and family resources.

Other research has examined whether specific aspects of romantic relationships are related to depression. Monroe *et al.* (1999) found that a romantic break up increases chances of experiencing a first major depressive episode in adolescence. Williams *et al.* (2001) found greater depressive mood reactivity among adolescent girls with low levels of intimacy in their romantic relationships. Among late-adolescent girls, Daley & Hammen (2002) found that lower emotional support and higher stress in romantic relationships were associated with depressive symptoms. Moreover, depressive symptoms were associated with partners' ratings of the girls as less interpersonally competent. Research also shows that more negative interactions in romantic relationships and romantic relationships characterized by inequality in the contribution of emotional resources and in decision-making are associated with greater depressive symptoms, especially for girls (Galliher *et al.*, 1999; La Greca & Harrison, 2005).

Research also has begun to examine the association between romantic functioning and depressive symptoms outside of involvement in romantic relationships. This is particularly important for studying younger adolescents who may not engage in relationships, but who may be developing ideas and feelings about romantic experiences. Davila *et al.* (2006) found that, among early-adolescent girls, poor romantic competence (i.e. maladaptive approaches to, thoughts and feelings about, and behaviors in romantic relationships) is associated with higher levels of past and current depressive symptoms. Furthermore, Steinberg and Davila found the association between poor competence and current depressive symptoms to be strongest among girls with emotionally unavailable parents.

In sum, romantic involvements, experiences, competencies, and behaviors are associated with depressive symptoms during all phases of adolescence, although there are few well-elaborated conceptual models to explain these associations. Next we discuss themes that might guide further conceptual and empirical development.

One theme is the role of emotion- and self-regulation processes. The association between depressive symptoms and romantic involvements across adolescence suggests that negotiating romantic experiences may be challenging or stressful, requiring adaptive emotion and self-regulation. Growing evidence suggests that such regulatory processes are key to successful development in a variety of domains and are important in understanding risk for depression (Chaplin & Cole, 2005). For example, the inability to experience happiness and the under-regulation of sad emotions are associated with depression (see Chaplin & Cole, 2005). To the extent that a challenging interpersonal experience elicits sadness, adolescents who are unable to contain such emotion may be at greater risk for becoming depressed. Similarly, potentially positive experiences may have little buffering effect on adolescents who have difficulty experiencing happiness. Evidence also suggests that adolescents may be less capable of high-level self-regulation as brain development in relevant areas is still in process (Sowell *et al.*, 1999). This may explain why even normative experiences are associated with depressive symptoms. Thus, it may be fruitful to consider the association between adolescent romantic relationships and depression from a stress and coping perspective, with an emphasis on self- and emotion-regulation processes.

Another theme is balancing intimacy and support with concerns about rejection and loss. Loss and fear of rejection are depressogenic, but intimacy and support may be protective. The ability to balance intimacy needs with concerns about rejection and to feel secure in relationships is a difficult developmental task that may affect risk for depression. Purdie & Downey (2000) found that, among early adolescent girls, greater rejection sensitivity was associated with greater insecurity about a boyfriend's commitment, and more hostility during romantic conflicts, which are exactly the types of experiences that may elicit rejection and increase risk for depression. Similarly, building on Coyne's (1976) model of how depressed people elicit rejection from others, dysphoric people who engage in excessive reassurance seeking, which is indicative of fear of rejection, are more likely to experience rejection by others, setting them up for further depression (Katz *et al.*, 1998; Joiner, 1999).

Attachment theory (Bowlby, 1969, 1973, 1980) also provides a useful framework for considering how concerns about rejection and capacity for intimacy affect interpersonal functioning and depression risk. Attachment theory also provides a framework for considering emotion regulation in the interpersonal context. The theory suggests that early relationships provide models for later ones, particularly with regard to expectations for caregiver availability, beliefs about self-worth in relationships, and strategies for regulating distress. People with negative models of self, who do not trust in the availability of others, and who cannot engage in adaptive support seeking and receipt in times of need, are at risk for interpersonal dysfunction and depression (Davila & Bradbury, 2001; Davila *et al.*, 1997), and the same may be true for adolescents. As such, attachment theory may inform understanding of how earlier relationship experiences, such as those in the family, as well as individual differences in rejection sensitivity, avoidance of intimacy, and emotion regulation can affect the association between adolescent romantic experiences and depression.

The themes described seem consistent with current literature, but several additional issues deserve consideration. The role of peer relationships in the association between romantic relationships and depression is an important avenue for research. The peer group plays a key role in the development of romantic relationships (Brown, 1999; Connolly & Goldberg, 1999) and can increase or decrease risk for depression. In addition, the role of assortative mating (the tendency to select romantic partners who are similar to oneself) deserves exploration, as partner characteristics may influence risk for depression. Daley & Hammen (2002) demonstrated that dysphoric late-adolescent girls tended to have partners with personality pathology that then limited the partners' ability to be supportive. Furthermore, data on depression contagion among adolescent peers and emerging-adult dating couples (Katz *et al.*, 1999; Stevens & Prinstein, 2005) suggests that regardless of assortative mating, dating partners may be vulnerable to depression by virtue of having a partner who is depressed.

The literature also raises the question of gender differences in the association between romantic relationships and depression. Many associations appear stronger for girls, although some studies only included girls. It is the case that depression is more prevalent among females beginning in adolescence (Nolen-Hoeksema & Girgus, 1994) and that females are more attuned to and affected by romantic experiences (Mayne *et al.*, 1997), suggesting the association may be stronger, but this is an empirical question.

It also is important to consider factors that may make romantic experiences more or less depressogenic. All adolescents have some type of negative romantic experience or disappointment, but not all get depressed. Identifying who is most likely to get depressed is a necessary goal. It also is necessary to recognize that some negative events (e.g. break-ups) are likely to be recurring given that adolescent romantic relationships are, typically, relatively temporary. Understanding how adolescents cope adaptively with this may shed light on how seemingly negative events may provide learning experiences that lead to positive rather than negative outcomes.

Critique and summary

The literature clearly documents an association between romantic experiences and depressive symptoms across adolescence and identifies several aspects of romantic functioning that increase risk. However, research is in its infancy and would benefit from further identification of the types of romantic experiences that affect depression, the mechanisms by which they do so, and the factors that increase or decrease the strength of their association. Finally, the association between adolescent romantic relationships and depression is almost certain to be bi-directional. Although this chapter focused more on how romantic experiences confer risk for depression, the best models will incorporate bi-directional associations.

Suggestions for research

Peer groups, friendships, and romantic relationships are important aspects of adolescents' interpersonal worlds that are associated with depressive symptoms and that may be instrumental in the development and maintenance of depression. Across these domains, studies suggest some consistency in risk factors. For instance, adolescents outside of the norm with regard to social relationships (in deviant or unpopular peer groups, in early romantic relationships), who have poor interpersonal skills, who experience negative interactions with peers, and who experience rejection are at greater risk for depression. There also are unique risks associated with each. For example, engagement in close friendships may be protective, whereas engagement in romantic relationships may be a risk factor. There also likely are ways in which the domains interact to confer risk or protection, although there is little research on this topic. We believe this is an important area for research, as each domain exists in the context of the others. For example, larger peer groups may serve as the source of close friendships and dating relationships, as well as the basis for evaluating partners and experiences. In addition, friends may play an important role in how romantic relationships are pursued, experienced, and managed.

Our review highlights areas for research across the domains. First, gender differences are relatively unexplored, but given gender differences in rates of depression during adolescence and in the role of and attunement to relationships, boys and girls may differ in how peer and romantic relationships affect risk for depression. Second, just as romantic relationships and friendships are likely to be embedded within and affected by peer groups, relationships with peers occur in the context of larger social structures, such as families and neighborhoods. Data have begun to suggest, that relations with parents may moderate associations between romantic functioning and depressive symptoms (Steinberg & Davila, 2008). Thus, it may be fruitful to examine how families and other social structures temper the effects of difficult peer relationships on depression. Third, although relationships confer risk for depression, depression can impair interpersonal functioning, thereby setting up the potential for a maladaptive, reciprocal cycle that leads to depression and troubled relationships. If this cycle is set in motion in adolescence, it may set the stage for impairment into adulthood.

Finally, we close by emphasizing that peer and romantic relationships in adolescence are both a source of stress and a source of strength that can both increase risk for depression or protect adolescents. A research agenda that includes a focus on when, how, and why these relationships play such roles and that further develops theory-driven models is necessary as we endeavor to understand what are likely to be a set of complex processes involving individual, dyadic, and social level factors.

REFERENCES

Ayduk, O., Downey, G., & Kim, M. (2001). Rejection sensitivity and depressive symptoms in women. *Personality and Social Psychology Bulletin*, **27**, 868–877.

Baker, M., Milich, R., & Manolis, M. (1996). Peer interactions of dysphoric adolescents. *Journal of Abnormal Child Psychology*, **24**, 241–256.

Bishop, J.A., & Inderbitzen, H.M. (1995). Peer acceptance and friendship: an investigation of their relation to self-esteem. *Journal of Early Adolescence*, **15**, 476–489.

Bowlby, J. (1969). *Attachment and Loss: Vol. 1. Attachment*. New York: Basic Books.

Bowlby, J. (1973). *Attachment and Loss: Vol. 2. Separation: Anxiety and Anger*. New York: Basic Books.

Bowlby, J. (1980). *Attachment and Loss: Vol.3. Loss: Sadness and Depression*. Harmondsworth, UK: Penguin.

Brendgen, M., Vitaro, F., Doyle, A.B., Markiewicz, D., & Bukowski, W.M. (2002). Same-sex peer relations and romantic relationships during early adolescence: interactive links to emotional, behavioral, and academic adjustment. *Merrill-Palmer Quarterly*, **48**, 77–103.

Brown, B.B. (1989). The role of peer groups in adolescents' adjustment to secondary school. In T.J. Berndt & G.W. Ladd (Eds.), *Peer Relationships in Child Development* (pp. 188–215). Oxford, UK: John Wiley & Sons.

Brown, B.B. (1999). "You're going out with who?": Peer group influences on adolescent romantic relationships. In W. Furman, B.B. Brown, & C. Feiring (Eds.), *The Development of Romantic Relationships in Adolescence* (pp. 291–329). Cambridge, UK: Cambridge University Press.

Brown, B.B. & Lohr, M.J. (1987). Peer-group affiliation and adolescent self-esteem: an integration of ego-identity and symbolic-interaction theories. *Journal of Personality and Social Psychology*, **52**, 47–55.

Brown, B.B., Eicher, S.A., & Petrie, S. (1986). The importance of peer group ("crowd") affiliation in adolescence. *Journal of Adolescence*, **9**, 73–96.

Carver, K., Joyner, K., & Udry, J.R. (2003). National estimates of adolescent romantic relationships. In P. Florsheim (Ed.), *Adolescent Romantic Relationships and Sexual Behavior: Theory, Research, and Practical Implications* (pp. 291–329). New York, NY: Cambridge University Press.

Chaplin, T.M., & Cole, P. (2005). The role of emotion regulation in the development of psychopathology. In. B.L. Hankin & J.R.Z. Abela (Eds.), *Development of Psychopathology: A Vulnerability-Stress Perspective* (pp. 49–74). Thousand Oaks, CA: Sage Publications.

Coie, J.D. (1990). Toward a theory of peer rejection. In S.R. Asher & J.D. Coie (Eds.), *Peer Rejection in Childhood* (pp. 365–398). New York, NY: Cambridge University Press.

Coie, J.D., Lochman, J.E., Terry, R., & Hyman, C. (1992). Predicting early adolescent disorder from childhood aggression and peer rejection. *Journal of Consulting and Clinical Psychology*, **5**, 783–792.

Collins, N.L., & Read, S.J. (1990). Adult attachment, working models, and relationship quality in dating couples. *Journal of Personality and Social Psychology*, **58**, 644–663.

Collins, W.A. (2003). More than myth: the developmental significance of romantic relationships during adolescence. *Journal of Research on Adolescence*, **13**, 1–24.

Compian, L., Gowen, L.K., & Hayward, C. (2004). Peripubertal girls' romantic and platonic involvement with boys: associations with body image and depression symptoms. *Journal of Research on Adolescence*, **14**, 23–47.

Connolly, J., & Goldberg, A. (1999). Romantic relationships in adolescence: the role of friends and peers in their emergence and development. In W. Furman, B.B. Brown, & C. Feiring (Eds.), *The Development of Romantic Relationships in Adolescence* (pp. 266–290). Cambridge, UK: Cambridge University Press.

Connolly, J., Geller, S., Marton, P., & Kutcher, S. (1992). Peer responses to social interaction with depressed adolescents. *Journal of Clinical Child Psychology,* **21**, 365–370.

Coyne, J.C. (1976). Toward an interactional description of depression. *Psychiatry: Journal for the Study of Interpersonal Processes,* **39**, 28–40.

Daley, S.E., & Hammen, C. (2002). Depressive symptoms and close relationships during the transition to adulthood: perspectives from dysphoric women, their best friends, and their romantic partners. *Journal of Consulting and Clinical Psychology,* **70**, 129–141.

Davila, J., & Bradbury, T.N. (2001). Attachment insecurity and the distinction between unhappy spouses who do and do not divorce. *Journal of Family Psychology,* **15**, 371–393.

Davila, J., Bradbury, T.N., Cohan, C.L., & Tochluk, S. (1997). Marital functioning and depressive symptoms: evidence for a stress generation model. *Journal of Personality and Social Psychology,* **73**, 849–861.

Davila, J., Steinberg, S.J., Kachadourian, L., Cobb, R., & Fincham, F. (2004). Romantic involvement and depressive symptoms in early and late adolescence: the role of preoccupied relational style. *Personal Relationships,* **11**, 161–178.

Davila, J., Steinberg, S.J., Ramsay, M. *et al.* (March, 2006). *Defining and Measuring Romantic Competence in Early Adolescence: The Romantic Competence Interview.* Poster presented at the biennial meeting of the Society for Research on Adolescence, San Francisco, CA.

De Los Reyes, A., & Prinstein, M.J. (2004). Applying depression-distortion hypotheses to the assessment of peer victimization in adolescents. *Journal of Clinical Child and Adolescent Psychology,* **33**, 325–335.

Doyle, A.B., Brendgen, M., Markiewicz, D., & Kamkar, K. (2003). Family relationships as moderators of the association between romantic relationships and adjustment in early adolescence. *Journal of Early Adolescence,* **23**, 316–340.

East, P.L., Hess, L.E., & Lerner, R.M. (1987). Peer social support and adjustment of early adolescent peer groups. *Journal of Early Adolescence,* **7**, 153–163.

Field, T., Diego, M., & Sanders, C. (2001). Adolescent depression and risk factors. *Adolescence,* **36**, 491–498.

Franzoi, S.L., & Davis, M.H. (1985). Adolescent self-disclosure and loneliness: private and self-consciousness and parental influences. *Journal of Personality and Social Psychology,* **48**, 768–780.

Furman, W., & Buhrmester, D. (1992). Age and sex differences in perceptions of networks of personal relationships. *Child Development,* **63**, 103–115.

Galliher, R.V., Rostosky, S.S., Welsh, D.P., & Kawaguchi, M.C. (1999). Power and psychological well-being in late adolescent romantic relationships. *Sex Roles,* **40**, 689–710.

Geller, B., Bolhofner, K., Craney, J.L. *et al.* (2000). Psychosocial functioning in a prepubertal and early adolescent bipolar disorder phenotype. *Journal of the American Academy of Child and Adolescent Psychiatry,* **39**, 1543–1548.

Graham, S., & Juvonen, J. (1998). Self-blame and peer victimization in middle school: an attributional analysis. *Developmental Psychology,* **34**, 587–599.

Hammen, C. (1991). Generation of stress in the course of unipolar depression. *Journal of Abnormal Psychology,* **100**, 555–561.

Harrison, H.M. (2006). *Peer Victimization and Depressive Symptoms in Adolescence.* Doctoral dissertation, University of Miami, Coral Gables, FL.

Hartup, W. (1992). Conflict and friendship relations. In W.W. Hartup & C.U. Shantz (Eds.), *Cambridge Studies in Social and Emotional Development* (pp. 186–215). New York: Cambridge University Press.

Hecht, D.B., Inderbitzen, H.M., & Bukowski, A.L. (1998). The relationship between peer status and depressive symptoms in children and adolescents. *Journal of Abnormal Child Psychology,* **26**, 153–160.

Hodges, E.V.E., Malone, M.J., & Perry, D.G. (1997). Individual risk and social risk as interacting determinants of victimization in the peer group. *Developmental Psychology,* **33**, 1032–1039.

Hussong, A.M. (2000). Perceived peer context and adolescent adjustment. *Journal of Research on Adolescence,* **10**, 391–415.

Joiner, T.E. (1999). A test of interpersonal theory of depression in youth psychiatric inpatients. *Journal of Abnormal Child Psychology,* **27**, 77–85.

Joyner, K., & Udry, R. (2000). You don't bring me anything but down: adolescent romance and depression. *Journal of Health and Social Behavior,* **41**, 369–391.

Katz, J., Beach, S.R.H., & Joiner, T.E. (1998). When does partner devaluation predict emotional distress? Prospective moderating effects of reassurance seeking and self-esteem. *Personal Relationships,* **5**, 409–421.

Katz, J., Beach, S.R.H., & Joiner, T.E. (1999). Contagious depression in dating couples. *Journal of Social and Clinical Psychology,* **18**, 1–13.

Kistner, J., Balthazor, M., Risi, S., & Burton, C. (1999). Predicting dysphoria in adolescence from actual and perceived peer acceptance in childhood. *Journal of Clinical Child Psychology,* **28**, 94–104.

Klein, D.N., Lewinsohn, P.M., & Seeley, J.R. (1997). Psychosocial characteristics of adolescents with a past history of dysthymic disorder: comparison with adolescents with past histories of major depressive and non-affective disorders, and never mentally ill controls. *Journal of Affective Disorders,* **42**, 127–135.

Kupersmidt, J.B., & Patterson, C.J. (1991). Childhood peer rejection, aggression, withdrawal and perceived competence as predictors of self-reported behavior problems in preadolescence. *Journal of Abnormal Child Psychology,* **19**, 427–449.

Ladd, G.W. (1999). Peer relationships and social competence during early and middle childhood. *Annual Review of Psychology,* **50**, 333–359.

La Greca, A.M., & Harrison, H.M. (2005). Adolescent peer relations, friendships, and romantic relationships: do they predict social anxiety and depression? *Journal of Clinical Child and Adolescent Psychology,* **34**, 49–61.

La Greca, A.M., & Prinstein, M.J. (1999). Peer group. In W.K. Silverman & T.H. Ollendick (Eds.), *Developmental Issues in the Clinical Treatment of Children* (pp. 171–198). Needham Heights, MA: Allyn & Bacon.

La Greca, A.M., Prinstein, M.J., & Fetter, M.D. (2001). Adolescent peer crowd affiliation: linkages with health-risk behaviors and close friendships. *Journal of Pediatric Psychology,* **26**, 131–143.

Larson, R.W., Clore, G.L., & Wood, G.A. (1999). The emotions of romantic relationships: do they wreak havoc on adolescents? In W. Furman, B.B. Brown, & C. Feiring (Eds.), *The Development of Romantic Relationships in Adolescence* (pp. 19–49). Cambridge, UK: Cambridge University.

Lewinsohn, P.M., Joiner, T.E., & Rohde, P. (2001). Evaluation of cognitive diathesis-stress models in predicting major depressive disorder in adolescents. *Journal of the American Academy of Child and Adolescent Psychiatry*, **10**, 203–215.

Little, S.A., & Garber, J. (1995). Aggression, depression, and stressful life events predicting peer rejection in children. *Development and Psychopathology*, **7**, 845–856.

Lopez, C., & DuBois, D.L. (2005). Peer victimization and rejection: investigation of an integrative model of effects on emotional, behavioral, and academic adjustment in early adolescence. *Journal of Clinical Child and Adolescent Psychology*, **34**, 25–36.

Mayne, T.J., O'Leary, A., McCrady, B., Contrada, R. & Labouvie, E. (1997). The differential effects of acute marital distress on emotional, physiological and immune functions in maritally distressed men and women. *Psychology and Health*, **12**, 277–288.

Monroe, S., & Simons, A.D. (1991). Diathesis-stress theories in the context of life stress research: implications for the depressive disorders. *Psychological Bulletin*, **110**, 406–425.

Monroe, S.M., Rohde, P., Seeley, J.R., & Lewinsohn, P.M. (1999). Life events and depression in adolescence: relationship loss as a prospective risk factor for first onset of major depressive disorder. *Journal of Abnormal Psychology*, **108**, 606–614.

Moran, P.B., & Eckenrode, J. (1991). Gender differences in the costs and benefits of peer relationships during adolescence. *Journal of Adolescent Research*, **6**, 396–409.

Nansel, T.R., Overpeck, M., Pilla, R.S. *et al.* (2001). Bullying behaviors among US youth: prevalence and association with psychosocial adjustment. *Journal of the American Medical Association*, **285**, 2094–2100.

Newcomb, A.F., & Bagwell, C.L. (1995). Children's friendship relations: a meta-analytic review. *Psychological Bulletin*, **117**, 306–347.

Newcomb, A.F., Bukowski, W.M., & Pattee, L. (1993). Children's peer relations: a meta-analytic review of popular, rejected, neglected, controversial, and average sociometric status. *Psychological Bulletin*, **113**, 99–128.

Nolen-Hoeksema, S., & Girgus, J.S. (1994). The emergence in gender differences in depression during adolescence. *Psychological Bulletin*, **115**, 424–443.

Parker, J.G., & Asher, S.R. (1987). Peer relationships and later personal adjustment: are low accepted children at risk? *Psychological Bulletin*, **102**, 357–389.

Parker, J.G., & Asher, S.R. (1993). Friendship and friendship quality in middle childhood: links with peer group acceptance and feelings of loneliness and social dissatisfaction. *Developmental Psychology*, **29**, 611–621.

Prinstein, M.J., & Aikins, J.W. (2004). Cognitive moderators of longitudinal association between peer rejection and adolescent depressive symptoms. *Journal of Abnormal Child Psychology*, **32**, 147–158.

Prinstein, M.J., & Cillessen, A.H.N. (2003). Forms and functions of adolescent peer aggression associated with high levels of peer status. *Merrill-Palmer Quarterly*, **49**, 310–342.

Prinstein, M.J., & La Greca, A.M. (2002). Peer crowd affiliation and internalizing distress in adolescence: a longitudinal follow-back study. *Journal of Research on Adolescence*, **12**, 325–351.

Prinstein, M.J., Boergers, J., & Vernberg, E.M. (2001). Overt and relational aggression in adolescents: social-psychological adjustment of aggressors and victims. *Journal of Clinical Child Psychology*, **30**, 479–491.

Prinstein, M.J., Borelli, J.L., Cheah, C.S.L., Simon, V.A., & Aikins, J.W. (2005). Adolescent girls' interpersonal vulnerability to depressive symptoms: a longitudinal examination of reassurance-seeking and peer relationships. *Journal of Abnormal Psychology*, **114**, 676–688.

Purdie, V., & Downey, G. (2000). Rejection sensitivity and adolescent girls' vulnerability to relationship-centered difficulties. *Child Maltreatment*, **5**, 338–349.

Quatman, T., Sampson, K., Robinson, C., & Watson, C.M. (2001). Academic, motivational, and emotional correlates of adolescent dating. *Genetic, Social, and General Psychology Monographs*, **127**, 211–234.

Rose, A.J. (2002). Co-rumination in the friendships of girls and boys. *Child Development*, **73**, 1830–1843.

Sowell, E.R., Thompson, P.M., Holmes, C.J., Jernigan, T.L., & Toga, A.W. (1999). In vivo evidence for post-adolescent brain maturation in frontal and striatal regions. *Nature Neuroscience*, **2**, 859–861.

Steinberg, S.J., & Davila, J. (2008). Adolescent romantic functioning and depression: the moderating role of parental emotional availability. *Journal of Clinical Child and Adolescent Psychology*, **37**, 350–362.

Stevens, E.A., & Prinstein, M.J. (2005). Peer contagion of depressogenic attributional styles among adolescents: a longitudinal study. *Journal of Abnormal Child Psychology*, **33**, 25–37.

Townsend, M.A.R., McCracken, H.E., & Wilton, K.M. (1988). Popularity and intimacy as determinants of psychological well-being in adolescent friendships. *Journal of Early Adolescence*, **8**, 421–436.

Umberson, D., & Williams, K. (1999). Family status and mental health. In C.S. Aneshensel & J.C. Phelan (Eds.), *Handbook of the Sociology of Mental Health* (pp. 225–253). New York, NY: Kluwer Academic/Plenum Publishers.

Vernberg, E.M. (1990). Psychological adjustment and experiences with peers during early adolescence: reciprocal, incidental, or unidirectional relationships? *Journal of Abnormal Child Psychology*, **18**, 187–198.

Vernberg, E.M., Jacobs, A.K., & Hershberger, S.L. (1999). Peer victimization and attitudes about violence during early adolescence. *Clinical Child Psychology*, **28**, 386–395.

Welsh, D.P., Grello, C.M., & Harper, M.S. (2003). When love hurts: Depression and adolescent romantic relationships. In P. Florsheim (Ed.), *Adolescent Romantic Relations and Sexual Behavior: Theory, Research, and Practical Implications* (pp. 185–212). Mahwah, NJ: Lawrence Erlbaum.

Whisman, M.A. (2001). The association between depression and marital dissatisfaction. In S.R.H. Beach (Ed.), *Marital and Family Processes in Depression: A Scientific Foundation for Clinical Practice* (pp. 3–24). Washington, D.C.: American Psychological Association.

Williams, S., Connolly, J., & Segal, Z.V. (2001). Intimacy in relationships and cognitive vulnerability to depression in adolescent girls. *Cognitive Therapy and Research*, **25**, 477–496.

Zimmer-Gembeck, M.J. (1999). Stability, change and individual differences in involvement with friends and romantic partners among adolescent females. *Journal of Youth and Adolescence*, **28**, 419–438.

18

Towards a developmental psychopathology of adolescent-onset depression: implications for research and intervention

Nicholas B. Allen and Lisa B. Sheeber

The substantial and reliable increase in the incidence of depressive disorder during the transition to adolescence suggests the importance of understanding the developmental changes that might contribute to this vulnerability. In this final chapter, we attempt to integrate key findings so as to shed light on the etiology of depressive disorder. As well, we will discuss the future directions that have been highlighted in the chapters, in terms of conceptual development, research questions and methodologies, and intervention design. These directions provide an agenda for research on adolescent depression, and also demonstrate the tremendous utility of taking a developmental psychopathology perspective on mental health problems during adolescence (Steinberg *et al.*, 2005).

Why is maturation during early adolescence associated with increased vulnerability to depression?

As would likely come as no surprise to parents of teenagers, research described by Larson and Sheeber in Chapter 2, indicates that on average adolescents have a wider emotional range than do adults. That is, they experience strong emotional states, both positive and negative, with greater frequency. It is notable, however, that contrary to conventional wisdom, this greater emotional range does *not* differentiate adolescents from younger children. Instead, the distinguishing feature of adolescent affectivity, relative to younger children, is a diminishing of positive moods and an increase in negative moods. This basic age trend, moreover, appears to be consistent across gender, ethnicity, and

Adolescent Emotional Development and the Emergence of Depressive Disorders, ed. Nicholas B. Allen and Lisa B. Sheeber. Published by Cambridge University Press. © Cambridge University Press 2009.

socioeconomic characteristics. Overall, the research indicates that the transition to adolescence is associated with a normative increase in the rate of daily negative emotion that slows down and plateaus in mid- to late-adolescence. Despite this downward dip in mood, however, most teenagers maintain the preponderance of positive affect that is associated with good mental health. In the third chapter, Seeley and Lewinsohn make clear that, simultaneous with these normative changes in affectivity, there is a dramatic increase in the incidence of depressive disorder, particularly among girls. This increase in the rate of disorder, moreover, is not a transitive epiphenomenon of adolescence. The occurrence of depressive disorder during adolescence connotes risk for further negative outcomes into adulthood, notably including the recurrence of depressive symptomatology and disorder.

In contrast to these affective changes, the overall trajectory of maturation across the lifespan is towards greater capacity for self-regulation. Notably, evidence on temperamental, cognitive, and neurobiological development indicates that this trend toward increased regulation is also true during the transition from childhood into adolescence. In Chapter 12, Sanson, Letcher, and Smart note that although there appears to be substantial continuity in the structure of temperament from childhood through adolescence, there are developmental changes characterized by decreasing negative reactivity and increasing self-regulation. Similarly Kesek, Zelazo, and Lewis (Chapter 8) review evidence indicating that there is a developmental trend throughout childhood and adolescence leading to increased ability to deal with complex or ambiguous situations that require more self-reflective, top-down control. This increased capacity is thought to be mediated by the maturation of the prefrontal cortex (PFC). Such changes might suggest that, as a cohort, adolescents would be *less* vulnerable to mood disorder than are younger children. These findings highlight a critical conundrum: how do normative developmental changes that appear to be associated with maturation of the capacity for self regulation result in population-wide increases in vulnerability to mood disorder and negative affective experiences? Below we discuss two models that might explain how adolescent maturation increases vulnerability to mood disorder.

First, as has been increasingly noted in the literature, and described by Kesek and colleagues in this volume, regulatory capacity and the neurological systems hypothesized to underlie it, continue to develop well into the early years of adulthood. Indeed, as noted in our introductory chapter, many authors have speculated that a potential explanation for increased vulnerability to mental disorder during early- to mid-adolescence may be the relative delay in PFC maturation as compared with the earlier, puberty-stimulated development of limbic areas, which result in greater sensitivity to affective and social stimuli (Nelson *et al.*, 2005; Steinberg, 2005). This sensitivity is perhaps best exemplified by the salience of romantic experiences as elicitors of strong emotions during adolescence (see Chapters 16 and 17). It may be particularly telling that engagement in romantic relationships is associated with increased depressive symptoms during adolescence, but not during adulthood. This suggests that the development of higher-order cognitive skills (as well, of course, as experience) may in time facilitate adaptive handling of these significant and complex relationships and the emotions they engender. In the short run, however, this association illustrates how the developmentally normative mismatch in the maturation of these brain regions and their associated functions, may lead to a period of relatively unregulated drives and emotions.

It should be noted as well that the *degree* of "mismatch" between the maturational trajectories of the PFC and the limbic areas may well be a variable on which there are individual differences. That is, until development of the PFC is complete, vulnerability may be especially high in individuals who experience a relatively high degree of discordance between these developmental processes. For instance, individuals who enter puberty early may be particularly vulnerable. This would be consistent with the greater risk for depressive symptoms and disorder associated with early pubertal timing in girls and perhaps, with the greater risk for girls who, on average, enter puberty earlier than boys (see Chapters 4 and 5). Hence, though the normative trajectory may be one of increasing resilience and self-regulation, there may be a significant minority of individuals who, as a function of greater discordance between relevant neurobiological systems, fail to show this pattern and are hence particularly vulnerable to disorder. A recent demonstration of such variability in developmental trajectories was provided by Johnson and colleagues (Johnson *et al.*, 2007), who used latent class analysis to establish three trajectory groups (i.e. "alright," "growing up," and "trouble") in girls aged 14 to 24. The psychosocial outcomes associated with each of these groups were significantly different, with the "trouble" group (about 11% of the total sample) showing the worst outcomes. These findings demonstrate that although there may be a normative pattern of positive development during adolescence, a significant minority of individuals may fail to show such development, and consequently be at risk of poor outcomes.

The consequences of this neurobiological mismatch for adolescent emotional functioning, moreover, may be exacerbated by the substantial and rapid changes in the social environment which also begin at the transition into adolescence, as has been described in a number of the previous chapters. For example, as described in Chapters 16 and 17, peer relationships not only become more salient, but substantially more complex as well. From a functional and evolutionary point of view it is, of course, not an accident that these biological and social changes co-occur. It is the very demands that are made by the adolescent's changing role (e.g. the increased need for independence and engagement with longer-term goals, the requirements of selecting, attracting, and competing for mates) that provided selective pressures that drove the changes in brain and sexual development that occur during adolescence (Weisfeld & Janisse, 2005). Nonetheless, the rapid changes in both social and biological trajectories, creates the possibility for discordance between social demands and maturational capacities. Indeed it may be that although adolescents' capabilities are maturing, the increased complexity and stressfulness of the contexts in which they find themselves can often outrun their biological, cognitive, and emotional maturation, and thus temporarily overwhelm their competencies.

Changes in family environments are particularly salient to the discussion of the developmental mismatch between demands and regulatory capacity. This is the case because a crucial change affecting family life is the normative withdrawal of parental regulatory controls as adolescents seek, and are permitted, greater autonomy in decision-making and social interactions, as well as in the management of their emotional lives (see Chapters 14 and 15). Hence, the increases in negative affect and depressive symptoms observed during adolescence may reflect the fact that external supports are being withdrawn at the same time that adolescents are experiencing increasing maturational and environmental challenges. As described in the chapters by Tompson and Hunter and their colleagues (Chapters 14 and 15), it appears that families' ability to maintain emotional attachments, as well as parents' ability to provide support and acceptance, are related to adolescents' emotional competence and inversely, to their risk for depression. It is also likely that, as described in these chapters, the quality of parent–child relationships and the early socialization of emotional behavior prior to adolescence influence adolescents' ability to navigate the challenges of this developmental period. Finally, both chapters on family processes highlight the importance of considering potential gender differences, with some evidence suggesting that girls may be more sensitive to the effects of family environments, perhaps because they continue to be more emotionally engaged with their families.

One challenge to the "mismatch" theory, however, is that to the extent that the upswing in depressive symptoms is attributable to a mismatch between affective reactivity, increased contextual demands, and regulatory capacity, one would expect to see declines in depressive phenomena with increased maturation, akin to the patterns observed in externalizing disorders (Davey et al., 2008). Contrary to this prediction, though, the incidence of first episode depressive disorder remains largely consistent through mid-adulthood (Burke et al., 1990). One possibility is that similar but etiologically distinct processes are responsible for onsets later in life. In other words, although poor regulatory control of affective processes may be a general vulnerability factor for depression across the lifespan, adolescence may represent a special case in the sense that these regulatory difficulties are linked to developmental processes particular to this phase of life, which act to potentiate the effects of more trait-like individual differences in vulnerability.

Another salient possibility is that the developing cognitive capabilities that emerge as a function of maturation lay the basis for *both* increased vulnerability and better self regulation. Larson and Sheeber (see Chapter 2) suggest that the emergence of new thinking skills means that emotions are more likely to be elicited by abstract ideas, as well as both anticipated and recalled events. Adolescents may hence be more prone than younger children to ruminating about adverse experiences, past and present, real and hypothetical. Moreover, their improved ability to take others' perspectives may render adolescents more vulnerable to experience distress brought about by events occurring to others (see Eisenberg *et al.*, Chapter 10). The possibility that the development of prefrontal structures may be associated with both maturation *and* increased vulnerability has been articulated more fully by Davey and colleagues (2008). They point out that substantial remodeling and maturation of both the dopaminergic reward system and the prefrontal cortex occur during adolescence, and that this remodeling coincides with adolescents beginning to enter the complex world of adult peer and romantic relationships, where the rewards that can be obtained (e.g. belonging, romantic love, status, and agency) are more abstract and temporally distant from the proximal context than are the rewards obtained during childhood. For example, as described by Gilbert and Irons (Chapter 11), adolescents are very focused on concerns related to social standing and acceptance – belonging to a group, being selected by a romantic partner, and being valued by friends. Development of the prefrontal cortex, which is thought to underlie increasing self-regulatory capacities, also makes it possible to pursue such complex and distal rewards. These rewards, however, are less certain and more readily frustrated than the more immediate rewards characteristic of childhood. The challenge of accessing these rewards may be amplified by the increasingly complex and competitive nature of adolescent social contexts (see Chapters 16 and 17). Davey and colleagues hypothesize that when these distant rewards are frustrated they suppress the reward system. Indeed, given the super-ordinate nature of the abstract and distal rewards that are being pursued, when these rewards are frustrated or disappointed there will tend to be a suppression of reward seeking not only of these super-ordinate rewards, but of all the motivated goals that are subsidiary to them. When such suppression is extensive and occurs for long enough, the clinical picture that results is one of depression. Hence, for example, a romantic break up could result in reduced motivation not only to date, but also to socialize with friends, to participate in large group situations (like school), and in the extreme, could result in an adolescent being unmotivated to even leave her room. This model is consistent with evidence that depression is very often precipitated by social rejection or loss of status during adolescence (Monroe *et al.*, 1999) as well as with the broader pattern of association between adverse social functioning (e.g. peer rejection or victimization; interactional stress in friendship) and depressive symptoms described in earlier chapters (e.g. Chapters 16 and 17). As such, the healthy maturation of brain systems might in fact simultaneously provide the basis for both improvements in functioning and increased vulnerability.

As has been noted, the gender difference in rates of depression also emerges at puberty. This is consistent with proposals that this difference emerges because of the heightened "affiliative need" of women that is driven by social and hormonal influences that operate from puberty (Allen *et al.*, 2006). The suggestion is that affiliative rewards have more salience for women, who are subsequently more likely to be disappointed by the frustration of these needs (Allen & Badcock, 2003, 2006). Interestingly, there is some evidence that the prefrontal gray matter changes that occur in adolescence begin earlier for females (Giedd *et al.*, 1999), which may account for some of the difference in vulnerability between the genders and is consistent with the notion that maturation of the prefrontal cortex may provide the basis for enhanced vulnerability to depressive states.

Directions for research on the developmental psychopathology of depression

Despite the diversity of topics covered in this volume, a number of common themes emerged. The fact that these themes were highlighted by a number of authors, working in both developmental and clinical areas, and across a variety of research domains, suggests that they are significant emergent issues with broad relevance for advancing research on the development of depression during adolescence. The broadest level issue that arose was the importance of research that will yield a more sophisticated understanding of the interaction between environmental factors, individual differences, and biological maturation. Numerous authors writing about both biological and social domains expressed this idea. For example, in Chapter 6, Paus noted that the environment is likely to exert a powerful influence on brain structure, not only during infancy and early childhood, but also into adolescence. Similarly, in the chapters on pubertal development, both DeRose and Brooks Gunn (Chapter 4) and Graber (Chapter 5) discuss the influence of the pre-pubertal environment on pubertal timing. They indicated, moreover, that we still have a limited understanding of how the various aspects of pubertal development (biological, sexual, psychological, interpersonal) interact to produce increased vulnerability to depression. Conversely, the authors of the chapters on family context (Chapters 14 and 15) indicate the need to understand the relations between social processes and individual differences in understanding risk. In particular, Hunter and colleagues (Chapter 14) called for more research on the moderating role of individual differences on children's response to parental emotion socialization. More generally, Tompson and colleagues (Chapter 15) highlighted the need to examine the interaction between family processes and genetic vulnerability to depression. These are but a few examples of potential research areas. As our knowledge of the biological, psychological, and social processes that underlie adolescent development increases, we will likely be in a position to ask more sophisticated questions about how they interact to produce vulnerability to depression. For example, not only will it be important to examine how developmental changes in various brain regions relate to depression, but also how contextual and individual factors like family processes and temperament moderate these relationships (Silk *et al.*, 2007). One challenge to studying the interaction between contextual and other biological, psychological and developmental factors is that such an approach requires mastery of a disparate range of complex methodologies and research literatures, suggesting the need to form teams of researchers with varied expertise.

A number of additional methodological and conceptual issues warrant attention. First, numerous authors indicated that longitudinal data was of critical importance in addressing key research foci, including those as varied as: the antecedents and consequences of pubertal timing (Chapter 4 by DeRose and Brooks-Gunn); the influence of brain development on depression (and visa versa; Chapter 7 by Forbes, Silk, and Dahl); the development and consequences of moral emotions in adolescence (Chapter 10 by Eisenberg, Sheffield Morris, and Vaughan); and the influence of temperament (Chapter 13 by Klein and colleagues), family factors (Chapter 15 by Tompson, McKowen, and Asarnow), and peer relations (Chapter 16 by Furman, McDunn, and Young; Chapter 17 by La Greca, Davila, and Siegel) on risk for depression and related outcomes.

A second issue was the need for multi-method studies. Though of significance throughout developmental psychopathology, this point is particularly salient in studies of affective development wherein the low convergence between different affective domains (e.g. behavior, experience, physiology) suggests that findings may be strongly affected by measurement approach (Cacioppo *et al.*, 1992). The time is particularly opportune for multi-method approaches given the substantial advances being made in assessing affective processes using neuroimaging, psychophysiological, acoustic, and observational methodologies (see Coan & Allen, 2007, for a summary), as well as the increased interest in experience sampling methods (see Chapter 2).

A related issue is the need to develop a more nuanced understanding of the relations between different types of affective phenomena (i.e. affective temperament, emotional responses, and mood), as well as the way in which they interact, both during development and in the context of mood disorder. Though some evidence indicates that similar affects potentiate each other across these levels, current research suggests this effect may not be as general as presumed (Gross *et al.*, 1998). For example, a recent meta-analysis indicated that depressed persons have inhibited emotional responses to sad stimuli, despite the clear evidence that they experience more dysphoric mood states (Rottenberg, 2005). To date, however, very little research examining the relations between affective phenomena have been conducted in adolescents, so this is a clear direction for future work. Furthermore, affect-related behaviors influence the contexts in which people find themselves, further eliciting or inhibiting affective tendencies. For example, adolescents who are under-responsive to emotional stimuli (i.e. easily bored) may engage in sensation-seeking behaviors (e.g. risk taking) that in turn create the conditions for increases in negative moods (e.g. social rejection, low perceived control). Hence, the role of affective processes in the emergence of depression will depend on the conceptual level at which the question is addressed. This point harkens back to the multi-method issue in that measurement approaches tap specific aspects of affective process, with for example, self-report methodologies often tapping moods and more long-lasting emotions, and physiological indices revealing relatively fleeting emotional responses of which the adolescent may not be aware.

Further research is also needed on the relative roles of positive and negative affects in vulnerability to depression. Clark and Watson's (1991) seminal psychometric work on the unique role of positive affects in depressive disorders spurred interest in the role of inhibited reward processing in risk for depression. This is the focus explicitly taken by Forbes, Silk, and Dahl in Chapter 7, who describe how understanding brain systems underlying positive, reward-related emotions might form a bridge between adolescent development and adolescent depression. This is particularly so given the fact that brain reward systems are undergoing particularly dramatic changes during adolescence (see Davey et al., 2008). However, despite the specific associations between inhibited response to reward and depressed states, evidence is less clear regarding the role of dispositional positive affect as a risk factor for the emergence of depression. Klein and colleagues point out that although the evidence for high levels of negative emotionality as a temperamental precursor to mood disorders is strong, evidence for low levels of positive emotionality as a precursor to depression is much less clear. Moreover, it is clear that that negative affect is a strong, if non-specific, component of depression. Larson and Sheeber (Chapter 2) report that experience-sampling studies reveal a robust relationship between negative affect and depression. As such, it seems clear that any complete understanding of depressed states is going to require an accurate modeling of the interaction between aversive and appetitive processes. This may be especially so in terms of their role in the unfolding of depressive phenomena over the course of the disorder. It may be, for example, that subtle developmental changes in reward sensitivity are more problematic in the context of high temperamental negative emotionality, resulting in a greater likelihood of escalation of negative affects and inhibition of positive affect as the symptoms of depressive disorder emerge. In short, an understanding of the interaction between these systems, and especially the temporal course of such relationships, will be an especially important agenda for future research.

Finally, a number of contributors have indicated the need to examine the extent to which the influence of risk and protective mechanisms may be moderated by gender or cultural identity (e.g. Seeley and Lewinsohn, Chapter 2). Though gender has received considerable attention in some research areas (e.g. research examining family processes), it has been underexplored in others. For example, LaGreca and colleagues indicate that this is an important area for future research on the influence of peer and romantic relationships on risk for depression (Chapter 17). Emerging evidence that the timing and nature of brain development varies as a function of sex (Paus, Chapter 6), moreover, emphasizes the potential significance of this moderator. Relatedly, DeRose and Brooks Gunn (Chapter 4) indicate that though many studies of pubertal influences have been conducted with only girls, available evidence suggests that pubertal effects may emerge for boys as well, and they argue for the inclusion of boys in future research on puberty and adjustment.

The authors of the chapters on family processes (Chapters 14 and 15) note the scarcity of research examining the influence of cultural and ethnic characteristics. They indicate that we need studies with large enough samples of ethnic minority youth to examine how family processes may relate to depression in diverse populations. It seems likely that cultural differences with regard to affective processes and expression may influence the nature of associations between family relationships and interactional processes and risk for adolescent psychopathology (e.g. Lopez et al., 2004). Cultural norms, values, and identity, moreover, undoubtedly influence adolescents' interactions in other contexts as well as the fit between intrapersonal characteristics and contextual demands (Harkness & Super, 2000) such that this is an issue for future research on adolescent affective development more broadly.

Critical intervention strategies

The ultimate goal of understanding the developmental and etiological issues relevant to adolescent depression is to reduce the suffering associated with this condition by designing and implementing effective treatment and prevention strategies. This is especially the case given the high level of continuity in depressive disorders from youth into adulthood (Harrington & Vostanis, 1995; Lewinsohn et al., 2000), and the fact that early onset of depression is associated with significant reductions in educational and vocational attainment in affected individuals (Berndt et al., 2000). It is, moreover, well established that depressive disorders are highly recurrent (Costello et al., 2002), and indeed, research suggests that in many individuals, depressive episodes show a worsening pattern, characterized by increased severity, frequency, and autonomy (i.e. episodes are less clearly precipitated by psychosocial stress), and by lack of responsiveness to initially effective treatments (Kendler *et al.*, 2000; Post, 1992). Given that by 18 years of age, approximately 20% of adolescents have had at least one depressive episode (Lewinsohn *et al.*, 1998), it is vital to design prevention and early intervention strategies that are effective, relevant, and engaging to adolescents.

As has been noted by other authors, treatments for adolescent depression have primarily consisted of downward extensions of interventions developed for adults (Weisz & Hawley, 2002), and have hence not benefited as much as they could have from the emerging literature on the adolescent affective development or the developmental psychopathology literature relevant to the emergence of depression. The current volume provides a wealth of information in these areas of relevance to researchers focused on treatment development and clinicians working with depressed youth as well as to health, school, and community professionals likely to come into contact with at-risk youth who might benefit from referral to mental health services.

Given that recent reviews on preventative work in child and adolescent depression indicate that selective and indicated prevention have been more effective than universal intervention strategies (Horowitz & Garber, 2006), a critical issue is how we can identify at-risk adolescents to whom we can direct preventative efforts, as well as what these efforts might look like. A number of salient suggestions have emerged from the chapters in this book. With regard to individual and contextual characteristics, there is a clear need to pay attention to adolescents who demonstrate subthreshold symptoms (Seeley and Lewinsohn, Chapter 3) as well as those at risk as a function of affective dispositions (Klein and colleagues, Chapter 13), early pubertal timing (DeRose and Brooks-Gunn, and Graber, Chapters 4 and 5), family history of affective disorder (Klein *et al.*, 2001), or the stress associated with adverse family interactions (Tompson, Chapter 15), challenging peer relationships, or early entry into romantic relationships (Furman and La Greca and colleagues, Chapters 16 and 17). Many of these risks may be especially predictive of difficulties for girls. Additional research is needed to evaluate whether these risks operate similarly in members of ethnic, racial, or sexual minority groups as well as to explore the additional stressors that may render members of these subgroups at additional risk. Finally, risk for relapse appears to be most acute in adolescent girls with multiple episodes, family conflict, or a family history of depressive disorder (Lewinsohn *et al.*, 2000).

The need to better integrate research and knowledge regarding biological and contextual risks, discussed earlier, was also reflected in suggestions regarding interventions. For example, Graber (Chapter 5) has suggested that because puberty is hypothesized to confer risk via interaction with social-contextual factors, a focus on issues such as relationships with parents and peers, and development of coping skills for managing stressful events, would likely be the most fruitful approach to prevention efforts. In particular, she has proposed gender-specific programming that focuses on developing effective strategies for addressing the unique social stressors faced by young pubescent girls, as well as for regulating the emotions engendered by them (Graber & Sontag, 2006). Similarly, DeRose and Brooks-Gunn (Chapter 4) have suggested that the spike in depression that occurs during the transition to puberty could perhaps be lessened with better preparation for pubertal onset via education and discussion within family, school, and community settings that could positively influence how adolescents affectively experience the transition. In a related vein, Sanson and colleagues (Chapter 12) proposed that there is a role for temperament-based parenting interventions, to help families to understand how parental responses can amplify or reduce the problems associated with certain high-risk temperament characteristics in their child. Though this approach has been used successfully with infants and young children (Sheeber & Johnson, 1994; van den Boom, 1994), it has received very little attention in work with adolescents and is clearly a promising area for further research. As affective temperament is a key aspect of temperament conferring risk, it is likely that such efforts would benefit from, and expand upon, initial work addressing parent socialization and coaching of adolescent affect (Chapter 14). Moreover, as noted by Sanson (Chapter 12), there would also be a role for interventions that assist adolescents in learning to both moderate their own predispositions and develop effective coping styles.

This last point, provides a segue to the critical issue of the extent to which treatments for adolescents should focus on the adolescent (either individually or in a group) or on the adolescent in the context of the family. There is an interesting disjoint in the literature whereby the role of family processes as a factor in adolescent affective development and depression appears quite compelling, yet the evidence for family-focused interventions is less so (see Chapters 14 and 15). However, promising family treatments that attend to the developmental demands and capabilities of adolescents are emerging (Diamond et al., 2003), and consistent with the recent practice parameters published by the American Academy of Child and Adolescent Psychiatry (Birmaher & Brent, 2007), cognitive-behavioral, interpersonal, and biological approaches to treatment all include parents in at least a psychoeducational component. It seems clear that the psychoeducational component could be broadened to include information about adolescent neurological, affective, cognitive, and social development, so as to facilitate parenting more likely to achieve a balance between facilitating the autonomy necessary for development and the regulatory support necessary for adaptive and healthy functioning. Moreover, it seems that the next step is to use our emerging knowledge base about adolescent development to develop and test hypotheses regarding which intervention components adolescents can benefit from on their own (i.e. where parental support could feel intrusive and demeaning to their efforts) and those where parental scaffolding, or collaboration remain necessary. The knowledge presented in this volume should place us in good stead to begin this task.

Conclusion

This volume had aims that were, in a sense, both substantive and methodological. On the substantive side the authors have provided an excellent series of up-to-date integrative reviews of various aspects of the development of emotion, and the emergence of depressive disorders, during adolescence. As noted in the opening chapter, the pairing of "developmental" and "clinical" chapters on each topic allows the reader to see the links (both actual and potential) between these perspectives; and therein lies the methodological aspect of the volume. The volume is based on the premise that when there is a substantial and reliable association between a phase of development and an increase in the incidence of disorder, then "drilling down" to understand the developmental changes that impinge on the core phenomena of that disorder (or risk for that disorder) will help to shed light on the etiology of the disorder – not only during that phase of life, but potentially revealing mechanisms that are relevant across the life span. In other words, this kind of developmental psychopathology approach can act as a "conceptual laboratory" in which to make fundamental discoveries about the nature of mental disorders. We believe that the issues outlined in this final chapter not only delineate a critical future agenda for scientific and clinical studies of adolescent depression, but also demonstrate the tremendous utility of taking a developmental psychopathology perspective on mental health problems during adolescence.

REFERENCES

Allen, N.B., & Badcock, P.B. (2003). The social risk hypothesis of depressed mood: evolutionary, psychosocial, and neurobiological perspectives. *Psychological Bulletin,* **129**(6), 887–913.

Allen, N.B., & Badcock, P.B.T. (2006). Darwinian models of depression: a review of evolutionary accounts of mood and mood disorders. *Progress in Neuropsychopharmacology and Biological Psychiatry,* **30**(5), 815–826.

Allen, N.B., Barrett, A., Sheeber, L., & Davis, B. (2006). Pubertal development and the emergence of the gender gap in mood disorders: a developmental and evolutionary synthesis. In D. Castle, J. Kulkarni, & K. Abel (Eds.), *Mood and Anxiety Disorders in Women.* Cambridge, UK: Cambridge University Press.

Berndt, E.R., Koran, L.M., Finkelstein, S.N. *et al.* (2000). Lost human capital from early-onset chronic depression. *American Journal of Psychiatry*, **157**(6), 940–947.

Birmaher, B., & Brent, D. (2007). Practice parameter for the assessment and treatment of children and adolescents with depressive disorders. *Journal of the American Academy of Child and Adolescent Psychiatry*, **46**(11), 1503–1526.

Burke, K.C., Burke, J.D., Regier, D.A., & Rae, D.S. (1990). Age at onset of selected mental disorders in five community populations. *Archives of General Psychiatry*, **47**(6), 511–518.

Cacioppo, J.T., Uchino, B.N., Crites, S.L. *et al.* (1992). Relationship between facial expressiveness and sympathetic activation in emotion: a critical review, with emphasis on modeling underlying mechanisms and individual differences. *Journal of Personality and Social Psychology*, **62**(1), 110–128.

Clark, L.A., & Watson, D. (1991). Tripartite model of anxiety and depression: psychometric evidence and taxonomic implications. *Journal of Abnormal Psychology*, **100**(3), 316–336.

Coan, J., & Allen, J.J. (2007). *Handbook of Emotion Elicitation and Assessment*. New York, NY: Oxford University Press.

Costello, E.J., Pine, D.S., Hammen, C. *et al.* (2002). Development and natural history of mood disorders. *Biological Psychiatry*, **52**(6), 529–542.

Davey, C.G., Yucel, M., & Allen, N.B. (2008). The emergence of depression in adolescence: development of the prefrontal cortex and the representation of reward. *Neuroscience and Biobehavioral Reviews*, **32**(1), 1–19.

Diamond, G., Siqueland, L., & Diamond, G.M. (2003). Attachment-based family therapy for depressed adolescents: programmatic treatment development. *Clinical Child and Family Psychology Review*, **6**(2), 107–127.

Giedd, J.N., Blumenthal, J., Jeffries, N.O. *et al.* (1999). Brain development during childhood and adolescence: a longitudinal MRI study. *Nature Neuroscience*, **2**(10), 861–863.

Graber, J.A., & Sontag, L.M. (2006). Puberty and girls' sexuality: why hormones are not the complete answer. *New Directions for Child and Adolescent Development*, **2006** (112), 23–38.

Gross, J.J., Sutton, S.K., & Ketelaar, T. (1998). Affective-reactivity views. *Personality and Social Psychology Bulletin*, **24**(i3), 279.

Harkness, S., & Super, C.M. (2000). Culture and psychopathology. In A.J. Sameroff, M. Lewis, & S.M. Miller (Eds.), *Handbook of Developmental Psychopathology* (pp. 197–216). New York, NY: Kluwer Academic/Plenum Publishers.

Harrington, R., & Vostanis, P. (1995). Longitudinal perspectives and affective disorder in children and adolescents. In I.M. Goodyer (Ed.), *The Depressed Child and Adolescent* (pp. 311–341). Cambridge, UK: Cambridge University Press.

Horowitz, J.L., & Garber, J. (2006). The prevention of depressive symptoms in children and adolescents: a meta-analytic review. *Journal of Consulting and Clinical Psychology*, **74**(3), 401–415.

Johnson, W., Hicks, B.M., McGue, M., & Iacono, W.G. (2007). Most of the girls are alright, but some aren't: personality trajectory groups from ages 14 to 24 and some associations with outcomes. *Journal of Personality and Social Psychology*, **93**(2), 266–284.

Kendler, K.S., Thornton, L.M., & Gardner, C.O. (2000). Stressful life events and previous episodes in the etiology of major depression in women: an evaluation of the "kindling" hypothesis. *American Journal of Psychiatry*, **157**(8), 1243–1251.

Klein, D.N., Lewinsohn, P.M., Seeley, J.R., & Rohde, P. (2001). A family study of major depressive disorder in a community sample of adolescents. *Archives of General Psychiatry*, **58**(1), 13–20.

Lewinsohn, P.M., Rohde, P., & Seeley, J.R. (1998). Major depressive disorder in older adolescents: prevalence, risk factors, and clinical implications. *Clinical Psychology Review*, **18**(7), 765–794.

Lewinsohn, P.M., Rohde, P., Seeley, J.R., Klein, D.N., & Gotlib, I.H. (2000). Natural course of adolescent major depressive disorder in a community sample: predictors of recurrence in young adults. *American Journal of Psychiatry*, **157**(10), 1584–1591.

Lopez, S.R., Nelson Hipke, K., Polo, A.J. *et al.* (2004). Ethnicity, expressed emotion, attributions, and course of schizophrenia: family warmth matters. *Journal of Abnormal Psychology*, **113**(3), 428–439.

Monroe, S.M., Rohde, P., Seeley, J.R., & Lewinsohn, P.M. (1999). Life events and depression in adolescence: relationship loss as a prospective risk factor for first onset of major depressive disorder. *Journal of Abnormal Psychology*, **108**(4), 606–614.

Nelson, E.E., Leibenluft, E., McClure, E.B., & Pine, D.S. (2005). The social re-orientation of adolescence: a neuroscience perspective on the process and its relation to psychopathology. *Psychological Medicine*, **35**(2), 163–174.

Post, R.M. (1992). Transduction of psychosocial stress into the neurobiology of recurrent affective disorder. *American Journal of Psychiatry*, **149**(8), 999–1010.

Rottenberg, J. (2005). Mood and emotion in major depression. *Current Directions in Psychological Science*, **14**(3), 167–170.

Sheeber, L.B., & Johnson, J.H. (1994). Evaluation of a temperament-focused, parent-training program. *Journal of Clinical Child Psychology*, **23**(3), 249–259.

Silk, J.S., Vanderbilt-Adriance, E., Shaw, D.S. *et al.* (2007). Resilience among children and adolescents at risk for depression: mediation and moderation across social and neurobiological contexts. *Development and Psychopathology*, **19**(03), 841–865.

Steinberg, L. (2005). Cognitive and affective development in adolescence. *Trends in Cognitive Science*, **9**(2), 69–74.

Steinberg, L., Dahl, R., Keating, D. *et al.* (2005). The study of developmental psychopathology in adolescence integrating affective neuroscience with the study of context. In D. Cicchetti & D.J. Cohen (Eds.), *Developmental Psychopathology* (pp. 710–741). New York, NY: John Wiley & Sons.

van den Boom, D.C. (1994). The influence of temperament and mothering on attachment and exploration: an experimental manipulation of sensitive responsiveness among lower-class mothers with irritable infants. *Child Development*, **65**(5), 1457–1477.

Weisfeld, G.E., & Janisse, H.C. (2005). Some functional aspects of human adolescence. In B.J. Ellis & D.F. Bjorklund (Eds.), *Origins of the Social Mind: Evolutionary Psychology and Child Development* (pp. 189–218). New York, NY: Guilford Press.

Weisz, J.R., & Hawley, K.M. (2002). Developmental factors in the treatment of adolescents. *Journal of Consulting and Clinical Psychology*, **70**(1), 21–43.

Index

Lightning Source UK Ltd.
Milton Keynes UK
UKOW050756261012

201226UK00004B/30/P